BREAST CANCER

Multidisciplinary Pathways for Cancer Care in the Community

BREAST CANCER

Multidisciplinary Pathways for Cancer Care in the Community

James L. Weese, MD, FACS
Vice President, Cancer Service Line
Advocate Health—Midwest Region
Clinical Adjunct Professor of Surgery
University of Wisconsin School of Medicine and Public Health
Milwaukee, Wisconsin

Elsevier
1600 John F. Kennedy Blvd.
Ste 1800
Philadelphia, PA 19103-2899

BREAST CANCER: MULTIDISCIPLINARY PATHWAYS FOR CANCER
CARE IN THE COMMUNITY   ISBN: 978-0-323-93249-3

Copyright © 2024 by Elsevier, Inc. All rights reserved.

No part of this publication may be reproduced or transmitted in any form or by any means, electronic or mechanical, including photocopying, recording, or any information storage and retrieval system, without permission in writing from the publisher. Details on how to seek permission, further information about the Publisher's permissions policies and our arrangements with organizations such as the Copyright Clearance Center and the Copyright Licensing Agency, can be found at our website: www.elsevier.com/permissions.

This book and the individual contributions contained in it are protected under copyright by the Publisher (other than as may be noted herein).

Notice

Practitioners and researchers must always rely on their own experience and knowledge in evaluating and using any information, methods, compounds or experiments described herein. Because of rapid advances in the medical sciences, in particular, independent verification of diagnoses and drug dosages should be made. To the fullest extent of the law, no responsibility is assumed by Elsevier, authors, editors or contributors for any injury and/or damage to persons or property as a matter of products liability, negligence or otherwise, or from any use or operation of any methods, products, instructions, or ideas contained in the material herein.

Executive Content Strategist: Nancy Anastasi Duffy
Senior Content Development Specialist: Sneha Kashyap
Publishing Services Manager: Shereen Jameel
Project Manager: Gayathri S
Design Direction: Ryan Cook

Printed in India

Last digit is the print number: 9 8 7 6 5 4 3 2 1

Working together
to grow libraries in
developing countries

www.elsevier.com • www.bookaid.org

Contributors

Jennifer Jarvey Balistreri, BA, MS
Senior Community Impact Coordinator
Aurora Health Care
Advocate Health—Midwest Region
Milwaukee, Wisconsin

Kenneth T. Bastin, MD, MBA
Adjunct Professor
Department of Human Oncology
University of Wisconsin School of Medicine and Public
  Health
Milwaukee, Wisconsin

Anna Berry, MD
Senior Vice President
Biomarker Data and Laboratory Medicine
Syapse
Seattle, Washington

Dhrubajyoti (Dhru) Bhattacharya, JD, MPH, LLM, EMBA
Chief Diversity, Equity, & Inclusion Officer
Human Resources
Banner Health
Phoenix, Arizona

Amy Bock, RN, MBA, BSN, OCN
Administrator
Radiation Oncology Associates
Milwaukee, Wisconsin

Jodi Leigh Brehm, MD, FACS
Breast Surgeon
Aurora Health Care
Advocate Health—Midwest Region
Mount Pleasant, Wisconsin

Jamie Cairo, DNP, AOCNP
Nurse Practitioner
Cancer Service Line
Aurora Health Care
Advocate Health—Midwest Region
Milwaukee, Wisconsin

Kendra Campbell, BSN, RN, OCN
Cancer Nurse Navigator Manager
Cancer Service Line
Aurora Health Care
Advocate Health—Midwest Region
Green Bay, Wisconsin

Aaron H. Chevinsky, MD, FACS
Oncology Service Line Chief and Medical
  Director for the Riverside Cancer Care
  Network
Newport News, Virginia

Elizabeth Duchac, RD, CSO
Clinical Oncology Dietitian
Cancer Service Line
Aurora Health Care
Advocate Health—Midwest Region
Milwaukee, Wisconsin

Armando E. Giuliano, MD, FACS
Chief, Surgical Oncology
Cedars-Sinai Medical Center;
Clinical Professor
Department of Surgery
UCLA School of Medicine
Los Angeles
California

Donald Allen Goer, PhD
Senior Scientist (retired)
IntraOp Medical, Inc.
Sunnyvale, California

Timothy Goggins, MD, MS, MBA
Hematology/Oncology, Hospice and
  Palliative Care
Cancer Service Line
Aurora Health Care
Advocate Health—Midwest Region
Germantown, Grafton and Milwaukee, Wisconsin

Ameer Gomberawalla, MD, FACS
Medical Director Breast Oncology
Advocate Health—Midwest Region;
Breast Surgical Oncologist
Surgery
Advocate Christ Medical Center
Oak Lawn, Illinois

Sigrun (Siggy) Hallmeyer, MD
Attending Physician
Medical Group of Advocate Health—Midwest Region
Advocate Lutheran General Hospital
Park Ridge, Illinois

Jay K. Harness, MD, FACS
Breast Surgeon
Providence St. Joseph Hospital
Orange, California

Carol Huibregtse, MSN, RN, OCN
Director Quality
Cancer Service Line
Advocate Health—Midwest Region
Milwaukee, Wisconsin

Greg Kauffmann, MD, MS
Radiation Oncologist
Department of Radiation Oncology
Aurora West Allis Medical Center
West Allis, Wisconsin

Paul Madsen, MD
Radiologist
Diagnostic Radiology
Medical Group of Advocate Health—Midwest region
Milwaukee, Wisconsin

Sara Madsen, DO
Physician
Department of Radiology
Medical Group of Advocate Health—Midwest Region
St. Luke's Medical Center
Milwaukee, Wisconsin

Ashley Marumoto, MD
Clinical Assistant Professor
Department of Surgery
University of Hawaii, John A. Burns School of Medicine
Honolulu, Hawaii

Shannon McCarthy, RD, CSO, CD
Oncology Dietitian
Nutrition Services
Aurora Health Care
Milwaukee, Wisconsin

Amanda Meindl, MD
Anatomic and Clinical Pathologist
Department of Pathology
Great Lakes Pathologists S.C.
West Allis, Wisconsin

Harry Nayar, MD
Plastic Surgeon
Aurora Health Care
Milwaukee, Wisconsin

Rubina Qamar, MD
Physician
Department of Hematology/Oncology
Aurora Health Care
Milwaukee, Wisconsin

Juliann Reiland, MD, FACS
Breast Surgeon, Retired
Columbia Falls, Montana

Corey J. Shamah, MD
Physician
Department of Hematology/Oncology
Aurora Health Care
Milwaukee, Wisconsin

Leslie J. Waltke, PT, DPT
Cancer Rehabilitation Coordinator
Aurora Physical Therapy
Aurora Health Care
Milwaukee, Wisconsin

Joseph John Weber, MD, FACS
Breast Surgical Oncologist
Surgical Oncology
Aurora Health Care, Milwaukee;
Clinical Adjunct Assistant Professor
University of Wisconsin School of Medicine and Public
     Health, Madison;
Assistant Clinical Professor of Surgery
Medical College of Wisconsin
Milwaukee, Wisconsin

James L. Weese, MD, FACS
Vice President
Cancer Service Line
Advocate Health—Midwest Region;
Clinical Adjunct Professor of Surgery
University of Wisconsin School of Medicine and Public
     Health
Milwaukee, Wisconsin

Deborah Wham, MS, CGC
Genetic Counselor, Manager
Genomic Medicine
Aurora Health Care
Milwaukee, Wisconsin

Nicole M. Zaremba, MD, FACS
Medical Director
Comprehensive Breast Care Center
Aurora St. Luke's Medical Center
Milwaukee, Wisconsin

Ellen L. Ziaja, MD, MS, BS
Radiation Oncology
Aurora Health Care
Summit, Wisconsin

Brad Zimmerman, MBA, MSW, APSW, OSW-C
Social Work Lead
Cancer Care
Aurora Health Care
Milwaukee, Wisconsin

Alyssa Zimny, MD
Resident
Diagnostic Radiology
Aurora St. Luke's Medical Center
Milwaukee, Wisconsin

Preface

Our approach to patients with breast cancer has changed dramatically during many of our careers. New discoveries and refinements now allow many of these patients to be cured. Even those who present with advanced disease can look forward to prolonged survival with an approach characteristic for a chronic disease. Operations have changed from radical approaches to local disease to a better understanding of the biology of breast cancer, which has encouraged focus on staging, local control, and multidisciplinary approaches to enhance both survival and quality of life. New surgical techniques have created better and more natural reconstructions. Operative techniques are now available to reduce the risk of lymphedema.

With newer understanding of the genetics of breast cancer we can give better advice to patients at increased risk of developing the disease and tailor therapy accordingly. We have increased our ability to prevent the development of breast cancer and new drugs focused on the mutations intrinsic to cancer cells have expanded the number of precision medicines available for treatment.

Clinical trials will be the mainstay of progress in the treatment of all cancers, but particularly those starting in the breast. In a system such as ours, where we treat thousands of patients with breast cancer each year, we feel the use of multidisciplinary pathways is a very important approach. Unlike guidelines that give multiple "approved" approaches, pathways allow us to prioritize clinical trials and then give prescribed recommendations based on efficacy, toxicity, and cost, in that order. Ultimately, this allows the data generated on our patients to have more value to move the field forward.

It has been an honor to work with my colleagues to produce this book. The beauty of current technology will allow us to continually update new changes in the e-book edition.

James L. Weese, MD, FACS

To my inspiration and motivation: Barbara, Scott, Brooke, Ben, and Eden, and the many patients with breast cancer who have entrusted us with their care.

Contents

PART 1: Breast Cancer Care in the Community

1 Breast Cancer in the Community, 2
JAMES L. WEESE

Introduction, 2
References, 4

2 Multidisciplinary Team Approach to the Management of Breast Cancer, 6
AARON H. CHEVINSKY and JOSEPH JOHN WEBER

Implementation of a Multidisciplinary
Care Program, 6
Program Components, 6
Value of Multidisciplinary Care, 6
Which Patients Should Participate?, 8
Decisions on Testing Prior to and After Multidisciplinary Evaluation, 8
High-Risk Patient Evaluation and
Management, 8
Ancillary Services to Assist the Breast
Cancer Patient, 9
Shared Decision Making, 9
Summary and Conclusion, 9
References, 9

3 Oncology Nurse Navigation in the Care of Breast Cancer, 11
KENDRA CAMPBELL and JAMIE CAIRO

Introduction, 11
History of Patient Navigation, 11
Program Accreditation, 11
Defining the Oncology Nurse Navigator Role, 12
Literature Review of Oncology Navigation, 12
Role Development, 13
Knowledge and Skills Requirements, 13
Specialty Certification in Breast Navigation, 13
Psychosocial Screening and Support, 14
Addressing Barriers to Care, 14
Multidisciplinary Team, 14
Survivorship and End of Life, 14
References, 15

PART 2: Patient Screening, Diagnosis, and Evaluation in the Community

4 Breast Cancer Screening, 18
PAUL MADSEN, SARA MADSEN, and ALYSSA ZIMNY

Early Use of Mammography for Cancer Detection
and Benefits of Screening Mammography 18
Screening Mammography Risks, 18
Standardization of Technique and Patient
Positioning, 19
Characterizing Breast Tissue Density, 19
Mammography Limitations/Incorporation of
Tomosynthesis, 21
Screening Guidelines for Average-Risk Women, 22
Higher-Than-Average Risk Populations, 25
Personal History, 25
Family History/Genetic Risk Factors, 25
Calculated Individual Risk, 27
Radiation History, 27
Race, 27
Special Patient Populations, 27
Male, 27
LGBTQ, 28
Pregnancy/Lactation, 28
Recent Vaccination, 28
Magnetic Resonance Imaging Screening for Breast
Cancer, 28
Screening Ultrasound, 29
References, 30

5 Outcomes and Quality Indicators, 33
JOSEPH JOHN WEBER, AARON H. CHEVINSKY, and CAROL HUIBREGTSE

Introduction, 33
Framework for Outcomes and Quality Indicators in
Breast Cancer Care, 33
System Initiatives and Management of Quality, 33
Quality Indicators, 36
Examples of Breast Quality Measures, 38
Implementation of an Outcomes and Quality
Management Team, 38
Ways to Improve Breast Cancer Treatment, 38
Summary and Conclusion, 39
References, 39

6 Evaluation and Treatment in the Underserved Community, 40
JENNIFER JARVEY BALISTRERI and DHRUBAJYOTI BHATTACHARYA
Introduction, 40
From Theory to Practice: No Community Left Behind, 42
References, 44

PART 3: Breast Cancer Treatment in the Community

7 Contemporary Surgical Approaches to Breast Cancer, 46
ASHLEY MARUMOTO, ARMANDO E. GIULIANO, AMEER GOMBERAWALLA , NICOLE M. ZAREMBA, and HARRY NAYAR

BIOPSY TECHNIQUES, 46
Key Points, 46
Historical Context, 46
Indications, 46
Fine Needle Aspiration Versus Core Needle Biopsy, 46
Types of Needles and Devices, 46
Palpable Lesions Versus Nonpalpable Lesions, 46
Considerations, 47
Stereotactic Biopsy, 47
Ultrasound Biopsy, 47
Magnetic Resonance Biopsy, 48
Postbiopsy Considerations and Concordance, 48
SURGICAL OPTIONS, 49
Key Points, 49
Historical Context, 49
Surgical Localization of the Biopsied Lesion, 49
Breast Conservation, 50
Margins Following Breast-Conserving Surgery, 51
Mastectomy, 51
Sentinel Node Biopsy, 52
Axillary Dissection, 53
Complications, 53
Operation After Neoadjuvant Chemotherapy, 54
Future Directions, 54
MANAGEMENT OF THE AXILLA AND LYMPHEDEMA, 54
Introduction, 54
Definition and Incidence, 54
Stages of Lymphedema, 54
Preoperative Assessment and Surveillance, 55
Reduction of Risk, 56
De-Escalating Axillary Surgery, 57
Axillary Surgery After Neoadjuvant Chemotherapy, 57

Axillary Reverse Mapping, 58
Lymphatic Microsurgical Preventive Healing Approach, 58
Less Radiation to Prevent Lymphedema, 60
Partial Breast Irradiation, 60
Omit Radiation in the Elderly and Neoadjuvant Responders, 60
Post-Lymphedema Treatment, 61
Nonsurgical Management of Arm Lymphedema, 61
Surgical Treatment of Arm Lymphedema, 61
Section Summary, 61
DCIS, LOBULAR CARCINOMA IN SITU, AND OTHER HIGH-RISK LESIONS, 62
Key Points, 62
Epidemiology, 62
Diagnosis, 62
Natural History, 62
Pathology, 62
Treatment, 62
Recurrence, 63
Prognostic Scores, 63
Future Perspectives, 63
Other High-Risk Lesions, 63
BREAST RECONSTRUCTION, 64
Key Points, 64
Introduction to Breast Reconstruction, 64
ONCOPLASTIC BREAST RECONSTRUCTION, 64
Key Points, 64
PREOPERATIVE CONSIDERATIONS, 64
Key Points, 64
BASIC ONCOPLASTIC APPROACH, 65
Key Points, 65
LEVEL 1 ONCOPLASTIC PROCEDURES, 66
Key Points, 66
UPPER POLE, 67
Key Points, 67
Crescent Mastopexy, 67
(Hemi)Batwing Mastopexy, 67
Circumareolar (Donut) Mastopexy, 67
Lower Pole, 67
Level 2 and Extreme Oncoplastic Procedures, 71
Vertical Mastopexy, 71
Wise Pattern Reduction Mammoplasty, 72
Split Wise Pattern Reduction Mammoplasty, 72
Conclusion, 72
BREAST RECONSTRUCTION, 72
Key Points, 72
Introduction, 73
Patient Selection, 74
Implant-Based Reconstruction, Technical Aspects, 74
Complications, 74
Tissue-Based Reconstruction, 75
Patient Selection, 75
Technique, 77
Complications, 78
Conclusion, 78
References, 78

8 Radiation Therapy, 87

KENNETH T. BASTIN, ELLEN L. ZIAJA, GREG KAUFFMANN, DONALD ALLEN GOER, JAY K. HARNESS, and JULIANN REILAND

Radiation Therapy Background, 87
Radiation Therapy Definitions, 88
Radiation Biology, 90
  Assessing Patients Appropriate for Radiation Therapy, 90
General Clinical Radiation Therapy Concepts, 91
  Radiation Side Effects Following Treatment of Breast Cancer, 91
  Radiation Therapy Technical Definitions, 91
Ductal Carcinoma In Situ, 92
Invasive Breast Cancer, Breast-Conserving Adjuvant Radiation Treatment, 93
Post-Mastectomy Radiation Therapy, 93
Other Radiation Therapy Indications, 94
Intraoperative Radiation Therapy as Adjunctive Treatment of Breast Cancer, 94
  IORT as a Boost, 95
  Clinical Results for IOERT as a Boost, 95
  Clinical Results for IORT as a Boost, 96
  IORT as the Sole Radiation Treatment (IORT APBI), 96
  Clinical Results for IORT/IOERT APBI, 98
  APBI Clinical Results: Orthovoltage (50-kV X-rays) Prospective Randomized Results, 98
Conclusion, 99
References, 99

9 Systemic Therapy for Breast Cancer, 101

SIGRUN HALLMEYER, RUBINA QAMAR, and COREY J. SHAMAH

Introduction, 101
Neoadjuvant Therapy for Breast Cancer, 101
  Introduction, 101
  Patient Selection for Neoadjuvant Therapy, 102
  Preoperative Evaluation, 103
  Neoadjuvant Systemic Therapy, 103
  Post-Treatment Assessment and Management, 109
  Adjuvant Therapy After Neoadjuvant Treatment, 109
Adjuvant Treatment of Breast Cancer, 110
  Hormone Receptor–Positive and HER2-Negative Subtype, 110
  Multigene Assays, 110
  Adjuvant Endocrine Therapy, 111
  Role of Ovarian Suppression in Premenopausal Women, 112
  Aromatase Inhibitors, 112
  Aromatase Inhibitors and Tamoxifen, 113
  Duration of Endocrine Therapy, 113
  Role of Cyclin-Dependent Kinase 4 and 6 Inhibitors, 113
  Adjuvant Chemotherapy, 115
  HER2-Positive Subtypes, 115

  Treatment of Smaller HER2-Positive Tumors, 116
  Management of Residual Disease After Neoadjuvant Therapy, 116
  Hormone Receptor and HER2-Negative Subtype, 117
  Role of PARP Inhibitors in Patients With BRCA Mutation, 118
  Adjuvant Bisphosphonate Therapy, 118
  Special Considerations, 118
Metastatic Breast Cancer, 119
  Biology of Metastatic Disease, 119
  Hormonal Therapy, 119
  HER2-Positive Breast Cancer, 121
  Triple-Negative Breast Cancer, 122
  Chemotherapy, 123
  Bone-Modifying Agents, 124
Summary, 124
References, 124

10 Breast Cancer Pathology for Precision Oncology, 131

ANNA BERRY and AMANDA MEINDL

Background, 131
Hormone Receptors and HER2, 131
Molecular Classification of Breast Cancer, 132
  Luminal Subtypes, 133
  HER2-Positive/HER2-Enriched Subtype, 133
  Basal-like Subtype, 133
Molecular Prognostic Tests—OncotypeDX and MammaPrint, 134
Biomarker Testing for Precision Oncology and Cancer Risk Assessment, 135
References, 138

11 Physical Therapy for Patients With Breast Cancer, 139

LESLIE J. WALTKE

An Introduction to Breast Cancer Physical Therapy, 139
An Overview of Breast Cancer Physical Therapy, 140
Referring to Breast Cancer Physical Therapy, 140
Breast Cancer Surgery: Implications for Physical Therapy, 143
  Section Key Points, 143
  Efficacy of Postoperative Breast Cancer Physical Therapy, 143
  Referral to Postoperative Breast Cancer Physical Therapy, 143
  Goals of Postoperative Breast Surgery Physical Therapy, 144
  Post–Breast Cancer Surgery Physical Therapy Subjective History, 144
  Post–Breast Cancer Surgery Objective Examination, 144
  Post–Breast Cancer Surgery Rehabilitation Assessment, 145
  Post–Breast Cancer Surgery Physical Therapy Plan of Care, Interventions, and Treatment, 145

Resolving the Postoperative Breast Cancer Physical Therapy Phase, 145
Lymphedema Risk Reduction and Risk Reduction Education, 145
Chemotherapy: Implications for Rehabilitation Physical Therapy, 147
Section Key Points, 147
Efficacy of Physical Therapy During Chemotherapy, 147
Breast Cancer Radiation Therapy: Implications for Physical Therapy, 149
Section Key Points, 149
Overview of Physical Therapy During Radiation Therapy for Breast Cancer, 149
Rehabilitation During Radiation Therapy for Breast Cancer, 149
Rehabilitation After Radiation Therapy for Breast Cancer, 149
Metastatic Breast Cancer: Implications for Physical Therapy, 150
Section Key Points, 150
Physical Therapy Efficacy in Metastatic Breast Cancer, 150
Physical Therapy Interventions in Metastatic Breast Cancer, 150
Physical Therapy Interventions for Late and End-Stage Metastatic Breast Cancer, 151
Breast Cancer Survivorship: Implications for Physical Therapy, 151
Section Overview, 151
Physical Therapy for Long-Term Side Effects, 152
Physical Therapy for Late Effects, 152
Team Phoenix—An Innovative Tool to Redefine Cancer Survivorship, 153
Chapter Summary 153
References 153

PART 4: Follow-Up and After care

12 Nutrition 158
ELIZABETH DUCHAC and SHANNON MCCARTHY
Introduction, 158
Role of Oncology Dietitians, 158
Medical Nutrition Therapy, 158
Soy, 160
Flaxseed, 161
Lymphedema, 161
Anti-inflammatory Diet, 161
References, 163

13 Breast Cancer Survivorship in Community Oncology Practice, 164
JAMIE CAIRO

Surveillance, 164
Imaging, 164
Mammography, 164

Magnetic Resonance Imaging, 164
Genetics, 165
Breast Cancer Tumor Marker Testing and Other Blood Tests, 165
Bone Density Testing, 165
Screening for Secondary Cancers, 165
Assessment and Management of Physical and Psychosocial Long-Term and Late Effects of Breast Cancer and Treatment, 166
Body Image, 166
Lymphedema, 166
Cardiotoxicity, 166
Cognitive Impairment, 167
Distress, Depression, and Anxiety, 167
Fatigue, 168
Pain and Neuropathy, 170
Infertility, 170
Sexual Health, 171
Menopausal Symptoms and Early Menopause, 171
Wellness Guidelines and Health Promotion, 171
Survivorship Care Plans and Care Coordination, 172
Models of Care, 173
Barriers to Survivorship Care, 174
Program Evaluation and Metrics, 174
References, 175

14 Breast Cancer Palliative Care, 179
TIMOTHY GOGGINS
Palliative Chemotherapy, 179
Symptom Management, 179
Nutrition, 182
Psychosocial, 183
Communication and Counseling, 183
Advance Directives/Living Will/Healthcare Power of Attorney, 183
Goals of Care, 184
References, 184

PART 5: Related Topics for Delivery of Care Today and Tomorrow

15 Genetics and Prevention, 188
JODI LEIGH BREHM and DEBORAH WHAM
Genetic Risk Factors, 188
Familial/Personal History/Lifestyle Risk Factors, 191
Risk-Reducing Interventions, 192
Tamoxifen, 192
Raloxifene, 192
Exemestane/Anastrozole Aromatase Inhibitors, 193
Managing Hot Flashes or Vasomotor Symptoms Caused by Risk-Reducing Medications, 193
Uterine Cancer, 193
Vaginal Atrophy/Dyspareunia, 193
Cardiac Events, 193
Osteopenia/Osteoporosis, 193
Musculoskeletal Complaints/Joint Ache, 194

Contents

Risk-Reducing Surgery, 194
Management of the High-Risk Patient, 194
References 194

16 Coping With the High Cost of Cancer, 197
BRAD ZIMMERMAN

The Significance Behind Recognizing Financial
Hardship in People With Cancer, 197
The Patient Experience, 198
Let's Talk Health Insurance, 198
Where Does Your Health Insurance Plan Come
From? 198
Plan Type, 198
Plan Premiums, Deductibles, Out-of-Pocket
Maximums, and Copays, 199
Seeking Transparency in Healthcare Costs, 199
Look Deeper Into the Healthcare System for
Financial Assistance, 199
The Role of the Healthcare Organization, 199
It Starts With Cancer Screenings, 200
Increase Community Outreach, 200
Employ a Prior Authorization Team, 200
Financial Counselors, 201
Financial Advocates, 201
Financial Navigators, 202

Oncology Social Workers, 202
Public Benefits Specialists, 202
The Pharmacy Team , 202
Financial Health Advisors, 202
Making the Healthcare Organization's Role More
Transparent, 202
Charity Care, 202
Understand Financial Assistance Resources, 203
Utilize a Software Tool to Identify Financial
Assistance Funding Sources, 203
Utilize a Quality Metric to Identify and Evaluate
Financial Assistance Need, 204
The Impact of Financial Hardship on the Country,
204
Cancer Policy Advocacy, 205
Conclusion, 205
References, 205

17 Expectations for the Future, 207
AMY BOCK and JAMES L. WEESE

References, 209

Index, 211

PART 1

Breast Cancer Care in the Community

1

Breast Cancer in the Community

JAMES L. WEESE

Introduction

The treatment of breast cancer has changed dramatically over the last generation. Treatment has gone from surgery only to complex interactions with surgeons, radiation oncologists, medical oncologists, and others. New treatments become available almost weekly at a time when there is increasing pressure to maximize quality of life as well as the potential for cure while keeping close reigns on the cost of care. As population health directives become more important, the question of how to pick the right treatment at the right time for any given patient is tantamount. As we explore the field moving forward, the use of evidence-based choices becomes increasingly important. Although there are many "correct" choices to provide optimal care, it is also important that physicians deliver the best evidence-based care in a way that moves the field of cancer therapy forward. We strongly believe that the use of evidence-based pathways is the best way to insure this happens.

There is much written about cancer guidelines—a collection of treatment choices based on historical and concurrent clinical trials and years of experience. Although we believe individual practitioners should have sufficient latitude to choose therapy for any given patient, often these choices are not based on the best available care as determined by published evidence. As we address the ever-expanding cost to provide cancer care, we feel strongly that a standardized approach to the treatment of breast and other cancers will allow us to make the most progress.

With this concept in mind, we believe that **pathways**, prioritized evidence-based choices for cancer treatment, are a better approach to move the field forward. The problem with this concept is who makes the decision regarding what is the best pathway. As a healthcare system, when we started to address this issue, we felt there were critical guiding principles that needed to be followed:

1. Appropriate clinical trials should always be the first recommended option.
2. Pathways should be determined by practicing clinicians from both academic and community centers so that data could be reviewed by the doctors actually caring for the patients. This is preferable to pathways selected by insurance companies, which tend to prioritize the least

expensive route rather than the best, evidence-based pathway.
3. After a clinical trial option, pathways should be selected prioritizing **efficacy** of treatment, **toxicity** of treatment, and **cost of care** in determining the order of prioritization. Specifically if two or more treatments were equally effective, they should be ranked by the least toxic to the patient, and if equally effective, and equally toxic, they should be ranked by the lowest cost of care.

Unlike guidelines, such as National Comprehensive Cancer Network (NCCN) where multiple recommendations are listed for any given stage of disease, we felt it was most important to have recommendations prioritized so that we could collect and evaluate the data of a large number of similarly staged patients treated the same way. This has also allowed us to offer and accrue a large number of patients to clinical trials to help move the field forward. It has also allowed us to create a standardized precision medicine program to be sure that appropriate patients receive genomic testing of their tumor, and are recommended to receive the newest molecular therapy that is appropriate to their specific tumor mutations.

Oncologists in our group are encouraged to follow the recommended pathways, always offering their patients the ability to participate in clinical trials, and to be involved in the decision-making process. The physicians have the opportunity to deviate from the recommended pathway if they believe there are reasons why the recommended treatment is not the best for a given patient. For most diseases, between 85% and 92% of patients are treated on pathway.

In many years as a practicing surgical oncologist, I have found few words scarier to patients than "You have cancer." In the United States, every year, 281,550 women and 2650 men are told they have breast cancer.[1] The treatment options have expanded dramatically since 1894 when William Halsted told patients their only option for potential cure was a radical mastectomy.[2] Treatment approaches for breast cancer have substantially moved from surgical approaches only to truly multidisciplinary care. Fortunately, surgical options are extensive including far less radical procedures. Radiation therapy has been highly refined, again giving patients numerous options for treatment. Now, with molecular testing of tumors, we have become much better at defining which patients will or will not benefit from chemotherapy or immunotherapy, and with recent discoveries, even patients with extensive metastatic disease can live many years after diagnosis.

When we evaluate where treatment is available, most patients prefer to receive their care close to home. With better-trained surgeons and surgical oncologists, availability of advanced radiation treatments in the community, and opportunities to participate in clinical trials, patients no longer need to travel to academic centers to receive truly state-of-the-art care.

With the many options that are available to patients, they can receive the right care at the right time in the right place—proximal to where they live. Applying methods of standardization utilizing evidence-based pathways, broad-based disease-specific conferences, and dissemination of appropriate information regarding the most innovative therapies, this care can be delivered across wide geographies allowing patients to receive their care closer to their families, home, and support structures. The questions frequently asked involve how to find such centers; what are the appropriate questions patients should be asking; and how can they get the best and most appropriate care to maximize their chance for cure, have the best quality of life, and, if not curable, live the longest, most comfortable survival.

This integration of care involves evaluation and treatment by a multidisciplinary team. Particularly with the use of "virtual telemedicine," this type of evaluation can be performed even in remote areas where patients live. Accelerated treatment options for radiation therapy,[3,4] greater use of outpatient surgery, and shortened chemotherapy cycles along with the increased use of some of the newer oral chemotherapy agents as well as hormonal and molecular treatments make innovative, evidence-based care available to almost all breast cancer patients.

Utilizing best-practice education and standardization of surgical techniques along with a significant quality program, operations performed need not be limited to surgeons doing the operation "the way I've always done this" at a time when studies have shown that newer, less deforming procedures provide comparable or improved chance for cure.[5–8] Many new reconstructive techniques have been added to community centers as well.[9,10] Radiation therapy for breast cancer in the past required a 7-week course for completion. With newer techniques, this can be reduced to $3\frac{1}{2}$ weeks to as little as 1 day for appropriately selected patients.[11,12] Chemotherapy duration has been reduced from years to several months in most patients. With more recent availability of molecular therapy, it can be administered orally with less frequent visits to the physician's office.

There is much confusion, particularly among patients, about how to determine the best treatment for their cancer. Although the internet provides an incredible amount of information, the wide range of sources makes it very hard for anyone, especially patients and their families, often under duress, to find and interpret what they are reading. Unfortunately, the most outlandish and unproven recommendations can be presented in a way that can give false hope and misinterpretation. In looking for accurate sources of information, patients frequently check the NCCN guidelines and get quite confused. NCCN is a consortium consisting of many of the National Cancer Institute Comprehensive Cancer Center teams.[13] Although this represents a highly knowledgeable group, it tends to be made up of members from academic centers rather than oncologists practicing in the community, where most patients are actually treated. The NCCN guidelines are very thorough and generally include all treatment options that have been shown to have efficacy against a specific tumor type. This provides an excellent reference list, but because of the large collection of recommendations, it can be very confusing, even to clinicians, regarding which is the best treatment to choose and is particularly confusing to patients.

With the large number of patients seen in our system, we prefer to rely on pathways rather than guidelines.[14] Introduction of evidence-based pathways has improved patient access to clinical trials but can also prioritize treatment based on the efficacy of drugs with the lowest toxicity and the lowest cost. In our system, pathways are selected by a national group of practicing academic and community oncologists who meet virtually on a quarterly basis. Additional meetings are held when game-changing new therapies are introduced for consideration of incorporation into pathways. This is possible while offering patients the best opportunity for cure when possible, and for long-term palliation focusing on quality of life when an individual patient does not have curable disease.

Guidelines (including NCCN), unlike pathways, provide physicians a wide range of "acceptable" treatments but generally do not prioritize the treatments in any order. Progress in medical oncology is made by comparing several treatments against "best available" but often take years and many thousands of patients to have the data to answer such questions. Particularly in a large system that sees thousands of new cancer patients each year, the use of pathways allows standardization, which improves care, reduces complications, but at the same time allows the flexibility to change treatments when new discoveries are made. This also provides better data to review and confirm efficacy of treatment and allows better quality controls. It also has the potential to save costs, particularly when very expensive therapies can be eliminated by more sophisticated molecular tests that can define their likely effectiveness.

It is our belief that oncology is a field that improves care and outcomes by continually seeking better, safer, less toxic, and hopefully less costly treatments. We strongly support clinical trials, as that is the best way to compare new treatments to the best available current care.[15,16] This should continue until cancer is ultimately irradicated as a disease. We feel that standardization of "best" care is an obligation of a system such as ours. Pathways should not be looked at as "cookbook" medicine, but should offer oncologists a way to select evidence-based care while continuing to allow them the flexibility to choose alternative approaches when they feel this is appropriate based on the specific characteristics of any given patient. By prioritizing clinical trials, this allows patients the flexibility to participate in studies designed to improve the care for their disease and may enhance their prognosis. We consider it a sign of appropriate success that, depending on the individual cancer type and stage, the on-pathway rate for treatment runs between 85% and 92% across our system.

In addition to helping select a clinical trial or the best evidence-based care, the use of pathways helps standardize cost of care.[17,18] The new molecular treatments, although potentially more effective and less toxic, are often outrageously expensive. By appropriately using molecular testing and careful evaluation of the evidence, as we have done though a sophisticated Precision Medicine program, we have found that these drugs are now selectively offered when we can suggest the highest likelihood that they will be effective. This also allows us to avoid expensive treatment that we feel will not be effective in any patient's particular tumor.[19–21]

Pathways allow us to standardize care offered to a large group of patents across a broad geography. Although we have not found that pathways themselves save large amounts of healthcare dollars, we have found that comparing treatment for patients treated on pathway versus those treated off-pathway has a smaller range of costs. With our high rate of compliance with pathways we can provide more predictable costs with less variation.

A further benefit of standardization and size has been our ability to leverage the knowledge and skills of our physicians and advanced practice clinicians (APC) to the benefit of our patients. Within medical oncology, all our physicians have selected two diseases of particular interest. We have also created system-wide disease-specific conferences where all new complex cases are presented to this large panel of physicians. In the case of breast cancer, the most common new cancer seen in the system, we have created five regional conferences in Wisconsin where new cases are presented for discussion. The advantage of this approach is that care is standardized across a wide geography, and even those practicing in our more remote locations can feel there is wide support for the care they are providing to their patients. Although oncologists in the smaller locations need to treat all patients with multiple diagnoses, they benefit from the expertise in the system, and more importantly, they also serve as valuable resources in the system. By selecting the diseases of interest, they agree to increase their continuing medical education in these areas, which helps provide focus at a time when new knowledge expands at an explosive rate. This subspecialization has also helped enhance engagement among our physician and APC teams. This has also allowed us to provide both in-person and virtual multidisciplinary disease-specific clinics. As an example, breast cancer patients can be evaluated by all appropriate specialists in one setting based around the patient, their family, and needs. Although this can be less convenient for the physicians, if done appropriately, it can be done in an efficient and timely manner. Patients and their families do not get overwhelmed, and they often can come to the clinic with a diagnosis and leave with a full plan as to their near-term care. This system also allows for appropriate evaluation by not only the breast surgeon, medical oncologist, and radiation oncologists but allows genetic counselors, plastic surgeons, dieticians, financial counselors, and other support professionals to create an all-encompassing care plan for the patient. A comprehensive program of disease-specific nurse navigators facilitates coordination of the many disciplines.

In 2007, 22.7% of patients diagnosed with breast cancer died from their disease while only 15.5% diagnosed in 2021 succumbed.[1,22] Although this is remarkable progress, it shows that there is tremendous progress still to be made. Standardization of evaluation and treatment will allow continued reduction in patient mortality from breast cancer.

This book has been developed by authors who are highly experienced in working in multidisciplinary teams utilizing evidence-based pathways, and offers how these types of treatments can be prioritized and standardized to provide all patients with the right care, in the right place, at the right time.

References

1. American Cancer Society. *Cancer Facts & Figures 2021*. Atlanta: American Cancer Society; 2021.
2. Lawrence W Jr, Lopez MJ. Radical surgery for cancer: a historical perspective. *Surg Clin N Am*. 2005;14:441–446.
3. Smith BD, Arthur DW, Buchholz TA, et al. Accelerated partial breast irradiation consensus statement from the American Society for Radiation Oncology (ASTRO). *Int J Radiat Oncol Biol Phys*. 2009;74(4):987.
4. Vicini FA, Cecchini RS, White JR, et al. Long-term primary results of accelerated partial breast irradiation after breast-conserving surgery for early-stage breast cancer: a randomised, phase 3, equivalence trial. *Lancet*. 2019;394(10215):2155.
5. Fisher B, Montague E, Redmond C, et al. Comparison of radical mastectomy with alternative treatments for primary breast cancer. A first report of results from a prospective randomized clinical trial. *Cancer*. 1977;39(suppl 6):2827–2839. https://doi.org/10.1002/1097-0142(197706)39:6<2827::aid-cncr2820390671>3.0.co;2-i.
6. Fisher B, Anderson S, Bryant J, et al. Twenty-year follow-up of a randomized trial comparing total mastectomy, lumpectomy, and lumpectomy plus irradiation for the treatment of invasive breast cancer. *N Engl J Med*. 2002;347:1233–1241.
7. Galimberti V, Cole BF, Viale G, et al. Axillary dissection versus no axillary dissection in patients with breast cancer and sentinel-node micrometastases (IBCSG 23-01): 10-year follow-up of a randomised, controlled phase 3 trial. *Lancet Oncol*. 2018;19(10):1385–1393. https://doi.org/10.1016/S1470-2045(18)30380-2.
8. Giuliano AE, Ballman KV, McCall L, et al. Effect of axillary dissection vs no axillary dissection on 10-year overall survival among women with invasive breast cancer and sentinel node metastasis: the ACOSOG Z0011 (Alliance) Randomized Clinical Trial. *JAMA*. 2017;318(10):918–926. https://doi.org/10.1001/jama.2017.11470.
9. Rizki H, Varghese JS. Surgical techniques in breast cancer: an overview. *Surgery*. 2022;40(2):121–131.

10. Platt J, Baxter N, Zhong T. Breast reconstruction after mastectomy for breast cancer. *CMAJ*. 2011;183(18):2109–2116.

11. Cernusco NLV, Bianco PD, Romano M, et al. Long-term outcomes using electron IOERT APBI for early stage breast cancer: the Verona University Hospital experience. *Clin Breast Cancer*. 2021S1526-8209(21)00143-9.

12. Vaidya JS, Baum M, Tobias JS, et al. Long-term results of targeted intraoperative radiotherapy (Targit) boost during breast conserving surgery. *Int J Radiat Oncol Biol Phys*. 2011;81(4):1091–1097.

13. National Comprehensive Cancer Network. *NCCN Guidelines, Version 2.2022*. www.nccn.org; 2022.

14. Zon RT, Frame JN, Neuss MN, et al. American Society of Clinical Oncology policy statement on clinical pathways in oncology. *J Oncol Pract*. 2016;12(3):261–266.

15. Unger JM, Cook E, Tai E, et al. The role of clinical trial participation in cancer research: barriers, evidence, and strategies. *Am Soc Clin Oncol Educ Book*. 2016;35:185–198. https://doi.org/10.1200/EDBK_156686.

16. Hirsch BR, Califf RM, Cheng SK, et al. Characteristics of oncology clinical trials: insights from a systematic analysis of ClinicalTrials.gov. *JAMA Intern Med*. 2013;173(11):972–979. https://doi.org/10.1001/jamainternmed.2013.627.

17. Weese JL, Citrin L, Shamah CJ, et al. Implementation of treatment pathways in a large integrated health care system. *J Clin Oncol*. 2016;34(15):6613–6613. https://doi.org/10.1200/JCO.2016.34.15_suppl.6613.

18. Weese JL, Shamah CJ, Sanchez FA, et al. Use of treatment pathways reduce cost and decrease ED utilization and unplanned hospital admissions in patients (pts) with stage II breast cancer. *J Clin Oncol*. 2019;37(suppl 15):e12012–e12012.

19. Cantenacci DVT. Expansion platform type II: testing a treatment strategy. *Lancet Oncol*. 2015;16(13):1276–1278.

20. Saltz LB. Precision oncology giveth and precision oncology taketh away. *Lancet Oncol*. 2019;20(4):464–445.

21. Meric-Bernstam F, Hurwitz H, Raghav KPS, et al. Pertuzumab plus trastuzumab for HER2-amplified metastatic Colorectal Cancer (MyPathway) an updated report from a multicentre, open-label, phase 2a, multiple basket study. *Lancet Oncol*. 2019;20:518–530.

22. American Cancer Society. *Cancer Facts & Figures 2007*. Atlanta: American Cancer Society; 2007.

2

Multidisciplinary Team Approach to the Management of Breast Cancer

AARON CHEVINSKY AND JOSEPH JOHN WEBER

Implementation of a Multidisciplinary Care Program

When setting up a multidisciplinary treatment program (Fig. 2.1), several areas must be evaluated, which include selecting the needed personnel, their proximity to the primary treatment site(s), and their ability to attend meetings in-person or virtually. The types of meetings that can be arranged include multidisciplinary tumor boards (case presentations) and multidisciplinary clinic conferences (patient seen and examined by the team) also known as multidisciplinary care centers (MDCC). The difference includes whether there is only a discussion of the patient's relevant history, physical examination, radiologic studies, and pathology versus the direct patient evaluation with the patient physically present to be examined by the team and participating in the treatment discussion. There are benefits and drawbacks of each approach. For tumor board presentations, clinicians may be present in one location, or may join remotely. The relevant history and findings can be shown to the group by radiology and pathology, and an agreement of the proper treatment pathway can be reached with one member of the team designated to convey the information to the patient and implement the treatment plan. The drawback is that the patient may need to make several visits to the clinicians, and therefore it may not be the most time-effective approach. Some recent studies[1–3] have recommended patients receive their first course of therapy within 30 days of diagnosis. Delays in treatment implementation may lead to earlier recurrence or reduction in cure rate. In the MDCC model, the patient is seen and examined by the relevant members of the team (typically surgery, medical, radiation oncology, and plastic surgery (when needed), and a decision about treatment is reached and implemented by the chosen team member.[4,5] Radiologists and pathologists with an interest in breast cancer may also be present or available upon request to review imaging and pathology and/or for surgical planning. Patients are also seen by a nurse navigator to assist in logistics of the treatment implementation, as well as referral to plastic and reconstructive surgeons, social workers, integrative and complementary medicine specialists, nutritionists, physical therapists, and genetic counseling as needed. Drawbacks of this approach include the potential for time inefficiency for the clinician who may need to wait for other members of the multidisciplinary team to complete their evaluations. Often a hybrid model can be effective where the patient's case is presented to the larger group of clinicians, and a smaller, select group then gathers to meet and examine the patient and have a discussion with the patient regarding the proposed treatment pathway.

Program Components

Multidisciplinary breast cancer treatment teams include the following physician specialties: surgery (breast surgery, surgical oncology, and/or general surgery), plastic and reconstructive surgery, medical oncology, radiation oncology, breast radiology, and pathology. The following ancillary service representatives are recommended to assist the core multidisciplinary team: tumor registry, nurse navigation, research, and genetics. Other areas may be added at the discretion of the site, including complementary and integrative health, fertility specialists, physical and occupational therapy, nutrition, pastoral care, as well as trainees in medicine, nursing, and other allied health fields. For the initial evaluation of the patient, the three major disciplines— surgery, medical oncology, and radiation oncology—should be available to assess and examine the patient. Residents and fellows of the appropriate disciplines are encouraged to attend as well.

Value of Multidisciplinary Care

In a system with a well-defined treatment paradigm and well-defined pathways for care, the implementation of multidisciplinary care teams and pathways allows for the most accurate, up-to-date evidence-based and cost-effective care (Fig. 2.1). Patients are seen by the key members of the treatment team, and treatment decisions are made in a collaborative format using the best evidence. Patients and their

CHAPTER 2 Multidisciplinary Team Approach to the Management of Breast Cancer 7

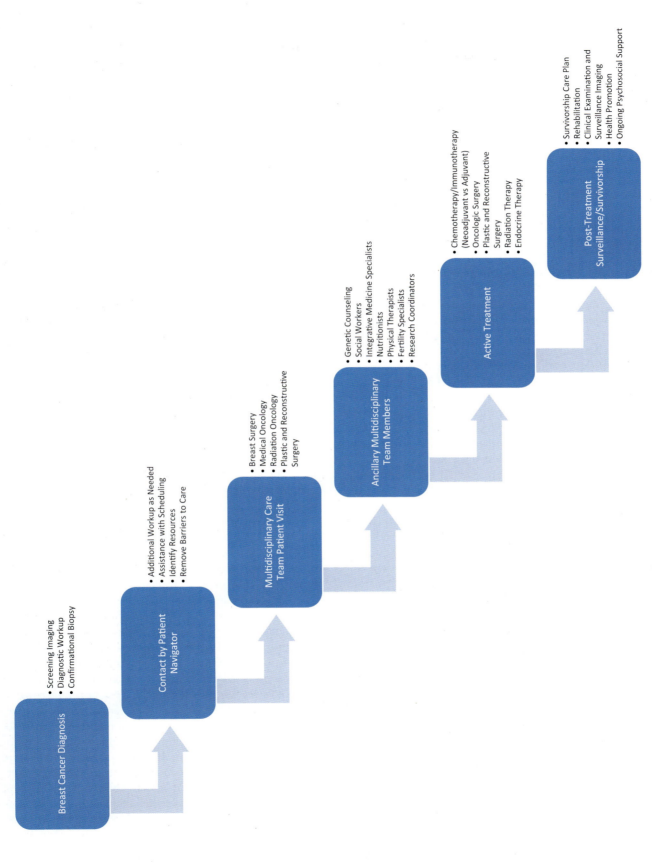

• **Fig. 2.1** Multidisciplinary Approach to the Management of Breast Cancer.

families can be part of the decision-making process and feel empowered by their inclusion. Multidisciplinary treatment teams provide a high level of patient and family satisfaction and allow patients to both participate and understand the scientific/medical basis for the treatment decisions. In this setting, patients are encouraged to participate in the shared decision-making process when options are presented. Patients can then be presented and evaluated again during times of treatment change, further allowing refinement and clarification of the individualized care plan.

Which Patients Should Participate?

In an optimal situation, all breast cancer patients would be treated in a multidisciplinary treatment environment. Certain patients should preferentially be seen in a multidisciplinary format (personnel and space permitting). All patients with newly diagnosed invasive or in situ cancer should be seen by a multidisciplinary team to assess the tumor extent and decide about the treatment pathway. Prior to the meeting, it is best that the following information be gathered and available for review: patient's history including prior breast biopsies and pathology (reviewed by in-house pathologists and radiologists), menstrual and pregnancy history, family history of breast and other cancers, any prior genetic testing, and what, if any, symptoms led to evaluation. In addition, all imaging of the breast should be available for review, including any prior films for comparison. The pathology should be available for in-house review, including all prognostic biomarker studies that have been performed (estrogen and progesterone receptor status, Her-2-neu status, and KI-67 if ordered). The nurse navigator plays a key role in reaching out to the patient/family and gathering this information to be available for the team's review. Other patients who are optimal for multidisciplinary format review and evaluation include patients who are being considered for neoadjuvant therapy, those completing neoadjuvant therapy, patients with suspected or documented recurrence, and any patient for which multidisciplinary evaluation may help in complex decision making. Some of these include patients with genetic mutations that increase the risk of breast cancer, patients with pre-malignant lesions, and patients in whom therapy is not taking the expected course. The goal is to be inclusive rather than exclusive.

Decisions on Testing Prior to and After Multidisciplinary Evaluation

When a patient presents for their multidisciplinary appointment, each member of the team should independently and then jointly review all the available data including available history and physical examination data, radiologic studies, and pathology including prognostic biomarkers. The team should then decide if any additional testing is required to recommend a treatment plan. These decisions may involve the request for additional biopsies of areas not originally sampled, the repeating of marker studies, and additional radiologic studies such as breast magnetic resonance imaging (MRI) to determine the extent of tumor within the breast or axilla, and staging studies such as computed tomography (CT), bone scintigraphy, and positron emission tomography (PET) scanning to determine if local or distant metastatic disease may be present. This may lead to additional studies being requested, such as second-look ultrasound and additional biopsies under MRI or ultrasound guidance. Referral for genetic evaluation and research study participation should also be an integral part of the multidisciplinary evaluation.

High-Risk Patient Evaluation and Management

The appropriate management of patients at elevated risk for developing breast cancer is a complex topic. These patients are appropriate for a multidisciplinary management panel when they have developed cancerous or precancerous findings. The management of these patients at elevated risk and discussion of risk reduction strategies will be covered more fully in Chapter 15 of this book.

Women born and residing in the United States have a breast cancer risk of approximately 12.5% (1:8). This risk increases with age and varies in different ethnic groups. Women considered at high risk are generally assumed to have a breast cancer lifetime risk of 20% on any of the commonly used calculation models (Tyrer-Cuzick, or Gail, or other models). These models utilize patient age; menstrual and pregnancy history; family history of breast, ovarian, and other cancers (and the age at which they were diagnosed); biopsy history (particularly with atypia seen); breast density; and prior exposure to radiation, among others, to calculate a risk score. Genetic evaluation and referral to our family cancer genetics program is offered for those patients whose personal or family history would make them appropriate for genetic testing.

Women who are found to be at high risk are referred to our high-risk breast program and are seen by the physicians and advanced practice clinicians and undergo a more in-depth risk assessment. If they are truly at high risk, then they are counseled about risk-reduction strategies as well as enhanced screening. Those at highest risk begin screening at age 35, or 10 years earlier than their earliest family member developed breast cancer. This enhanced screening includes biannual in-person evaluation and alternating mammogram/ultrasound and MRI at 6-month intervals. Patients are counseled regarding risk-reducing strategies including exercise; diet; healthy living and avoiding obesity, smoking, and excess alcohol; and other behaviors that will further increase their risk. They are also offered risk-reducing anti-estrogen therapies when appropriate. Those at the highest level of risk are offered risk-reducing surgeries (mastectomy and oophorectomy) as appropriate.

When a patient at high risk does develop invasive or in situ breast cancer, they are evaluated in a multidisciplinary setting to discuss appropriate treatment options. The patients are included in this joint decision-making process to allow their input into the treatment options. This complex decision making often needs to take into consideration genetic syndromes that increase the risk of subsequent cancers, patient's reproductive desires, and their concerns regarding the ability of screening tests to discover other cancers if they should develop. The team assesses the patient's risks of recurrence, and of developing a subsequent cancer, and makes recommendations based on the best available information. Based on the extent of the cancer, breast-conserving surgery may or may not be recommended or given as an option. Overall, the patient partners with the team to develop the best individual treatment strategy within the parameters of our treatment protocols.

Ancillary Services to Assist the Breast Cancer Patient

Although the implementation and management of care for the patient with breast cancer may largely be driven by the surgical, medical, and radiation oncology specialists, there are several other ancillary services functioning in the multidisciplinary team to improve patient care. Support groups, both in-person and virtual, have been cited as being particularly helpful for navigating the long- and short-term impact of breast cancer. Emotional support benefits of support groups included a feeling of connectedness as well as understanding, which provided hope and healing to participants.[6] Social workers may also help connect patients to support groups and aid with additional resources, including psychosocial support.[7] Furthermore, breast cancer patient navigators are an essential part of the multidisciplinary team to help provide timely access to services and ensure completion of diagnosis and follow-up of care.[8]

Physical medicine and rehabilitation specialists are also important assets to the multidisciplinary team for the patient with breast cancer. Rehabilitation, which may be facilitated by physical and occupational therapists, includes improving strength and cardiovascular conditioning, alleviating pain, and reducing fatigue.[9] Given the increased risk of lymphedema following axillary surgery and radiation therapy for breast cancer, rehabilitation may also help with both its prevention and management.[10] Furthermore, exercise provides an important role to help women physically recover from treatment and potentially prevent cancer recurrence.[11]

Complementary and integrative medicine therapies may be used for supportive care during breast cancer treatment and to manage treatment-related side effects. Specialists who can facilitate such modalities as music therapy, meditation, yoga, and massage may help with depression as well as improve quality of life. Treatment-related nausea and vomiting may be improved by acupuncture and acupressure, and dietitians help with adequate nutrition and weight management during breast cancer treatment and survivorship. Integrative practices may help as effective supportive care strategies for the care of patients with breast cancer.[12]

Shared Decision Making

Once all the information has been reviewed, the multidisciplinary team reconvenes to discuss the treatment recommendations, which usually will involve a recommendation for surgery or neoadjuvant therapy as the initial modality (Fig. 2.1). As you will see in the subsequent chapters, decision making regarding upfront surgery versus neoadjuvant therapy (chemotherapy, immunotherapy, and/or anti-estrogen therapy) is complex and nuanced. Patients with more advanced disease generally will be selected for neoadjuvant therapy along with patients with more worrisome histologic findings including triple-negative and HER-2-neu positive breast cancers.

Summary and Conclusion

Multidisciplinary input in the care of the patient with breast cancer is essential to provide coordinated, evidence-based, and continuous cost-effective care. Using a team-based approach and shared decision making allows the patients and their families a feeling of participation in the process and will allow for greater compliance in the treatment plan. All members of the team contribute to the patient's treatment and recovery and should be valued for the important contributions they make to the overall treatment process.

References

1. Ho PJ, Cook R, Mohamed NKB, et al. Impact of delayed treatment in women diagnosed with breast cancer: a population-based study. *Cancer Med*. 2020;9:2435–2444.
2. Hanna TP, King WD, Thibodeau S, et al. Mortality due to cancer treatment delay: systematic review and meta-analysis. *BMJ*. 2020;371:m4087. https://doi.org/10.1136/bmj.m4087.
3. Smith EC, Ziogas A, Anton-Culver H. Delay in surgical treatment and survival after breast cancer diagnosis in young women by race/ethnicity. *JAMA Surg*. 2013;148(6):516–523. Published online April 24, 2013. https://doi.org/10.1001/jamasurg.2013.1680.
4. Murthy KR, Ferguson SE, Tereffe W, et al. Effect of a new model for multidisciplinary breast cancer care on clinical metrics leading to efficiency and timeliness of access. *J Clin Oncol*. 2014;32(suppl 2):107–107.
5. Kesson EM, Allardice GM, George WD, et al. Effects of multidisciplinary team working on breast cancer survival: retrospective, comparative, interventional cohort study of 13,722 women. *BMJ*. 2012;344:e2718. https://doi.org/10.1136/bmj.e2718.
6. Gray RE, Fitch M, Davis C, et al. A qualitative study of breast cancer self-help groups. *Psycho-Oncol*. 1997;6:279–289.
7. Kauffmann R, Bitz C, Clark K, et al. Addressing psychosocial needs of partners of breast cancer patients: a pilot program using

social workers to improve communication and psychosocial support. *Support Care Cancer*. 2016;24:61–65.

8. Budde H, Williams GA, Winkelmann J, et al. The role of patient navigators in ambulatory care: overview of systematic reviews. *BMC Health Serv Res*. 2021;21(1):1166.

9. Silver JK. Rehabilitation in women with breast cancer. *Phys Med Rehabil Clin N Am*. 2007;18(3):521–537.

10. Merchant SJ, Chen SL. Prevention and management of lymphedema after breast cancer treatment. *Breast J*. 2015;21(3):276–284.

11. Pinto BM, Maruyama NC. Exercise in the rehabilitation of breast cancer survivors. *Psychooncology*. 1999;8(3):191–206.

12. Greenlee H, DuPont-Reyes MJ, Balneaves LG, et al. Clinical practice guidelines on the evidence-based use of integrative therapies during and after breast cancer treatment. *CA Cancer J Clin*. 2017;67(3):194–232.

3

Oncology Nurse Navigation in the Care of Breast Cancer

KENDRA CAMPBELL AND JAMIE CAIRO

Introduction

A breast cancer diagnosis can be highly stressful and traumatic, not only for the patient but also for their family and support systems. The experience of moving through the breast cancer continuum from diagnosis to treatment and beyond is a complex process that can be alleviated by the guidance and support of an Oncology Nurse Navigator (ONN). An ONN is defined by the Oncology Nursing Society (ONS) as "a professional RN with oncology-specific clinical knowledge who offers individualized assistance to patients, families, and caregivers to help overcome healthcare system barriers."[1] The ONN works to help overcome healthcare system barriers and facilitate timely access to quality medical and psychosocial care from pre-diagnosis through all phases of the cancer experience. Using the nursing process, the ONN provides education and resources to cancer patients to better facilitate informed decision making and timely access to care. This chapter will focus on oncology nurse navigation in breast cancer care.

History of Patient Navigation

In 1989, the American Cancer Society (ACS) published the *Report to the Nation on Cancer in the Poor*, which summarized a series of national hearings that looked at patient access and barriers to care for those who live in poverty. The report found that poor Americans face significant barriers to obtaining cancer care. Those who live in poverty received substandard healthcare that they had difficulty paying for and were made to "endure assaults on their personal dignity when seeking treatment for cancer."[2] The report identified that cancer education programs were often "culturally insensitive and irrelevant."[3] Then president of the ACS, Dr. Harold Freeman, subsequently developed the first patient navigator program to address the elimination of barriers to care in Harlem in 1990. Freeman recognized that cancer care for poor, underinsured, and uninsured people faced unique barriers to care, which led to the development of a patient navigation program for the underserved. From this, Freeman was able to prove that cancer survival rates can improve with increased screening and reducing barriers to healthcare for cancer patients. Initially this navigation program was focused on breast cancer patients and staffed by lay community case workers. They worked to facilitate access by addressing financial barriers, such as no health insurance, as well as communication, information, and medical system barriers.[4] Over time the scope of patient navigation has expanded beyond just breast cancer and across the entire healthcare continuum including prevention, detection, diagnosis, treatment, and survivorship to the end of life.[3]

In 2005, the Patient Navigator and Chronic Disease Prevention Act added Section 340a of the Public Health Service Act (PHSA) that encouraged the development of programs to improve health outcomes for patients with cancer and other chronic diseases, with the goal of improved access to high-quality coordinated care. In 2012, the American College of Surgeons Commission on Cancer created a new standard addressing patient navigation to be implemented by 2015 for cancer programs seeking accreditation.

Program Accreditation

Healthcare accreditation validates that a cancer program meets or exceeds a set of quality and care standards set by an "accrediting" body of experts. Many accrediting bodies require that the cancer program have a navigation program in place. The National Cancer Institute defines a standard of care as "treatment that is accepted by medical experts as a proper treatment for a certain type of disease and that is widely used by healthcare professionals."[5] In breast cancer care, the standards that define and measure quality of care involve multiple organizations but are largely driven by the National Comprehensive Cancer Network (NCCN), the National Accreditation Program for Breast Centers (NAPBC) offered by the American College of Surgeons, and the American Society of Clinical Oncology (ASCO).

NAPBC represents a consortium of national, professional organizations dedicated to the quality of care of patients with diseases of the breast. In 2018, NAPBC published navigation standard 2.2, which states that, "A patient navigation process is in place to guide the patient with a breast abnormality through provider and referred services. The patient navigation process includes consistent care coordination throughout the continuum of care and an assessment of the physical, psychological, and social needs of the patient. The anticipated results are enhanced patient outcomes, increased satisfaction, and reduced costs of care. Patient navigation is provided by a professional (for example, nurse, social worker) who has documented training to provide individualized assistance to breast disease patients, families, and caregivers at risk. If patient navigation is provided by a lay navigator, then he or she is required to have documented patient navigation training."[6]

In 2021, ASCO developed Oncology Medical Home (OMH) standards, which provide a comprehensive road map for oncology practices to deliver high-quality, evidence-based cancer care including access to equitable, comprehensive, and coordinated team-based care including a process for patient navigation.

Defining the Oncology Nurse Navigator Role

Patient navigation can be performed by different types of professionals, including trained lay personnel, social workers, advanced practitioners, as well as nurses. Table 3.1 outlines the different navigation roles. There is variability in workflow by institution, but typically the ONN is one of the first points of contact for a newly diagnosed patient, often from the radiology department after the patient has an abnormal mammogram. The ONN completes a nursing assessment to identify the patient's unique, individualized needs. They offer emotional support, advocate for patients and their loved ones, provide continuity of care, address psychosocial needs, provide education, and assess barriers to care.

Literature Review of Oncology Navigation

According to ONS, patient navigation in oncology provides many benefits for patients, including a shorter time to diagnosis and start of treatment, increased patient and caregiver knowledge, better adherence to recommended care, and improved quality of life.[1] A randomized pilot study done in 2013[7] found that ONN's who specialize in breast cancer were more likely to provide the right amount of support and resources compared to other healthcare providers. Breast navigators also helped give patients their results as soon as possible, provided much needed emotional support, and helped them get accurate information from an expert in a timely manner. Randomized navigation studies

TABLE 3.1 Oncology Navigator Role Delineation

Oncology Nurse Navigator	Registered nurse with oncology expertise based around the core competencies of navigation, including the facilitation of timely and coordinated care, education and empowerment of patients and caregivers, promotion of patient- and family-centered care, and effective communication within the multidisciplinary team.
Social Work Navigator	Oncology social workers perform comprehensive psychosocial assessments, counseling, education, patient navigation, case management, resource coordination, and program development.
Financial Navigator	Maximize health insurance benefits, reduce economic barriers to care, and accurately explain insurance coverage. Do assessments for risk for and help mitigate financial toxicity.
Lay Navigator	A trained non-professional or volunteer who provides guidance and support to patients to overcome healthcare system barriers and facilitate timely access to care. Lay navigators can take on more "concrete" tasks such as completing paperwork, finding local or statewide resources, providing information on clinical trials or survivorship programs, while triaging the more clinical questions.

From Rua K The importance of role delineation in navigation. J Navig Surviv. 2018;9(8).

on resolution of breast abnormal screening demonstrate that navigated patients experienced a shorter time to results versus those in a non-navigated group.[8] Patient navigation improves timeliness in diagnosis and treatment of patients in underserved populations and was found to be more efficacious when utilized shortly after screening or diagnostic testing.[9]

In terms of improved coordination of care and communication, assessment, and adherence of treatment recommendations, it has been demonstrated that there is a decrease in time to definitive therapy and a higher percentage of newly diagnosed patients who start treatment within 30 days.[10] Hoffman et al.[11] found that women with breast cancer who received patient navigation, in particular those requiring biopsy, "reached their diagnostic resolution" significantly faster than those who did not have a navigator.[11]

There are organizational benefits as well. A study done by Kline et al. demonstrated that navigation resulted in increased patient retention and improved physician loyalty with downstream increase in revenue.[12] It was also associated with a reduction in unnecessary resource utilization, such as emergency department visits and hospitalizations, thus decreasing burdens on oncology providers, potentially reducing burnout, errors, and costly staff turnover. One of the benefits of using nurses with high levels of knowledge and expertise is that they can proactively reference NCCN guidelines, thereby facilitating appropriate staging studies in collaboration with the oncology provider, which can save time and also lead to positive financial returns on investment.[13] Bernardo et al. reviewed 113 published articles that assessed oncology navigation between 2010 and 2018 and found that the majority of studies identified favorable outcomes for oncology navigation, including increased uptake of and adherence to cancer screenings, timely diagnostic resolution and follow-up, higher completion rates for cancer therapy, and higher rates of attending medical appointments.[14]

Role Development

ONS recognized the need for oncology nurse navigators to have a defined scope and role as they serve not only the patient but the cancer care system in which they work. This led to the development of core competencies, first issued in 2013 and later revised and published in 2017, as a way to standardize the role. They identified priorities, including the development of a standardized job description and orientation as well as professional certification.

The ONN care model describes navigator interventions in the following categories:

- Assess and address barriers to care.
- Provide education, resources, and referral to local and national resources (i.e., physical/occupational therapy, dietitians, home health, financial counselors, and foundations).
- Participate in promotion of shared decision making, an important strategy to facilitate patient-centered care where patients are faced with complicated treatment decisions that require them to weigh efficacy and safety, quality of life, and cost.[15]
- Promote advanced care planning by encouraging patients to talk about their treatment wishes and overall goals of care.
- Support palliative care by assessing for late and long-term side effects and other physical barriers to patients' quality of life and educating patients about the differences between palliative care and hospice.[1]

Knowledge and Skills Requirements

ONS provides a set of recommendations for the ONN in terms of experience and skill set.

- Strong oncology knowledge and experience.
- Basic knowledge of insurance reimbursement systems
- Working knowledge of financial hardships and payer coverage
- Working knowledge of national, regional, and community resources
- Knowledge of self-care strategies and resources

TABLE 3.2	Novice Versus Expert Oncology Nurse Navigator
Novice ONN	An oncology nurse navigator who has 3 years or less of experience in the ONN role and is building on his or her academic preparation, nursing knowledge, and oncology experience to develop in the ONN role.
Expert ONN	An ONN who has worked at least 3 years, is proficient in the role, and has the education and experience to use critical thinking and decision-making skills pertaining to the evolution of navigation processes and the individual ONN.

From 2017 ONS Core Competencies by Oncology Nursing Society.

- Critical-thinking skills
- Strong leadership skills
- Strong interpersonal skills
- Ability to develop collaborative relationships both internally and externally
- Ability to work in teams
- Ability to work autonomously
- Strong verbal and written communication skills
- Strong organizational skills
- Ability to prioritize and reprioritize quickly
- Basic computer skills[1]

ONS also defines the differences between the expert and novice ONN (Table 3.2).

Specialty Certification in Breast Navigation

Obtaining specialty certification reflects an individual's achievement beyond licensure requirements and a basic level of knowledge and expertise. There are two breast-specific specialty certifications available. The Breast Patient Navigator Certification (BPNC) is a specialty certification offered by the National Consortium of Breast Centers. This program offers six types of breast navigator certifications:

- CN-BI (breast imaging) for those working in diagnostic imaging
- CN-BM (breast management) for those working in management or social services
- CN-BA (advocates) for volunteer and lay navigators
- CN-BC (clinical) for certified Medical Assistants and Licensed Practical/Vocational Nurses
- CN-BP (providers) for physicians and advanced practice providers
- CN-BN (RN) for all registered nurses

The Certified Breast Care Nurse (CBCN) is a specialty certification offered by the Oncology Nursing Certification Corporation and is a nationally accredited breast care nursing certification that is available exclusively to registered nurses. It requires a minimum of 2 years of experience as an RN within the 4 years prior to application, and a minimum of 2000 hours of breast care nursing practice, which can be clinical practice, nursing administration, education, research, or consultation. Applicants must also complete a minimum of 10 contact hours of nursing continuing education in breast care nursing or an academic elective in breast care nursing.

Psychosocial Screening and Support

Cancer patients are at increased risk of psychosocial distress, which can negatively impact their quality of life and ability to deal with their treatment regimen. Ng et al. found that 50.2% of breast cancer patients had perceived high levels of distress at diagnosis, and 51.6% still had high levels at 6 months after diagnosis.[16] Therefore, timely access to support services is essential during cancer treatment. Psychosocial distress is defined by the NCCN[17] as an "unpleasant emotional experience of psychological, social, and/or spiritual nature that may interfere with the ability to cope effectively with cancer, its physical symptoms, and its treatment" that can be a significant barrier along the continuum of care. Oncology nurse navigators provide important support in distress management by integrating psychosocial assessment with validated tools like the NCCN Distress Thermometer as a means to identify individual patient needs and assist in addressing those areas through intervention or referral.

Addressing Barriers to Care

ONNs work with the entire cancer care team to assess their patients for barriers to care and then to make appropriate referrals to supportive care resources. Some of the barriers to care that may be addressed by navigation include:

- Access to care, which can include difficulty in scheduling appointments because of knowledge or language barriers as well as lack of healthcare coverage.
- Financial and economic issues including being uninsured or inadequately insured, and not being able to make copayments or take time off of work to seek screening and/or treatment.
- Language barriers and health literacy issues that prevent patients from understanding the treatment recommendations and plan of care.
- Cultural and ethnic diversity that can lead to mistrust of the healthcare system, requiring tailored interventions and communication.
- Fragmented and poor communication among the patient's healthcare team and with the patient and their caregivers.
- Transportation barriers that can impede a patient's ability to get to appointments.
- Emotional and psychosocial issues including distress and fear, which can interfere with timely care.[18]

Multidisciplinary Team

The evolution of cancer care involves new and emerging technologies and treatments, leading to increasingly complex care. The care of breast cancer involves multiple specialties including surgical, medical, and radiation oncology, along with diagnostic radiology, pathology, genetic/risk counseling, clinical research, and other supportive services. The multidisciplinary approach has a number of advantages and allows for the tailoring of treatment based on the individual's tumor biology and sensitivity to therapy.[19] The ONN as the first point of patient contact plays an important role in coordinating the patient's multidisciplinary care, working in collaboration with the interdisciplinary team to contribute to and coordinate the presentation of the patient's case at breast case conference, and facilitate their attendance at a multidisciplinary breast clinic. Fig. 3.1 outlines the workflow of the breast multidisciplinary program at Aurora Cancer Care in Wisconsin and highlights the role of the Breast Care Navigator.

Once a treatment plan has been established, the ONN may continue to stay in contact with the patient to offer emotional support and address any barriers to care that could arise. Most often a cancer patient requires multimodality treatment of their disease. Transitioning from each type of treatment can be overwhelming for a cancer patient. With treatment transitions comes new information to learn, new potential side effects, new schedule of appointments, etc. From this, cancer patients have ongoing unanswered questions and concerns, and the ONN can be a valuable resource. Having an ONN to provide guidance throughout the process of their treatment journey can be very meaningful for patients and their loved ones, resulting in high levels of patient satisfaction. Having a single point of contact for support can prove to be invaluable to patients. In addition, the ONN can also function as a resource for the treating team.

Survivorship and End of Life

The care of a cancer patient does not end when their treatment does. The ONN provides support to patients into survivorship, palliative care, or end-of-life care as well. Transitions from acute to continuing care can be difficult and are prone to fragmentation. The nurse navigator can also be instrumental in addressing challenges during these transitions of care, leading to improved quality of life, decreased utilization of emergency department services and hospital readmission, duplicated tests, and fragmented care that can lead to increased healthcare costs and suboptimal overall patient outcomes.[20] For patients with curative intent cancers, survivorship care and support are important, and they can be instrumental in coordinating a cancer survivorship visit and making any other necessary referrals for the cancer patient to obtain essential ongoing follow-up care.

Patients diagnosed with metastatic breast cancer benefit from specialized care. It is important for them to be

CHAPTER 3 Oncology Nurse Navigation in the Care of Breast Cancer

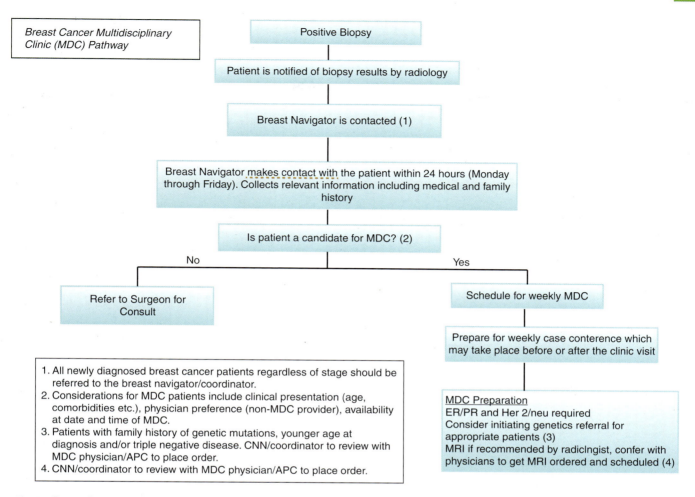

• **Fig. 3.1** Breast Cancer Multidisciplinary Clinic Pathway.

educated about the differences between palliative care and hospice. ONNs who serve as a patient advocate can not only educate patients and their families about the differences and advantages of such care but can also advocate for patients with the oncology team to encourage them to consider offering palliative care services in a timely manner as a way to manage symptoms caused by the cancer itself or side effects caused by the treatment.[21]

References

1. *2017 Oncology Nurse Navigator Core Competencies.* ons.org. https://www.ons.org/sites/default/files/2017ONNcompetencies.pdf.
2. A summary of the American Cancer Society Report to the nation: cancer in the poor. *CA Cancer J Clin.* 1989;39(5): 263–265. https://doi.org/10.3322/canjclin.39.5.263.
3. Freeman HP, Rodriguez RL. History and principles of patient navigation. *Cancer.* 2011;117(suppl 15):3539–3542. https://doi.org/10.1002/cncr.26262.
4. Cantril C, Christensen D, Moore E. Prime Pubmed: standardizing roles: evaluating oncology nurse navigator clarity, educational preparation, and scope of work within two healthcare systems. *PRIME PubMed | Standardizing Roles: Evaluating Oncology Nurse Navigator Clarity, Educational Preparation, and Scope of Work Within Two Healthcare Systems.* 2020. http://bjp.sagepub.unboundmedicine.com/medline/citation/30681989/Standardizing_Roles:_Evaluating_Oncology_Nurse_Navigator_Clarity_Educational_Preparation_and_Scope_of_Work_Within_Two_Healthcare_Systems_.
5. National Cancer Institute. *NCI Dictionary of Cancer Terms.* 2021. http://www.cancer.gov/publications/dictionaries/cancer-terms/def/standard-of-care.
6. National Accreditation Program for Breast Centers. 2018. https://accreditation.facs.org/accreditationdocuments/NAPBC/Portal%20Resources/2018NAPBCStandardsManual.pdf.
7. Mertz BG, Dunn-Henriksen AK, Kroman N, et al. The effects of individually tailored nurse navigation for patients with newly diagnosed breast cancer: a randomized pilot study. *Acta Oncol.* 2017;56(12):1682–1689. https://doi.org/10.1080/0284186X.2017.1358462.
8. Markossian TW, Darnell JS, Calhoun EA. Follow-up and timeliness after an abnormal cancer screening among underserved, urban women in a patient navigation program. *Cancer Epidemiol Biomarkers Prev.* 2012;21(10):1691–1700. https://doi.org/10.1158/1055-9965.EPI-12-0535.
9. Bush ML, Kaufman MR, Shackleford T. Adherence in the cancer care setting: a systematic review of patient navigation to traverse barriers. *J Cancer Educ.* 2018;33(6):1222–1229. https://doi.org/10.1007/s13187-017-1235-2.

10. Ramirez AG, Perez-Stable EJ, Penedo F, et al. Reducing time-to-treatment in underserved Latinas with breast cancer: the Six Cities Study. *Cancer Treat Outcomes*. 2014. https://doi.org/10.1158/1538-7755.disp13-c54.

11. Hoffman HJ, LaVerda NL, Levine PH, et al. Patient navigation significantly reduces delays in breast cancer diagnosis in the District of Columbia. *Prev Res*. 2011. https://doi.org/10.1158/1055-9965.disp-11-b90.

12. Kline RM, Rocque GB, Rohan EA, et al. Patient navigation in cancer: the business case to support clinical needs. *J Oncol Pract*. 2019;15(11):585590. https://doi.org/10.1200/JOP.19.00230.

13. Christensen D. Using a nurse navigation pathway in the timely care of oncology patients. *J Oncol Navig Surviv*. 2014;5(3):13–18.

14. Bernardo BM, Zhang X, Beverly Hery CM, et al. The efficacy and cost-effectiveness of patient navigation programs across the cancer continuum: a systematic review. *Cancer*. 2019;125(16):2747–2761. https://doi.org/10.1002/cncr.32147.

15. Covvey JR, Kamal KM, Gorse EE, et al. Barriers and facilitators to shared decision-making in oncology: a systematic review of the literature. *Support Care Cancer*. 2019;27(5):1613–1637. https://doi.org/10.1007/s00520-019-04675-7.

16. Ng CG, Mohamed S, Kaur K, et al. Perceived distress and its association with depression and anxiety in breast cancer patients. *PLoS One*. 2017;12(3):e0172975. https://doi.org/10.1371/journal.pone.0172975.

17. National Comprehensive Cancer Network (NCCN). *Distress Management Version 2.2020*. 2020. https://www.nccn.org/guidelines/category_1.

18. Shockney LD. The evolution of breast cancer navigation and survivorship care. *Breast J*. 2014;21(1):104–110. https://doi.org/10.1111/tbj.12353.

19. Tripathy D. Multidisciplinary care for breast cancer: barriers and solutions. *Breast J*. 2003;9(1):60–63. https://doi.org/10.1046/j.1524-4741.2003.09118.x.

20. Bellomo C. Survivorship/end-of-life care. *J Oncol Navig Surviv*. 2017;8(3). https://www.jons-online.com/issues/2017/march-2017-vol-9-no-3/1602-survivorshipend-of-life-care.

21. Shockney L. The value of palliative care early in the treatment process. *J Oncol Navig Surviv*. 2018. https://jons-online.com/special-issues-and-supplements/2018/best-practices-in-breast-cancer-october-2018-vol-9?view=article&artid=2036%3Athe-value-of-palliative-care-early-in-the-treatment-process.

PART 2

Patient Screening, Diagnosis, and Evaluation in the Community

4

Breast Cancer Screening

PAUL MADSEN, SARA MADSEN, AND ALYSSA ZIMNY

Early Use of Mammography for Cancer Detection and Benefits of Screening Mammography

Screening mammography is the practice of using radiologic imaging to evaluate breast tissue in otherwise asymptomatic patients in an effort to find clinically occult cancers. With regular screening exams, cancers may be detected at an earlier stage. This reduces the risk of advanced regional and metastatic disease while increasing the overall survival and cure rate for the patient. Routine screening also enables patients to have both improved surgical and oncological outcomes with the added benefit of potentially improved cosmetic outcomes if findings are small.

Radiography of the breast started in the early 20th century. One of the first published articles was from Stafford Warren, a radiologist, in 1930 using an in vivo stereoscopic mammographic technique prior to breast cancer surgery.[1] Of the 119 patients he imaged, interpretive errors based on his mammographic techniques (both those benign and malignant) were made in only 8 patients.[1] In Warren's report, he found "in many of the cases, there was no unanimity of opinion in the pre-operative clinical diagnosis … the opinion from the mammogram, on the other hand, was very often definitive and most frequently correct."[1]

Later in the 1960s, several landmark studies were performed solidifying mammography's influence and impact on breast cancer screening.[2] One of them was an early randomized controlled study headed by Philip Strax, Sam Shapiro, and Louis Venet from 1963 to 1967.[3] In its initial year evaluating screening mammography, Strax studied 20,211 women aged 40 to 64 from the Health Insurance Plan of Greater New York (HIP). During that trial, preliminary results established mammography found 21 breast cancers in clinically normal women. Meanwhile, 24 cancers were found only by physical exam, with 20 of those cases not visualized on mammography. Ten of the 55 detected cancers were visualized by both mammography and clinical exam. Meanwhile, the control group of 29,694 developed 46 cancers during the first year of observation.[4] An earlier study from 1966, by Griesbach and Eads, had similar results without a control.[5] A third study from Wolfe found 16 carcinomas in 3891 clinically normal women with routine mammograms in 1965.[6]

These early trials demonstrated that mammography had the potential to find as many if not more cancers than generalized medical care at the time.

The researchers (Strax, Shapiro, and Venet) evaluating patients from the HIP had the benefit of following patients for several years, sometimes up to a decade, if not longer. A follow-up report published in 1982 using data from the HIP demonstrated a 38.1% reduction in mortality from breast cancer in the first 5 years after starting at, minimum, annual screening mammography.[6] At 10 years after initially beginning screening, the reduction in mortality was found to be 24%. However, after the first 3 to 4 years, annual screening mammography was not required for the study, but rather at the discretion of the patient. Because of this, the study authors felt that if screening mammography was performed at a rate similar to what was performed during the first 5 years of the study, during years 6 to 10, the overall decreased mortality rate would be higher. The study authors subsequently estimated the 10-year mortality rate to be 32.4%.[7] The HIP study also revealed that those patients who were in the study group had a higher rate of no axillary involvement (56.4%) versus those in the control group (46.3%).[7] Screening only detected cancers had an even higher proportion without nodal involvement at 70.5%.[7]

More recently, using data from 550,000 women in nine Swedish counties from the Swedish Cancer Register, Duffy et al. in 2020 calculated a decrease in the 10-year breast cancer–related mortality rate by 41% when screening mammography was utilized. Additionally, among those diagnosed with breast cancer, those diagnosed through screening practices were 25% less likely to be of an advanced stage.[8] Earlier, in 2019, Tabár et al. published similar results from a study of one Swedish county, which demonstrated a 60% decrease in 10 years in the breast cancer death rate and a 47% decrease at 20 years for women diagnosed through screening mammography compared to those who did not participate in a standard screening program.[9]

Screening Mammography Risks

Despite demonstrating significant benefits with mammography, there are some associated downsides. Often, the biggest concern from both patients and ordering practitioners is the overall radiation dose from the exam itself. The estimated dose of radiation for a standard two-view screening mammogram is approximately 3 mGy (milligray) in total. Comparatively, this is equivalent to approximately 6 weeks of natural background radiation.[10] With the often-standard incorporation of digital breast tomosynthesis (often referred to as DBT or 3D imaging) as part of the annual screening exam, the glandular tissue is potentially exposed up to double this amount. Recent developments in technology have enabled manufacturers to reconstruct standard 2D images from tomosynthesis acquisitions, often referred to as "synthesized views." This technology was approved by the Federal Drug Administration (FDA) in 2013 and helps reduce the overall radiation dose for the patient.[11] Synthesized views preserve the added benefit of DBT while maintaining high image quality.

Not only may patients sometimes worry about the radiation dose from mammography, but there may also be psychological effects. Patients may dread the actual physical compression of the breast tissue during image acquisition. This, combined with the fear of possibly getting called back for further imaging, can create anxiety for the patient. The potential for psychological effects associated with anxiety surrounding screening mammograms is a patient risk that should be considered and discussed with patients as needed. There is no evidence to suggest less frequent examination would reduce patient anxiety. In a survey published by Radiological Society of North America (RSNA), over 70% of women showed preference for annual screening exams compared to biennial evaluation.[12] Additionally, only a minority (17%) of women believed biennial screening would reduce exam-related anxiety. Not every woman will perceive the same risks and benefits.[13] Therefore, it is important to have individualized clinical discussions with each patient.

Another possible downside to screening mammography is the potential cost of the exam itself and the potential added expenses for follow-up testing. Specifically, for breast imaging, many advancements have been made to reduce or eliminate out of pocket costs for screening mammography. Despite these changes, some private insurance patients are still charged for their examinations. In a study performed by Tran et al., approximately 5% of patients included in their analysis paid an out-of-pocket expense for their baseline screening mammogram.[14] Those charged for a screening mammogram were found to have delayed subsequent screening examinations compared to those who were not charged by their insurance provider. Although not specifically addressed in this analysis, these possible delays due to cost concerns, risk potential future delays in cancer diagnoses. This highlights the importance for all to have adequate medical coverage for annual screening exams if desired.

Standardization of Technique and Patient Positioning

Screening mammography consists typically of two images, the cranio-caudal (CC) and the medial-lateral oblique (MLO) views (Fig. 4.1). Ideally, the nipple should be in profile on both views, but is only required to be in profile on a single view. To ensure that enough tissue is included on both images, radiologists often assess the posterior nipple line. A line is drawn posteriorly and perpendicularly from the nipple toward the pectoralis muscle on the MLO view. A similar line is drawn on the CC view, extending posteriorly from the nipple toward the central posterior portion of the CC film. The two measurements should be within 1 cm of each other to make sure that enough tissue is included (Fig. 4.2).

Sometimes there is not enough tissue included laterally on the CC view. If this is the case, an exaggerated cranio-caudal (XCCL) view should then be obtained. In this view, the breast is positioned similarly to a CC view but, as the name suggests, the technologist exaggerates and includes more lateral breast tissue (Fig. 4.3). Ideally, the XCCL should be obtained in less than 10% of all screening exams.[15] It should not be part of the standard mammogram unless it is a baseline exam and prominent tissue is missing on the regular CC view, or an area of concern is seen in the lateral posterior breast tissue.

Characterizing Breast Tissue Density

In response to the increased utilization of mammography and the need for standardization of reporting and management recommendations, the American College of Radiology (ACR), along with support from various other medical groups, drafted the first version of the Breast Imaging-Reporting and Data System (BI-RADS) atlas with the most recent BI-RADS atlas published in 2013.[16] This updated atlas provides radiologists with a specific lexicon for each imaging modality and with guidelines regarding report format and patient management. This creates a foundation for all interpreting radiologists to essentially speak the same language and establish standards of care for mammography.

When reviewing mammograms, tissue density is characterized into one of four categories: predominantly fatty, scattered areas of glandular tissue, heterogeneously dense, and extremely dense (Fig. 4.4). On mammography, glandular tissue composed of breast stroma appears "white" and fat appears "dark." Previous BI-RADS guidelines had quantified the different classifications of breast tissue density as follows: Non-dense breasts such as predominantly fatty breasts have less than 25% of glandular tissue with scattered areas of glandular tissue containing roughly 25% to 50% of glandular tissue. Meanwhile dense breasts such as those that are heterogeneously dense have approximately 50% to 75% of glandular tissue, and those with extremely dense breasts have greater than 75% of glandular tissue. These quantifiers were established to help more evenly divide women amongst each of the tissue densities.[17] However, more recent literature suggests that these quantifiers are not needed, and they have been removed from current published reporting standard guidelines. Regardless of whether or now the quantifiers were used, breast tissue density remained unevenly distributed among screening

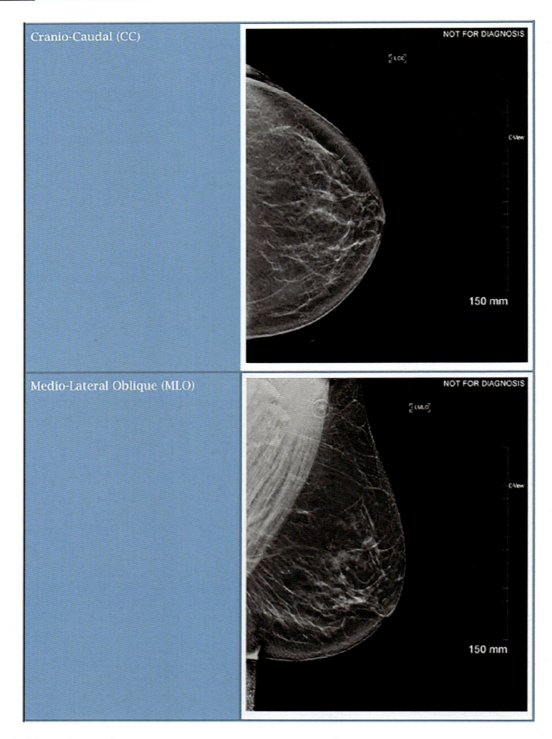

• Fig. 4.1 Standard views of a screening mammogram.

mammograms, with approximately 10% of mammograms having fatty tissue, 40% scattered, 40% heterogeneous, and 10% dense.[17] It is important to acknowledge that a woman's breast tissue density is not stagnant and may be variable over their lifetime. Often younger women have dense breasts, with more fatty changes in tissue density noted in postmenopausal patients. Besides aging, tissue density changes have been noticed with hormonal usage and weight fluctuations, among other etiologies. Technical variances in compression during image acquisition have also been shown to have an impact on breast tissue density. With dense breast tissue, mammography becomes less sensitive and there is increased potential for obscuring areas of interest including small masses.[18] Those women with dense breasts have been reported to have a 1.2- to 2.1-fold higher risk of breast cancer.[19] The interval cancer rate for dense

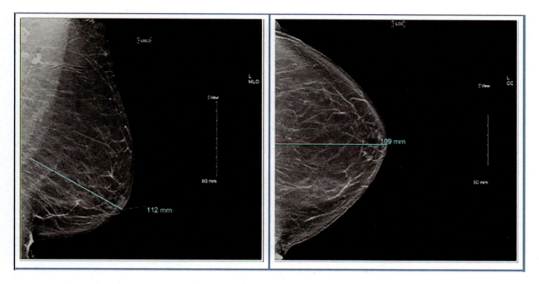

• **Fig. 4.2** Posterior nipple line: cranio-caudal *(CC)* and medio-lateral oblique *(MLO)* views demonstrating posterior nipple line showing equal amounts of tissue on both images. The difference in length between images should ideally be not greater than 1 cm.

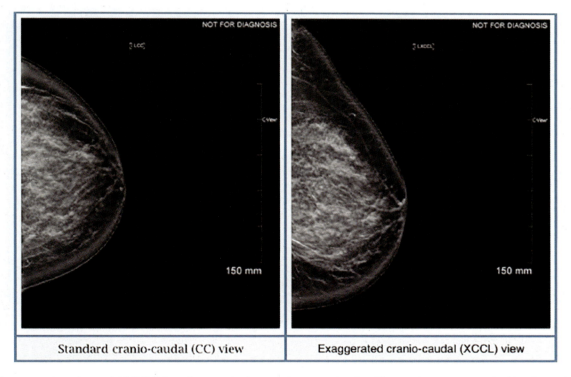

• **Fig. 4.3** Exaggerated cranio-caudal *(XCCL)* View: Comparative images demonstrating the difference between a standard cranio-caudal *(CC)* view and an XCCL view. In a CC view, tissue approaches the lateral side of the film while on an XCCL view tissue is exaggerated and pulled laterally.

breasts may be as much as 17-fold higher as compared to women with fatty breasts.[19]

Mammography Limitations/Incorporation of Tomosynthesis

One of the biggest limitations of standard 2D mammography is the possibility for overlapping tissue. If the breast tissue is dense, or there are denser islands of tissue, possible areas of interest may be inadvertently obscured on 2D mammography and create a false-negative assessment for the patient. Alternatively, areas of normal tissue may also overlap, creating a false area of interest (often referred to as summation artifact). This may lead to increased patient callbacks and higher patient anxiety. DBT, approved by the FDA for use in 2011, addresses some of those limitations. While each tomosynthesis manufacturer has a slightly different technique, the overall

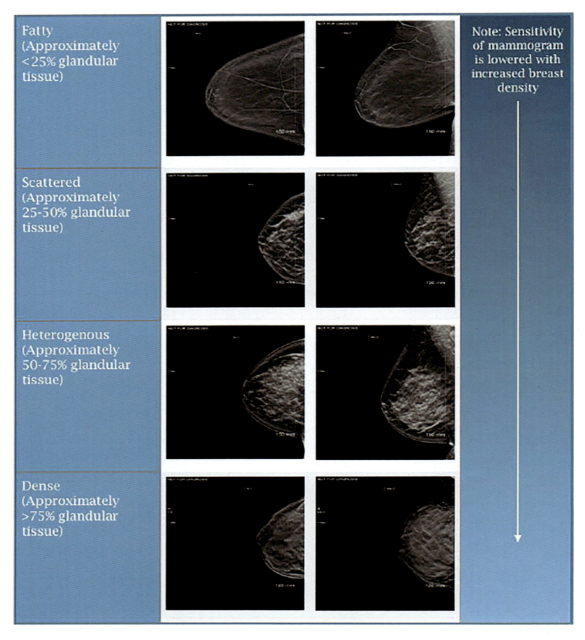

• **Fig 4.4** Characterizing glandular tissue on mammography using Breast Imaging-Reporting and Data System *(BI-RADS)* terminology (cranio-caudal *[CC]* and medio-lateral oblique *[MLO]* views).

concept is similar throughout. The breasts are positioned, compressed, and held stationary, exactly the same as a standard 2D mammogram. Images are obtained most often in CC and MLO views. The x-ray tube moves in an arc taking several low-dose images, which are then reconstructed into thin sections parallel to the detector. Images are then reconstructed into a 3D plane for the radiologist to "scroll through." The ability to "scroll through" dense islands of tissue helps the interpreting radiologist better assess for possible underlying areas of interest that may otherwise be missed on standard 2D mammography (Table 4.1). Since its approval, tomosynthesis has shown to reduce recall rates and improved cancer detection rates, up to 40%.[19] Given its profound impact and integral usage on mammography, tomosynthesis manufacturers have recently developed a "synthesized" 2D image reducing the need for "standard 2D" imaging. This technology was approved by the FDA in 2013 and helps reduce the overall radiation dose for the patient while maintaining high image quality.[20]

Screening Guidelines for Average-Risk Women

The American College of Radiology (ACR), in conjunction with the National Comprehensive Cancer Network (NCCN)

TABLE 4.1 Representative Cases of Screening/Diagnostic Mammography With Sonographic Correlates

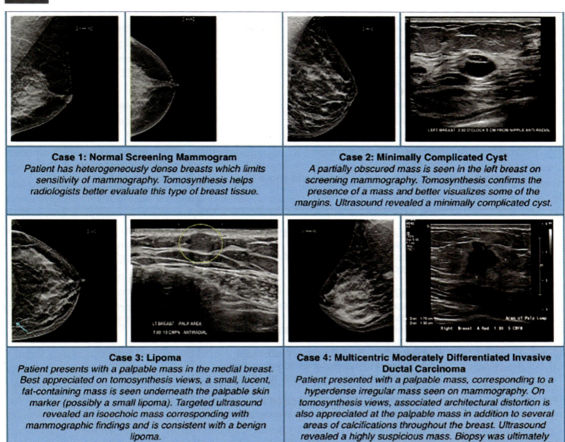

and the American Society of Breast Surgeons (ASBrS), recommends women of an average risk for breast cancer be screened using mammography annually beginning at the age of 40 (Fig. 4.5).[21–24] These guidelines recommending that screening begin at the age of 40 are further supported in populations of minority ethnicities where there are higher rates of cancer detection and lower survival rates below the age of 50. With screening beginning annually at the younger age of 40, cancers can be detected at earlier stages and treated with improved therapy response and survival (Table 4.2).

Biennial screening is discouraged by the ACR, NCCN, and ASBrS due to more advanced cancers at the time of diagnosis and increased mortality for the patient. Based on 2009 CISNET models, mortality reduction is as low as 23.2% for biennial screening (compared to approximately 40% for annual screening; Table 4.2).[25–27] Within the same analysis, 189 life-years are gained per 1000 women screened annually, while only 110 life-years are gained in women screened biannually (Table 4.2).[26] More recent CISNET models in 2017 continue to affirm that annual screening mammography offers the largest reduction in mortality from breast cancer at approximately 40%.

The ACR, NCCN, and ASBrS do not recommend terminating screening at a particular age in the absence of significantly reduced life expectancy from severe preexisting comorbidities. The importance of early detection and opportunity for treatment remains in older patient populations, as approximately 20% of breast cancers are diagnosed in patients 75 or older.[18,28] This is also confirmed with data from the National Cancer Institute (NCI) demonstrating that of all recorded breast cancers from 2015-2019, approximately 18.9% were patients aged 75 and above.[29] Using data from the National Cancer Institute's Surveillance, Epidemiology and End Results (SEER) database, Sanderson demonstrated that women aged 69-84 years had lower 10-year breast cancer mortality if screened annually than those who were screened biannually or sporadically, reaffirming the continued need for annual screening in this age group.[26]

Contrary to the recommended screening guidelines for average-risk women set forth by NCCN, ACR, and ASBrS, the American Cancer Society (ACS) has established its own guidelines regarding screening mammography for average-risk women. Per the ACS Guidelines, patient's between ages of 40 and 44 have the option to start or delay annual

TABLE 4.3 Summary of Recommendations for High-Risk and Special Patient Populations

		Annual Screening Mammography	Annual Screening Contrast-Enhanced MRI
Personal history of breast cancer or lobular neoplasia		Recommended, beginning at time of diagnosis but not before age 25	Can be considered, beginning at time of diagnosis but not before age 25
Family history of breast cancer		Recommended, beginning 10 years before age of onset of youngest affected relative (but not before age 30) or at age 40	Recommended, beginning 10 years before age of onset of youngest affected relative (but not before age 25) or at age 40
Genetic mutations/ syndromes	BRCA	Recommended, beginning at age 30	Recommended, beginning at age 25
	TP53 (Li-Fraumeni syndrome)	Recommended, beginning at age 30	Recommended, beginning at age 20
	PTEN (Cowden syndrome)	Recommended, beginning at age 35	Recommended, beginning at age 35
	CHEK2	Recommended, beginning at age 40	Can be considered, beginning at age 40
Calculated elevated lifetime risk >20% (Modified Gail model, IBIS tool, etc.)		Recommended, beginning 10 years before age of onset of youngest affected relative (but not before age 30) or at age 40	Recommended, beginning 10 years before age of onset of youngest affected relative (but not before age 25) or at age 40
History of radiation therapy		Recommended, beginning 8 years after completion of radiation therapy (but not before age 30)	Recommended, beginning 10 years before age of onset of youngest affected relative (but not before age 25)
Male		Can be considered if other risk factors are identified	Not generally indicated unless other risk factors exist
Transgender		Male-to-female: begin at age 40 if >.5 years of hormone therapy Female-to-male: begin at age 40 if have not undergone mastectomy	Not generally indicated unless other risk factors exist
Pregnancy/lactation		Recommended, begin at age 40	Not generally indicated unless other risk factors exist
Recent vaccination		Recommended, begin at age 40	Not generally indicated unless other risk factors exist

IBIS, International Breast Cancer Intervention Study.

screened using contrast-enhanced MRI with recommendations to begin MRI examinations 10 years before the age at which the youngest affected relative was diagnosed, but not before the age of 25 (see Table 4.3).[22]

Underlying BReast CAncer gene (*BRCA*) mutations are a well-known genetic risk factor for developing breast cancer. The estimated lifetime risk in BReast CAncer gene 1 (*BRCA1*) carriers is on the order of 50% to 85%, while BReast CAncer gene 2 (*BRCA2*) carriers have a less, yet still significantly higher than average, lifetime risk of developing cancer at approximately 45%.[35,36] Breast cancers diagnosed in *BRCA* carriers account for 6% of all cancers diagnosed.[37] For all known *BRCA* mutation carriers, annual screening via contrast-enhanced MRI should commence at age 25, and screening mammography is recommended to begin at the age of 30 (see Table 4.3).[38] This recommendation is based on the earlier average onset of breast cancer in *BRCA* carriers at 40 years of age compared to 61 years for average-risk individuals.[39]

Additional genetic mutations associated with higher breast cancer risks include *TP53*, *PTEN*, and *CHEK2* variants, among others. The *TP53* mutation is associated with Li-Fraumeni syndrome. These patients have a very high risk of breast cancer with incidence rates as high as 85% by the age of 60.[40] Guidelines from NCCN regarding screening practices recommend annual MRI for these patients beginning as early as age 20, with both MRI and mammography recommended from ages 30 and above (see Table 4.3).[38] Early initiation of screening in Li-Fraumeni syndrome patients is critical as the average age at time of diagnosis is only 34 years.[41]

The *PTEN* mutation is associated with Cowden syndrome. Women with *PTEN* mutations are recommended to have MRI and mammography annually. Screening should begin at age 35; however, in the setting of early-onset family history of breast cancer screening should begin 10 years earlier than the youngest age of diagnosis among those affected (see Table 4.3).[38]

Those with *CHEK2* mutations should begin annual mammography at the age of 40, similar to average-risk individuals, with possible addition of annual MRI evaluation (see Table 4.3).[38] Further recommendations for these and many more genetic variants are available within the NCCN's guideline for breast cancer screening and diagnosis.

Calculated Individual Risk

Several models have been developed to provide an individualized lifetime risk of developing breast cancer based on the presence of specific underlying independent factors, several of which have already been discussed in this section. The Modified Gail model is an eight-question risk assessment tool used for women over the age of 35. Its components include age, ethnicity, hormonal-based factors, personal history of lobular neoplasia, prior radiation therapy and previous benign breast biopsy, presence of genetic predisposition, and family history of breast cancer in first-degree relatives. This model functions to provide clinicians with a personalized patient risk assessment to guide screening recommendations and risk reduction strategies. It is important to note, however, that this model is not valid for patients with a positive history of lobular neoplasia or breast cancer, and is also not recommended as the best risk assessment tool for patients with *BRCA1/2* mutations or other higher-risk genetic syndromes.[42] Screening recommendations for these specific populations are described in detail above.

The International Breast Cancer Intervention Study (IBIS) tool, also known as the Tyrer-Cuzick Model, is another calculator that can estimate a woman's lifetime risk of breast cancer. This tool utilizes additional factors including ovarian cancer history, and an extended family history to include both first- and second-degree relatives.[43] One particular advantage of the IBIS tool is that its latest version includes the patient's breast tissue density to recognize that mammography has lower sensitivity in patients with higher-density tissue patterns. This model is one of several endorsed by the ACS for determining if MRI should be incorporated into a patient's screening regimen.[44] NCCN guidelines state that a calculated risk of 20% or greater using a model that includes family history is a reasonable indication to include annual screening MRI in addition to mammography beginning at age 40 or 10 years earlier than the age of diagnosis of the youngest affected family member.[22]

Another available resource is the BRCAPRO model developed by the Bayes Mendel Lab at Harvard University. The BRCAPRO tool is used to determine the likelihood of a patient being a carrier of the *BRCA1* or *BRCA2* mutation and is based on the patient's personal and family histories.[45] The Claus model is yet another statistical model available to clinicians. It was developed by the Centers for Disease Control and Prevention and includes family history extending to at least second-degree relatives. A modified version also accounts for family history of ovarian malignancies.[45]

Radiation History

A woman with a history of chest (mantle) radiation received between the ages of 10 and 30 should begin screening 8 years after the radiation therapy, but not before the age of 25 (see Table 4.3).[22] These guidelines are based on an elevated risk of developing breast cancer in patients who received radiation therapy for Hodgkin lymphoma. In a long-term follow-up study by Batia et al., Hodgkin lymphoma survivors were found to have an 18.5-fold increase in the development of a primary malignancy, with breast cancer being the most common type in this patient population.[46] Patients characterized as high risk based on prior radiation therapy are those who received a cumulative dose of 10 Gy or more prior to the age of 30.[47] The risk of breast cancer following treatment of Hodgkin lymphoma in a patient before the age of 25 is estimated to be 11.1% by age 45 and 29.0% by age 55.[48]

Race

African American women are diagnosed with stage 1 cancers less often than non-African American patients.[49] Minority women (including African American) are 58% more likely to be diagnosed with advanced-stage disease before the age of 50.[50] Invasive breast cancer in particular affects younger minority populations 72% more than non-Hispanic White patients.[50] Beyond higher risks of diagnosis and more aggressive cancers, minority women also are at a higher risk of dying at an earlier age from breast cancer.[42,51] In an evaluation of data from 2019, the percentage of deaths related to breast cancer was highest for Asian/Pacific Islanders (5.6%), followed by non-Hispanic Black (4.5%) and Hispanic (4.4%) populations.[52] These rates were higher than non-Hispanic White women (4.1%) and much greater than that of American Indian/Alaska Native women (2.6%). Women of color have higher rates of mortality with triple-negative, highly aggressive breast cancers.[53] These findings are just a few examples supporting the need for early detection in higher-risk patients so that aggressive cancers can be detected at an earlier stage and treated more effectively.

Recent attention has been brought to Asian populations and gaps in screening and diagnostic follow-up. An evaluation by Miller et al. describes Asian women as having the highest rise in breast cancer incidence over a 10-year period relative to other racial groups.[54] Only an estimated 66% of United States Asian women receive breast cancer screening with mammography.[55] Contributing barriers to screening examinations include language differences, other cultural factors, and socioeconomic backgrounds.[56]

Special Patient Populations

Male

Male breast cancers are rare and account for 1% of diagnosed breast cancers.[57] For this reason, generalized screening mammography is not recommended. As with female patients, increasing age is a risk factor for the development of breast cancers in men. Additional risk factors include a family history of breast or ovarian cancer and presence of a known underlying genetic mutation. Male patients with known *BRCA* mutations are at an increased risk for developing breast cancer. NCCN guidelines suggest consideration of annual mammography in male patients with gynecomastia beginning at age 50, or 10 years before the age of diagnosis of the earliest diagnosed male breast cancer in the patient's family (see Table 4.3).[38] Additional risk factors in men for the development of breast cancer include elevated estrogen and/or low androgen levels, both of which have several possible underlying etiologies.[58] Klinefelter syndrome, a genetic disease characterized by an additional X chromosome, is an example of a potential etiology that confers a significantly higher risk of developing breast cancer. While no specific guidelines exist, screening mammography in these populations should be considered.

LGBTQ

Patients identifying within one of the Lesbian, Gay, Bisexual, Transgender, Queer/Questioning (LGBTQ) subgroups may be more vulnerable to missed screening appointments and therefore at risk for delayed diagnosis of breast cancers.[59] In an updated set of guidelines released in 2021 by the ACR, special attention was made to address these groups. Recommendations suggest screening be based on the patient's sex assigned at birth, while taking into account previous surgeries and use of exogenous hormones. Male-to-female patients should begin annual screening at the age of 40 if hormones have been used for at least 5 years duration.[60] Female-to-male patients who have not undergone prior mastectomy should follow standard guidelines with annual screening beginning at age 40 (see Table 4.3).[60]

Pregnancy/Lactation

With the increasing average age of first pregnancies in the United States, timing overlap between screening examinations and family planning is sometimes inevitable for patients. While patients and providers may have concerns regarding the risk of radiation exposure to a growing fetus, mammography-related exposures are low and examinations otherwise indicated are recommended to not be postponed (see Table 4.3).[22]

Pregnancy-associated breast cancer includes cancers diagnosed during pregnancy, within the first year after delivery, or during breastfeeding.[22] Breast cancer is diagnosed in 1 out of every 3,000 to 10,000 pregnancies.[61] Some studies have suggested that the 7- to 10-year period following delivery may also be associated with a higher risk of breast cancer compared to nulliparous patients.[62] This increased risk is further worrisome, as breast cancers during pregnancy and in the postpartum period tend to be more aggressive and have higher mortality rates.[63] If otherwise indicated, performance of screening mammography should not be postponed/deferred in lactating patients. Patients may be recommended to breastfeed or pump breast milk prior to the examination in order to reduce breast density and therefore maximize the examination's sensitivity for cancer detection.[64]

Recent Vaccination

During the COVID pandemic, otherwise indicated screening mammograms were postponed by 4 to 6 weeks for fear of identifying axillary lymphadenopathy and possible further unnecessary workup. In a guideline published in February of 2022, the Society of Breast Imaging now recommends against altering screening schedules in asymptomatic patients recently vaccinated against the COVID virus who are of an average risk for breast cancer (see Table 4.3).[65]

Magnetic Resonance Imaging Screening for Breast Cancer

MRI imaging of the breast has become an important adjunct to screening mammography, particularly in those patients who are at high risk for malignancy. While mammography is a form of structural imaging, MRI is a form of functional imaging.[66] Several different sequences are obtained with the patient in the prone position. A gadolinium-based contrast is administered via an intravenous (IV) injection, and typically several sequentially run postcontrast sequences are obtained (usually between 3 and 5). Images are examined for the patterns of enhancement (both the shape and distribution) in addition to the kinetics of the contrast within the breast itself (i.e., areas of rapid washout, persistent or plateau kinetics). This helps determine the blood flow to the breast parenchyma and to any pathology that may be present in the breast. Most often on MRI, breast cancers are found to have areas of rapid washout likely caused by increased blood flow or angiogenesis, often peaking with early enhancement (likely 1 to 2 minutes) after contrast administration.[66]

Unlike mammography, a patient's tissue density does not mask a potential underlying malignancy on breast MRI. Rather, it is the background parenchymal enhancement (BPE) of a patient's normal fibroglandular tissue that can muddle interpretation. Current BI-RADS lexicon separates BPE into four categories: Minimal, Mild, Moderate, and Marked (Fig. 4.6). The amount of BPE identified on MRI is independent of the amount of fibroglandular tissue in the patient's breast. For those patients who have moderate or marked BPE, it can be hard to discern benign enhancement from small concerning areas of enhancement as they often may appear similar with similar kinetics.

While the sensitivity of MRI at detecting breast cancer is higher than that of mammography, the specificity is decreased. This creates a higher false-positive rate, with an increase of indeterminate findings. In turn, this can lead

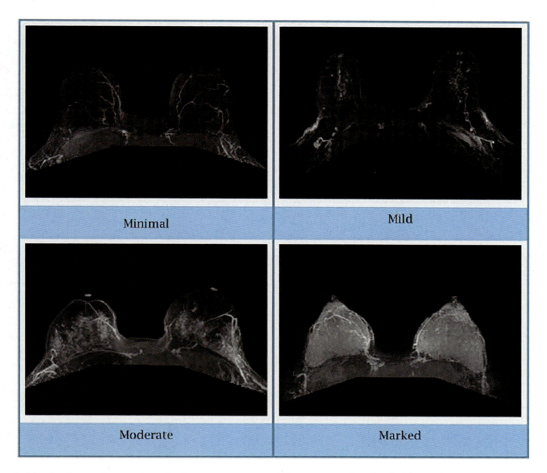

• **Fig 4.6** Characterizing background parenchymal enhancement on magnetic resonance imaging (MRI) using Breast Imaging-Reporting and Data System (BI-RADS) terminology.

to more patient anxiety with more benign breast biopsies being performed. Additionally, calcifications at times are not well visualized on MRI, but rather better visualized on mammography. This highlights the importance of using both mammography and MRI together to complement one another as screening modalities.

In 2015, a safety alert was issued by the FDA warning of possible adverse effects of repeat gadolinium contrast administration (a minimum of four doses) and possible deposition in patient's brain.[67] Two years later in 2017, the FDA released a communications bulletin confirming that sometimes trace amounts of gadolinium may be retained in the body long term; however, no definitive adverse health effects have been associated with the trace deposition.[68] The FDA stated that "the benefit of all approved GBCAs [Gadolinium based contrast agents] continues to outweigh any potential risks" in this updated bulletin.[68] Also in the 2017 communications bulletin, the FDA established a new "Medication Guide" to be provided to patients prior to receiving a GBCA explaining and acknowledging the differences between some of the contrast agents and their respective safety profiles. In high-risk breast cancer patients, annual screening MRI is often recommended. Over the course of a patient's lifetime, this may account for a significant amount of IV gadolinium administration. Subsequently, it is important to have an appropriate risk assessment for breast cancer to justify the need for annual screening breast MRI while acknowledging the possibility for trace long-term gadolinium deposition.

Screening Ultrasound

Ultrasound has often been used as an adjunct to mammography, particularly in the diagnostic setting. However, similar to screening MRI, screening ultrasound has been explored to help offset some of the limitations of screening mammography, particularly in those women who have dense breasts.[69] Ultrasound is often widely available at multiple institutions and does not require radiation or contrast administration. However, the overall quality of the exam and the images obtained relies on the expertise of the technologist performing it. Several studies evaluating hand held screening ultrasound in intermediate to high-risk women demonstrate a higher overall recall rate up to 119.9 per 1000 people with decreased specificity. Despite the high recall rate, studies demonstrate an increased cancer detection rate up to 4.3 additional cancers per 1000 women screened using ultrasound.[70]

Recent technological advancements have led to the development of automated breast ultrasound (ABUS). This helps establish consistent reproducibility and limits dependency on the performing technologist. Varying systems are currently on the market; however, the overall concepts are similar. Whole breast images are obtained by an automated system, which can then be reformatted in multiple planes establishing reproducible findings. Several ABUS screening studies have been performed demonstrating a higher recall rate similar to hand held ultrasound screening images, up to 134.6/1000 in those women who are average to high risk. They also demonstrate an increased cancer detection rate up to 7.7 per 1000, depending on the study.[70] Despite demonstrating an increased cancer detection rate, ultrasound is not good at evaluating ductal carcinoma in situ (DCIS). This most commonly presents as calcifications on mammography with false-negative results for ABUS ranging from 9% to 22%.[70] This highlights the importance of using both mammography and ultrasound to complement each other. At this time, given the high additional recall rates with decreased specificity, NCCN, ASBrS, and the ACR recommend that screening breast ultrasound is an adjunct to annual screening mammography if clinically indicated.[16,17,70]

REFERENCES

1. Gold RH, Bassett LW, Widoff BE. Highlights from the history of mammography. *Radiographics*. 1990;10:1111–1131.
2. Feig SA. Decreased breast cancer mortality through mammographic screening: results of clinical trials. *Radiology*. 1988;167(3):659–665.
3. Shapiro S, Strax P, Venet L. Periodic breast cancer screening in reducing mortality from breast cancer. *JAMA*. 1971;215(11):1777–1785.
4. Strax P, Venet L, Shapiro S, et al. Mammography and clinical examination in mass screening. *Cancer*. 1967;20:2184.
5. Griesbach AA, Eads WS. Experience with screening for breast carcinoma. *Cancer*. 1966;19:1548.
6. Wolfe JN. Mammography as a screening examination in breast cancer. *Radiology*. 1965;84:703.
7. Shapiro S, Venet W, Strax P, et al. Ten to fourteen year effect of screening on breast cancer mortality. *J Natl Cancer Inst*. 1982;69:349–355.
8. Duffy SW, Tabár L, Yen AM, et al. Mammography screening reduces rates of advanced and fatal breast cancers: results in 549,091 women. *Cancer*. 2020;126:2971–2979.
9. Tabár L, Dean PB, Chen TH, et al. The incidence of fatal breast cancer measures the increased effectiveness of therapy in women participating in mammography screening. *Cancer*. 2019;125:515–523.
10. Hendrick RE. Radiation doses and risks in breast screening. *J Breast Imaging*. 2020;2(3):188–200.
11. Park JM, Franken EA Jr, Garg M, et al. Breast tomosynthesis: present considerations and future applications. *Radiographics*. 2007;27:S231–S240.
12. Copit DS, Overcash JR. *Women prefer getting mammograms every year. RSNA Press Release*. https://press.rsna.org/timssnet/media/pressreleases/14_pr_target.cfm?ID=1982. November 21, 2017. Accessed April 16, 2022.
13. Kopans DB. *Breast Imaging*. Philadelphia, PA: Lippincott Williams & Wilkins; 1997. 2nd ed.
14. Tran L, Chetlen AL, Leslie DL, et al. Effect of out-of-pocket costs on subsequent mammography screening. *J Am Coll Radiol*. 2022;19:24–34.
15. Cardenosa G. *Breast Imaging Companion*. Philadelphia, PA: Lipponcott Williams & Wilkin; 2007.
16. D'Orsi CJ, Kopans DB. Mammography interpretation: the BI-RADS method. *Am Fam Physician*. 1997;55:1548–1550.
17. Freer PE. Mammographic breast density: impact on breast cancer risk and implications for screening. *Radiographics*. 2015;35:302–315.
18. Characteristics of Breast Cancer Cases. Breast Cancer Surveillance Consortium. https://www.bcsc-research.org/statistics/chars_cases. Accessed April 30 2022. The Breast Cancer Surveillance Consortium and its data collection and sharing activities are funded by grants from the National Cancer Institute (P01CA154292, U54CA163303), Patient-Centered Outcomes Research Institute (PCS-1504-30370), and Agency for Health Research and Quality (R01 HS018366-01A1).
19. Bicchierai G, Di Naro F, De Benedetto D, et al. A review of breast imaging for timely diagnosis of disease. *Int J Environ Res Public Health*. 2021;18(11):5509.
20. Ratanaprasatpron L, Chikarmane SA, Giess CS. Strengths and weaknesses of synthetic mammography in screening. *Radiographics*. 2017;37(7):1913–1927. https://pubs.rsna.org/doi/10.1148/rg.2017170032. November 13, 2017. Accessed April 17, 2022.
21. D'Orsi CJ, Sickles EA, Mendelson EB, et al. *ACR BI-RADS® Atlas, Breast Imaging Reporting and Data System*. Reston, VA: American College of Radiology; 2013.
22. National Comprehensive Cancer Network. Breast Cancer Screening and Diagnosis (Version 1.2021). https://www.nccn.org/professionals/physician_gls/pdf/breast-screening.pdf.
23. DePolo, J. American Society of Breast Surgeons Issues Updated Breast Cancer Screening Guidelines. BreastCancer.org. https://www.breastcancer.org/research-news/asbrs-issues-updated-screening-guidelines. May 10, 2019. Updated February 22, 2022. Accessed April 18, 2022.
24. Position Statement on Screening Mammography. The American Society of Breast Surgeons. https://www.breastsurgeons.org/docs/statements/Position-Statement-on-Screening-Mammography.pdf. Published 2019. Accessed April 30, 2022.
25. Lee CS, Moy L, Joe BN, et al. Screening for breast cancer in women age 75 years and older. *AJR Am J Roentgenol*. 2018;210(2):256–263.
26. SEER Cancer Stat Facts: Female Breast Cancer. Bethesda, MD: National Cancer Institute. https://seer.cancer.gov/statfacts/html/breast.html.
27. Arleo EK, Hendrick RE, Helvie MA, et al. Comparison of recommendations for screening mammography using CISNET models. *Cancer*. 2017;123(19):3673–3680.
28. Monticciolo DL, Newell MS, Moy L, et al. Breast cancer screening in women at higher-than-average risk: recommendations from the ACR. *J Am Coll Radiol*. 2018;15(3):408–414.
29. Fowble B, Hanlon A, Freedman G, et al. Second cancers after conservative surgery and radiation for stages I–II breast cancer: identifying a subset of women at increased risk. *Int J Rad Oncol Biol Phys*. 2001;51(3):679–690.
30. Group EC, Darby S, McGale P, et al. Effect of radiotherapy after breast-conserving surgery on 10-year recurrence and 15-year breast cancer death: meta-analysis of individual patient

data for 10,801 women in 17 randomized trials. *Lancet.* 2011;378(9804):1707–1716.

31. Arpino G, Laucirica R, Elledge RM. Premalignant and in situ breast disease: biology and clinical implications. *Ann Intern Med.* 2005;143(6):446.

32. Siu AL U.S. Preventive Services Task Force. Screening for Breast Cancer: U.S. Preventive Services Task Force Recommendation Statement. Ann Intern Med. 2016;Feb 16;164(4):279–296. Epub 2016 Jan 12. Erratum in: Ann Intern Med. 2016 Mar 15;164(6):448. PMID: 26757170. doi:10.7326/M15-2886.

33. U.S Preventive Services Task Force. Breast Cancer: Screening (May 09,2023 drafted version). https://www.uspreventiveservicestaskforce.org/uspstf/draft-recommendation/breast-cancer-screening-adults.

34. Bever L. Health panel recommends women get screening mammograms at age 40. The Washington Post. https://www.washingtonpost.com/wellness/2023/05/09/mammogram-age-40-breast-cancer-screening/, May 9, 2023. [Accessed 27 June 2023].

35. Chen S, Parmigiani G. Meta-analysis of BRCA1 and BRCA2 penetrance. *J Clin Oncol.* 2007;25(11):1329–1333.

36. Antoniou A., Pharoah PD, Narod S, et al. Average risks of breast and ovarian cancer associated with BRCA1 or BRCA2 mutations detected in case series unselected for family history: a combined analysis of 22 studies. 2003;72(5):1117–1130. [Published correction appears in *Am J Hum Genet* 2003;73(3):709.]

37. Kurian AW, Ward KC, Howlader N, et al. Genetic testing and results in a population-based cohort of breast cancer patients and ovarian cancer patients. *J Clin Oncol.* 2019;37(15):1305–1315.

38. National Comprehensive Cancer Network. Genetic/Familial High-Risk Assessment: Breast, Ovarian, and Pancreatic (Version 2.2022). https://www.nccn.org/professionals/physician_gls/pdf/genetics_bop.pdf.

39. Lee MV, Katabathina VS, Bowerson ML, et al. BRCA-associated cancers: role of imaging in screening, diagnosis, and management. *Radiographics.* 2017;37(4):1005–1023.

40. Bharucha PP, Chiu KE, François FM, et al. Genetic testing and screening recommendations for patients with hereditary breast cancer. *Radiographics.* 2020;40(4):913–936.

41. Schon K, Tischkowitz M. Clinical implications of germline mutations in breast cancer: TP53. *Breast Cancer Res Treat.* 2018;167(2):417–423.

42. Breast Cancer Risk Assessment Tool: About the Calculator. National Cancer Institute. https://bcrisktool.cancer.gov/about.html. Version 4.1, updated December 2017. Accessed March 31, 2022.

43. Ikonopedia. IBIS (International Breast Cancer Intervention Study): Online Tyrer-Cuzick Model Breast Cancer Risk Evaluation Tool. https://ibis.ikonopedia.com/. Accessed March 31, 2022.

44. Saslow D, Boetes C, Burke W, et al. American Cancer Society guidelines for breast screening with MRI as an adjunct to mammography. *CA Cancer J Clin.* 2007;57(2):75–89.

45. BRCAPRO. BayesMendel Lab. Harvard University. https://projects.iq.harvard.edu/bayesmendel/brcapro. Accessed March 31, 2022.

46. Bhatia S, Yasui Y, Robison LL, et al. High risk of subsequent neoplasms continues with extended follow-up of childhood Hodgkin's disease: report from the Late Effects Study Group. *J Clin Oncol.* 2003;21(23):4386–4394.

47. Mariscotti G, Belli P, Bernardi D, et al. Mammography and MRI for screening women who underwent chest radiation therapy (lymphoma survivors): recommendations for surveillance from the Italian College of Breast Radiologists by SIRM. *Radiol Med.* 2016;121(11):834–837.

48. Travis LB, Hill D, Dores GM, et al. Cumulative absolute breast cancer risk for young women treated for Hodgkin lymphoma. *J Natl Cancer Inst.* 2005;97(19):1428–1437.

49. Iqbal J, Ginsburg O, Rochon PA, et al. Differences in breast cancer stage at diagnosis and cancer-specific survival by race and ethnicity in the United States. *JAMA.* 2015;313(2):165.

50. Hendrick RE, Monticciolo DL, Biggs KW, et al. Age distributions of breast cancer diagnosis and mortality by race and ethnicity in United States women. *Cancer.* 2021;127(23):4384–4392.

51. U.S. Cancer Statistics Working Group. U.S. Cancer Statistics Data Visualizations Tool, based on 2020 submission data (1999–2018): U.S. Department of Health and Human Services, Centers for Disease Control and Prevention and National Cancer Institute. www.cdc.gov/cancer/dataviz. Released in June 2021.

52. Trentham-Dietz A, Chapman CH, Bird J, et al. Recent changes in the patterns of breast cancer as a proportion of all deaths according to race and ethnicity. *Epidemiology.* 2021;32(6):904–913.

53. Cho B, Han Y, Lian M, et al. Evaluation of racial/ethnic differences in treatment and mortality among women with triple-negative breast cancer. *JAMA Oncol.* 2021;7(7):1016–1023.

54. Miller BC, Bowers JM, Payne JB, et al. Barriers to mammography screening among racial and ethnic minority women. *Soc Sci Med.* 2019;239:112494.

55. Xie H, Li Y, Theodoropoulos N, et al. Mammography screening disparities in Asian American women: findings from the California Health Interview Survey 2015–2016. *Am J Health Promot.* 2022;36(2):248–258.

56. Sohn YJ, Chang CY, Miles RC. Current gaps in breast cancer screening among Asian and Asian American Women in the United States. *J Am Coll Radiol.* 2021;18(10):1376–1383.

57. Miao H, Verkooijen HM, Chia KS. Incidence and outcome of male breast cancer: an international population-based study. *J Clin Oncol.* 2011;29(33):4381–4386.

58. Gao Y, Heller SL, Moy L. Male breast cancer in the age of genetic testing: an opportunity for early detection, tailored therapy, and surveillance. *Radiographics.* 2018;38(5):1289–1311.

59. Haviland KS, Swette S, Kelechi T, et al. Barriers and facilitators to cancer screening among LGBTQ individuals with cancer. *Oncol Nurs Forum.* 2020;47(1):44–55.

60. Monticciolo DL, Malak SF, Friedewald SM, et al. Breast cancer screening recommendations inclusive of all women at average risk: update from the ACR and society of breast imaging. *J Am Coll Radiol.* 2021;18(9):1280–1288.

61. Ayyappan AP, Kulkarni S, Crystal P. Pregnancy-associated breast cancer: spectrum of imaging appearances. *Br J Radiol.* 2010;83:529–534.

62. Asztalos S, Pham TN, Gann PH, et al. High incidence of triple negative breast cancers following pregnancy and an associated gene expression signature. *SpringerPlus.* 2015;4:710.

63. Johansson AL, Andersson TM, Hsieh CC, et al. Increased mortality in women with breast cancer detected during pregnancy and different periods postpartum. *Cancer Epidemiol Biomarkers Prev.* 2011;20(9):1865–1872.

64. Vashi R, Hooley R, Butler R, et al. Breast imaging of the pregnant and lactating patient: imaging modalities and pregnancy-associated breast cancer. *AJR Am J Roentgenol.* 2013;200(2):321–328.

65. Grimm L, Srini A, Dontchos B, et al. Revised SBI recommendations for the management of axillary adenopathy in patients with recent COVID-19 vaccination. *Society of Breast Imaging.* https://www.sbi-online.org/Portals/0/Position%20Statements/2022/SBI-recommendations-for-managing-axillary-adenopathy-post-COVID-vaccination_updatedFeb2022.pdf. Updated February 2022. Accessed April 20, 2022.

66. Gao Y, Moy F, Heller SL. Digital breast tomosynthesis: update on technology, evidence, and clinical practice. *Radiographics*. 2021;41:321–337.

67. FDA Drug Safety Communication: FDA evaluating the risk of brain deposits with repeated use of gadolinium-based contrast agents for magnetic resonance imaging (MRI). US Food and Drug Administration. Published July 27, 2015. Updated May 18, 2017. Accessed April 20, 2022.

68. FDA Drug Safety Communication: FDA Drug Safety Communication: FDA warns that gadolinium-based contrast agents (GBCAs) are retained in the body; requires new class warnings. https://www.fda.gov/drugs/drug-safety-and-availability/fda-drug-safety-communication-fda-warns-gadolinium-based-contrast-agents-gbcas-are-retained-body. Published May 22, 2017. Updated May 16, 2018. Accessed April 20, 2022.

69. ACR Practice Parameter for the Performance of Whole-Breast Ultrasound for Screening and Staging. American College of Radiology. https://www.acr.org/-/media/ACR/Files/Practice-Parameters/USWholeBreast.pdf. Published 2019, Accessed April 30, 2022.

70. Van Zelst JCM, Mann RM. *Automated three-dimensional breast US for screening: technique*, artifacts, and lesion characterization. *Radiographics*. 2018;38:663–683.

5

Outcomes and Quality Indicators

JOSEPH JOHN WEBER, AARON H. CHEVINSKY, AND CAROL HUIBREGTSE

Introduction

Given the complexity of the care of patients with breast cancer, outcomes assessment and improvement in the quality of care delivered have become essential.[1] Quality of cancer care may be difficult to define and assess precisely; however, given the variability of morbidity and mortality of patients with breast cancer based on different characteristics, quality metrics become a way to help achieve a standard of care.[2] *Ensuring Quality Cancer Care*, published by the Institute of Medicine in 1999, was prompted by the variability of quality in cancer care and need for standardizing quality of care and quality monitoring.[3] Since that time, standardized measures have been used by both payers and purchasers of healthcare to ensure that beneficiaries are receiving high-value care, and Medicare payments are tied to reporting of quality metrics and level of performance achieved on quality measures.[4] Moreover, professional organizations and provider groups have established quality measures that capture important processes of care that could be used for pay-for-reporting and other systems, helping with feasibility of system implementation. The aim of these processes includes increasing quality of care, reducing risks, enhancing efficiency, and improving patient satisfaction. Furthermore, creation of quality indicators helps with continuous multidisciplinary improvement and helps assure high-quality outcomes.[5–7] Implementation of quality indicators is feasible for breast centers to help achieve excellence in breast cancer care. All systems will be required to demonstrate their commitment to quality of care and show demonstrable achievements in care improvement in the upcoming years. Medicare and many other payers are already "bundling" episodes of care, and it is crucial for each hospital system or breast center to be efficient, standardized, and responsible for providing consistent, measurable, and demonstrable quality outcomes.

Framework for Outcomes and Quality Indicators in Breast Cancer Care

Outcomes and quality of care are important in the evaluation of breast cancer care from a patient, provider, and system levels. On all levels, indicators are used to monitor the quality of breast cancer care, make comparisons over time,

and support quality improvement for all practitioners and centers involved in the care of these patients. The Center for Medicare and Medicaid Services (CMS), the Commission on Cancer of the American College of Surgeons (CoC), and the National Accreditation Program for Breast Centers (NAPBC) are already requiring these measures and are performing comparisons between regional and national centers during their accreditation processes. The Institute of Medicine has identified six attributes of quality healthcare.[8] These are:

1. Effectiveness: Provide services based on scientific knowledge with success in producing the desired or intended result.
2. Patient-centeredness: Respectful care, responsive to patient needs, clinical and psychosocial.
3. Timeliness: Delivering care without unnecessary delay.
4. Safety: Avoiding harm and ensuring patients are protected from undue danger, risk, or injury.
5. Efficiency: Avoiding waste while achieving the desired clinical result.
6. Equitability: Fair and equal care to all patients.

These attributes are useful in identifying potential quality care initiatives to help quality directors select topics of importance for their patient populations, clinicians, and system leaders. By creating a grid with these attributes, and considering the patient, provider, and system levels as potential focus points, it allows for a framework to enable community cancer program leaders to evaluate their breast cancer quality initiatives. Table 5.1 lists these attributes, along with a sample of potential Breast Cancer Quality Care Initiatives that community cancer program leaders may find useful to investigate within their own programs.

Utilizing this framework, community cancer program leaders can initiate improvement measures best suited for their patient community, clinicians, and organization.

System Initiatives and Management of Quality

System initiatives relevant to breast cancer quality can be retrieved from accrediting bodies such as the CoC, the NAPBC, and Quality Oncology Practice Initiative (QOPI).

33

TABLE 5.1 Different Quality Attributes and Some Potential Breast Cancer Care Quality

Quality Attribute	Potential Breast Cancer Care Quality Initiatives

Effectiveness	• Patient care level
	  • i.e., Mammography screening volumes and results
	• Provider level
	  • i.e., Treatment process measures and pathways
	• System level
	  • i.e., Referral policies and navigation resources to ensure patients access available services

Patient-centeredness	• Patient care level
	  • i.e., Management of psychosocial distress and appropriate support
	• Provider level
	  • i.e., Management of treatment-related complications such as postmastectomy lymphedema
	• System level
	  • i.e., Coordination of care among modalities and sites of service

Timeliness	• Patient care level
	  • i.e., Time from symptoms to diagnosis
	• Provider level
	  • i.e., Time from diagnosis to treatment
	• System level
	  • i.e., Timeliness of referrals

Safety	• Patient care level
	  • i.e., Monitoring of flap viability after breast reconstruction
	• Provider level
	  • i.e., Morbidity from surgery and chemotherapy
	• System level
	  • i.e., Appropriate specialists' referrals

Efficiency	• Patient care level
	  • i.e., Timeliness of scheduling patients for biopsy after abnormal screening examinations
	• Provider level
	  • i.e., Appropriate utilization of testing
	• System level
	  • i.e., Length of stay for surgical procedures

Equitability	• Patient care level
	  • i.e., Ethnic or racial minorities access to care
	• Provider level
	  • i.e., Recruitment of a diverse population of providers
	• System level
	  • i.e., Underserved service areas and appropriate outreach to community leaders

Accreditation provides the framework for delivering high-quality cancer care through specific standards, quality measures, clinical trial accruals/participation, and professional education.[9]

Managing quality initiatives in a large healthcare system can be a challenging task, since best practices and treatment regimens may change at a rapid rate. Furthermore, recruiting physician involvement can be difficult. In a study done by the *Journal of Oncology Practice*, 97% of oncologists surveyed believed quality improvement was important, but only 49% participated in quality improvement projects in the last 5 years.[10]

Having a strong platform based on multidisciplinary input is crucial in selecting and implementing quality measures. Recruiting champions in multidisciplinary roles is one of the first steps in establishing a robust quality review program. Just like building a house, the foundation is one of the most important aspects of building a successful breast quality program, since these multidisciplinary champions are vital to the success of the program. Developing a systematic, explicit method of prioritizing a set of measures based on how well they identify high-priority targets for quality improvement could offer significant advantages.[11] Fig. 5.1 provides an example of a vertical cancer quality program structure that we use within our healthcare system. A breakdown of the breast quality council is displayed below. This model is then duplicated across all disease sites listed.

Fig. 5.1 adds to the foundation that encompasses a course of action for multidisciplinary quality measure selection, data analysis, data distribution, and development of process improvement plans ultimately leading to increased engagement in a group of caregivers. The coordinated process to provide quality metric feedback to front-line providers has shown greater enthusiasm for the data, engages behavior modification, and encourages more accountability

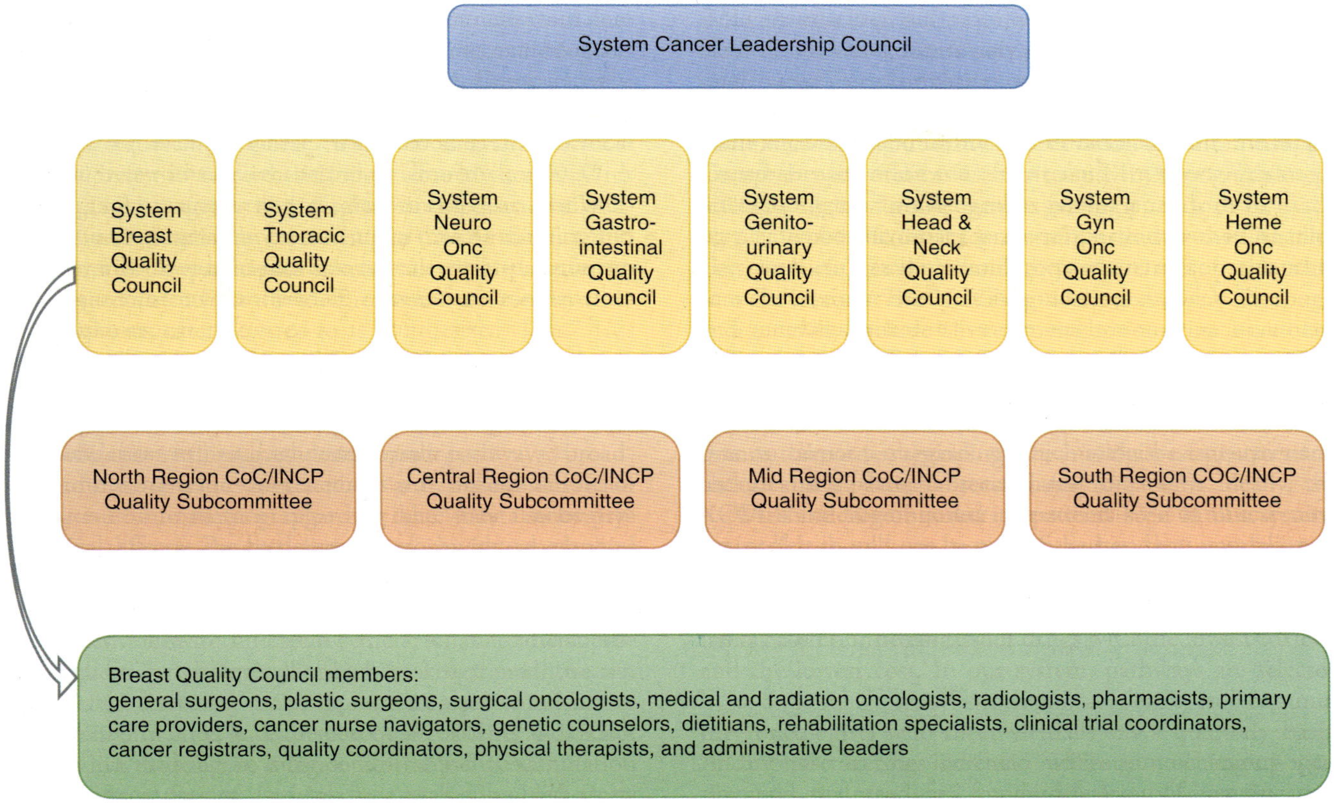

CHAPTER 5 Outcomes and Quality Indicators

• **Fig. 5.1** Example of a Vertical Cancer Quality Program Structure. *CoC*, Commission on Cancer of the American College of Surgeons; *INCP*, Integrated Network Cancer Programs.

Cancer Type	2020 System Cancer Quality Measures					Data here would be sites A - N, Named by location on dashboard					
	Measure	System Score	Cases	Data Range		Site A		Site B		Site C	
Breast Cancer	% of re-excision rates for newly diagnosed breast cancer patients who have undergone lumpectomy or partial mastectomy (lower is better)	9%	30/323	03 & 04 2019		5%	2/40	14%	1/7	0%	0/1

• **Fig. 5.2** An Example of Actual Data Representation in Quality Measure Dashboard.

with process improvement plans that are integral to establishing the best patient outcomes.[12]

Clinicians learn through science and best-practice standards. Expertise evolves with years of experience, training, and staying abreast of newly emerging practices. Thus, variability in practice may be demonstrated based on characteristics such as training or years of experience. Reporting and monitoring quality of care, quality of practice, and discussing outliers help practitioners standardize and improve their practice. Closing the loop is part of a successful quality process.[13] Using a dashboard to share the system's quality data as well as site/local data promotes that accountability and engagement. Color coding gives a quick visual on how a site is performing, mimicking a report card. Fig. 5.2 is an example of actual data in the quality measure dashboard. The system dashboard is shared biannually with all relevant providers as well as local and system leadership. Outliers are reviewed and results are disseminated to the System Cancer

Leadership Council as well as the hospitals' regional cancer quality subcommittees.

While the distribution of data and the tools used to assemble the data are important, establishing an organizational structure to ensure the data gets into the hands of the provider may provide the best opportunity to "close the loop," take ownership of the data, and ensure best practice. Healthcare organizations worldwide use quality dashboards to provide feedback to clinical teams and managers, monitor care quality, and stimulate quality improvement. However, there is limited evidence regarding the impact of quality dashboards and audits. Feedback research focuses on providing guidance to individual clinicians rather than to clinical and managerial teams.[14]

Accountability can also be facilitated with the use of quality charters. Charters can further define the scope of work of the system breast cancer quality council as well as ensure that it falls under the umbrella of the quality committee hierarchy. All quality councils within our system work under charters that have been approved by the hospital and local market management committees. Information discussed during council meetings should be protected health information (PHI) and not discussed in any forum other than the quality council meetings. There should also be boundaries that are clearly defined in the charter when defining the scope of work. The quality council should focus on identifying potential areas of quality improvement opportunities within the applicable service line/clinical program. Outlier cases may need to be referred for peer review after inquiry at the quality committee.

Quality Indicators

Some quality measures overlap between various organizations, yet that does not necessarily mean they are the most important. There are no guiding factors as to which measures are most important, because many factors can affect quality measure selection. It is unclear if any previous efforts that use explicit criteria to prioritize a set of measures in a systematic way help identify which measures are most likely to help achieve a particular outcome.[11]

Quality indicators for breast cancer can be systematically developed and used as a quality measurement tool for breast cancer care.[15] One option for prioritizing a set of quality measures includes the use of a weighted tool. The weighted tool describes and scores each quality measure against its performance improvement opportunity, ease in data collection, organizational endorsement and national benchmark, regulatory and reimbursement impact, value to the patient, and consideration of the resources required to implement change. The final score is then used to prioritize and select quality measures. The higher the score, the more impactful the measure (Table 5.2).

TABLE 5.2 **Example of Weighted Tool for Selecting Measures**

Name of Measure	
Measure is aligned with Cancer Quality Council's stated objectives (Yes = continue, No = stop)	Yes
Performance Improvement Opportunity	
Site's current performance	73%
National benchmark at top quartile (grade A)	>85%
Opportunity for improvement from current performance	15 points
≥15 points = 20	
≥10 but <15 points = 15	
≥5 but <10 points = 10	
<5 points = 5	
Total (20 points possible)	**15 points**
Data Collection	
Data can be gathered electronically (Yes = 15, No = 0)	15 points
Additional resources required to collect data (Yes = 0, No = 15) defined by specialty services, i.e., biostatistician, data analyst	15 points
Total (30 points possible)	**30 points**
Organizational Endorsement/National Benchmark (5 pts to each applicable line)	
ACoS/CoC (American College of Surgeons/Commission on Cancer)	5 points
ASCO (American Society of Clinical Oncology)/QOPI (Quality Oncology Practice Initiative)	5 points
ASBS (American Society of Breast Surgeons)	5 points
CAP (College of American Pathologists)	
NQF (National Quality Form)	
NAPBC (National Accreditation Program for Breast Centers)	5 points
NCBC (National Consortium of Breast Centers)	
PQRS (Physician Quality Reporting System)	
Total (40 points possible)	**20 points**

(Continued)

TABLE 5.2 Example of Weighted Tool for Selecting Measures—cont'd

Regulatory and Reimbursement Considerations

CMS quality measure (*Yes = 30*, No = 0) — 30 points

The Joint Commission reporting requirement (Yes = 30, No = 0)

Reported performance affects reimbursement (Yes = 30, No = −0)

Contributing to decreased healthcare cost (Yes = 30, No = 0)

Total (120 points possible) — **30 points**

Affected Patient Volume

Volume of patients affected (defined by specific disease/procedure)

   >50% = 30 points

    >30% and <50% = 20 points — 30 points

    >10% and <30% = 10 points

    <10% = 0 points

Total (30 points possible) — **30 points**

Value to Patient as Defined by Advisory Board[16]

Early diagnosis (5 points)

Delivering appropriate treatment at lowest cost (5 points) — 5 points

Limiting inpatient and emergency department visits (5 points)

Improved patient quality of life (5 points) — 5 points

End-of-life planning (5 points)

Positive patient experience (5 points) — 5 points

Total (30 points possible) — **15 points**

Resources Required to Implement Change

Modify behavior = 20 points — 20 points

Change to EMR (Electronic Medical Record) = 15 points

Operational Expenses (salary/supplies) = 10 points

Capital Expenses = 5 points

Total (20 points possible) — **20 points**

Total Points — **160 points**

Fictitious values inserted for educational value only. Highlights in italics indicate how points are calculated/achieved.
CMS, Centers for Medicare and Medicaid Services.

In Table 5.2, 160 points is the total weighted score (total of those points highlighted in bold). This is a measure with high points, meaning it accommodates multiple requirements from accrediting bodies, has an ease of data collection, impacts a large patient population, influences patient satisfaction, and needs limited resources to implement change. Using this points system helps prioritize the quality measures based on a weighted score. Of note, many of the categories in the weighted tool reflect the Institute of Medicine attributes mentioned earlier in this chapter.

Once multidisciplinary quality measures have been selected, establishing the quality measure methodology is imperative to ensure successful auditing and consistent data review. Inclusion and exclusion criteria set a clear definition of both the numerator and denominator. These data are then captured, reviewed, validated, and introduced at regular intervals. It is encouraged that with a vertically integrated community healthcare system, this data capture be completed and distributed at a system, regional, and a site-specific levels to clearly identify opportunities for

6

Evaluation and Treatment in the Underserved Community

JENNIFER JARVEY BALISTRERI AND DHRUBAJYOTI BHATTACHARYA

Introduction

It is of no surprise that the efforts behind community outreach and health equity have many layers. There are ever-evolving pieces as well as variables that remain consistent. Within this chapter, we will take a look at experiential approaches and best practices to fostering effective and sustainable community outreach and health equity. An example from the field is offered to illustrate the utility of this approach in practice. All of the approaches covered in this chapter include some of the same principles too. These principles first and foremost begin with building and sustaining a relationship with the community. These practices include, but are not limited to, ensuring that an under-empowered community is being supported through collaboration with internal and external stakeholders, connecting to community passion, understanding disparities and barriers to care, respect, and being aware of potential historical traumas or stigmas, letting the community share their needs versus assuming them, active listening, accountability, process/program transparency, understanding the role of a healthcare institution, and fostering overall collective efficacy for health advocacy. All of these practices have the common goal of health equity, meaning each member of the community is given an opportunity to obtain high-quality healthcare regardless of their differences from one another. In practice, this requires the removal of unjust disparities. What makes a disparity unjust, however, requires an intentional engagement of stakeholders to identify blind spots that may compromise the delivery of care.

Ensuring that an under-empowered community is being supported through collaboration with internal and external stakeholders is, in other words, gathering those who have complementing resources to provide a full spectrum of support for health education and screening. Also, identifying these stakeholders will help with a comprehensive look at who will be involved or affected by outreach goals and outcomes. By proactively researching and evaluating current programming within the targeted area or population, the community outreach strategy can better define what improvements need to be made and what best practices may

need further support for sustainability. The internal stakeholders one would review are what the health institution is providing to the community at large. This can take the shape of monetary support, in-kind donations, educational resources, screening, cultural competency, ethics, advocacy, representation, or how inclusive the culture is within the health institution. This can also include ensuring various team members are heard when deciding the groups or external disease sites to focus on and support.

The external stakeholders include the general public, specific community identifiers such as race, ethnicity, or identity, the local government support programming, government policy connected to health access and coverages, local events that support health and wellness, community-based organizations, citizenship, refugee status, educational institutions, community leaders, faith and spiritual influencers, research within the department of health, and employers. Although it is nearly impossible to keep a day-to-day update on each of these variables, a general understanding is essential to the impact they each have on the community at large and specific groups within.

Connecting to community passion is another way that community outreach can create realistic strategies, reach goals, and obtain successful outcomes. In other words, the health institution and community will have a shared vision and value for the same results. This can be obtained by primary or secondary research on a specific population or community's values, shared interests, behaviors, providing resources for primary needs, and micro-culture expectations. Once these are identified, community outreach can be paired with sustainable programming and education.

Moving forward beyond just connecting to a community then leads to the importance of screening and having a support system within the community. One way we have been able to connect to a community through this approach is through our work with the lesbian, gay, bisexual, transgender, queer, and/or questioning (LGBTQ+) community regarding breast health/cancer screening. There is a stigma from some of the LGBTQ+ that medical providers need to be aware of and accept additional training for transgender patients. Nonetheless, knowing there are higher risks for various diseases and health habits, such as tobacco use and drinking, our outreach team had focused efforts to support health and wellness by providing clinical breast exams at Pride events. Also, by bringing these efforts to a space where a community is gathering brings the internal social support needed to build trust and share or show representation.

Not only does screening provide potential life-changing and life-saving resources, but it may also create a need for social support and navigation of the health system. Our organization has identified this need and fosters the team member roles of community health workers, social work navigators, and cancer nurse navigators. These play a crucial role in supporting the patient's needs, beyond the screening or medical care to follow.

Understanding a population's health disparities and barriers to care are generally data-driven approaches to community outreach and health equity. Although objective data is important to establish a clear strategy with measurable outcomes, subjective data and feedback are also vital to the big picture and create an interconnected approach to supportive and collaborative change. As many know, the objective data will provide an assessment of a community's general health status and access to care. Subjective feedback will aid in understanding perceptions, the influence of social roles and norms, previous experiences, and willingness to engage in programs such as screening. Stepping into a specific population's shoes is a necessary first step toward genuine support, care, and help for others.

With these approaches in mind, a best practice of how feedback and subjective data have been used within our organization can be reviewed throughout our human papilloma virus (HPV) education program for youth. Our initial goal was to provide HPV Education to children ages 13 to 17 within an urban population to see whether this can impact the self-reported HPV vaccination rate, increased knowledge of HPV contraction, and impact decisions on safe sex behaviors. Although Wisconsin HPV vaccination rates were slowly rising at the time, there were still glaring gaps in education and vaccination access throughout the state. Only 13 of our 72 counties have reached vaccination rates of 15% or higher for eligible 11- to 12-year-old boys and girls.[1] Milwaukee County vaccination completion rates still hover around 40%. It was clear more work needs to be done.

In summary, this education program was brought to a public school system in Wisconsin after objective data was reviewed and found to be understated in the ninth-grade curriculum at the time. Through evaluation, subjective and objective data review, and feedback from providers, teachers, and health education specialists were able to support a revised HPV education program. Within 4 years, we educated over 4000 freshmen in health education classrooms in Milwaukee, WI. We took program feedback from students and tailored our presentation and education to their needs. We continue to ask the students questions to ensure the program is taught at a level that could be easily understood if they know whether their HPV vaccination series was completed, and if they believe they have enough HPV vaccination access resources going forward. We also give students the opportunity to ask questions of the healthcare provider present. In 2019, our data reflected that 74% of the students knew what HPV was before our lesson, yet only 32% knew if they had completed the vaccine, 22% reported they did not have the vaccine series completed and the rest were unsure. Table 6.1 shows there has been an increase in vaccination rates within the zip codes of the schools where the program was presented. By tailoring our work to educate and influence HPV behaviors, including vaccination rates, we were able to see an increase in vaccination utilization in Milwaukee, WI. The largest increases were within 53,221 with 8.19% and 53,204 with a 7.03% increase in vaccination rates.

Unfortunately, the program has been paused due to the pandemic and other internal health education barriers. This program also allowed the introduction of the importance of cancer screening and prevention to these students earlier in their lives.

The subjective and feedback-fueled approach we took to allowing students and cultural competence to influence program changes reflected the practice of empathy. Empathy acknowledges your own and others' emotions in both social and healthcare settings. Empathy requires active listening. Empathy is sensitive to nonverbal cues that a community may share yet go unnoticed. Having empathy is being more aware of a group's feelings, not solely focused on the ideas created within the health institution.

By practicing empathy, the health institution strategy will actively acknowledge various perceptions, stigmas, and

TABLE 6.1 Data Representing Vaccination Rates Within the Zip Codes of the Schools

Zip Code	2015 HPV Completion Rates	2016 HPV Completion Rates	2017 HPV Completion Rates
53215	N = 8978 43.45%	N = 9073 47.81%	N = 9147 50.83%
53211	N = 2206 24.61%	N = 2144 25.21%	N = 2081 29.61%
53221	N = 3643 34.96%	N = 3715 38.78%	N = 3800 43.15%
53206	N = 4070 39.1%	N = 4063 42.24%	N = 4009 43.83%
53204	N = 7205 39.76%	N = 7147 43.52%	N = 7117 46.79%

HPV, Human papilloma virus.

influences of mental health, and not be built on solely objective data-driven approaches alone. Empathy helps a community feel fairly heard, understood, and validated. In other words, empathetic assessments and evaluations are where the subjective data can be used to benefit a fully comprehensive strategy.

Respecting feedback and being aware of potential historical traumas or stigmas go hand in hand with letting the community share their needs versus assuming what they need after objective data review. This can be acquired through active listening, empathy, research on the community's experiences, evaluating historical contexts, and requesting feedback. The accountability for creating a foundation of support also lies within this space. Stakeholders need to be assured and shown that the feedback collected will be used to create, evolve, change, or expand a strategy with a mindful approach. This can be evaluated by how a health institution's cultural competency is being trained and practiced and the perception of its functionality from patients and team members.

The partnership and process/program transparency of a health institution create a strong level of morale and connectedness for various communities. This approach can also foster a positive and trustworthy reputation of providers, team members, and the organization as a whole. By including both internal and external stakeholders with clear communication, there is a sense of collaboration versus disjointed or counterproductive gatekeeping of information and decision-making. It is also important to understand the level of engagement among stakeholders as well when communicating various changes or updates.

Community outreach and health equity lastly need to foster overall collective efficacy for health advocacy. The continued and ever-evolving goal is to create new social norms on how various communities not only interact with health institutions but also how they will encourage others to do the same. Community outreach and health equity can often be negatively represented or entangled within the specific top-down measures, skewed expectations, miscommunicated intentions, or superficial approaches to connecting resources to communities. Instead, truly effective community outreach and health equity is a genuine, impactful collaboration to educate, support, and prevent disparities in healthcare. By providing education, screening, and support within an unbiased and empathetic approach, collective efficacy will be built organically.

From Theory to Practice: No Community Left Behind

In January 2020, amid scarce COVID vaccine, health systems were required to prioritize individuals to receive the vaccine and reduce their risk for severe illness from COVID-19. Our Patient Prioritization Team was specifically convened to generate a list of patients in accordance with federal and state guidelines, including those issued by the Centers for Disease Control and Prevention (CDC) and the Advisory Committee on Immunization Practices (ACIP). Additional state guidelines were offered by the Wisconsin Department of Health

Services and State Disaster Medical Advisory Committee (SDMAC) and the Illinois Department for Public Health (IDPH). Patient prioritization was a necessary but insufficient step in a process that began with identifying individuals at the highest risk of severe illness from COVID. Prioritization was a *process* guided by equity, flexibility, and agility. Equitable identification of eligible high-risk populations meant that patients would be initially identified and scored based on clinical and social general risk criteria, and ranked by higher scores to generate an eligibility list, as discussed below.

Flexibility was cited in reallocating vaccines to ensure no doses were wasted. The list would be refined based on site-specific considerations (e.g., excess vaccine supply, vaccine expiration) to advance herd immunity and protect patients. Agility was imperative in response to improving workflows and messaging. Feedback loops were established to track vaccination uptake, and share trends with system leadership to inform the broader vaccine distribution strategy.

A combination of medical and social vulnerability captured the sensitivity of the prioritization process to identify eligible persons.

Patients, age 65+, were prioritized based on clinical indications (CDC's high-risk comorbid conditions), social vulnerability (Area Deprivation Index),[1] and age group.[2] Those with CDC high-risk comorbid conditions were at heightened risk of severe illness from COVID; the Area Deprivation Index (ADI) was a measure validated to census blocks that allow rankings of neighborhoods by socioeconomic disadvantage, which has been positively associated with COVID risk (and includes factors like income, education, employment, and housing quality) and offered targeted prioritization because it is centered on the census block (neighborhood). According to the CDC, older adults, age 75+ (third condition), were up to a 23-fold higher risk of hospitalization or up to a 480-fold higher risk of death compared to those individuals, ages 18 to 29.[1]

Adults of any age with certain underlying medical conditions were at increased risk for severe illness from COVID-19. Severe illness included hospitalization, ICU admission, intubation or ventilation, or death. The more underlying medical conditions someone had, the greater their risk for severe illness. In other words, more conditions equated to greater risk.

Patients were scored according to a tally of the CDC conditions, age, and residing in an ADI decile group corresponding to a more disadvantaged block group/neighborhood. Older patients with more conditions and residing in areas of greater social disadvantage are ranked higher than younger patients with fewer conditions, and residing in areas of less social disadvantage.[2] For example, a patient with chronic obstructive pulmonary disease (COPD) and diabetes living in an area with a lower ADI (≤7) would have a **score of 2** (1 point for each condition). A patient with COPD, diabetes, ***and*** living in an area with a higher ADI (8 to 10) would have a **score of 3** (one extra point for higher ADI). A patient with COPD, diabetes, living in an area with a higher ADI (8 to 10), and age 75+, would have a **score of 4** (one extra point for older age group).

Amid scarce resources, sub-prioritization based on socio-economic vulnerability was also appropriate based on the higher risk of severe illness from COVID-19. We used the ADI,[3] which allowed for rankings of neighborhoods by socioeconomic disadvantage. Notably, reliance on the ADI enabled us to identify a larger population of eligible, underrepresented populations than the social vulnerability index (SVI),[4] which was being used by other systems at the time.

There is an inextricable linkage between equity and belonging, which is easily overlooked in the design and review of interventions. After the prioritization list was generated, a different division would take responsibility for extending invitations to eligible persons. Emails were deployed and individuals were invited to get vaccinated at a system facility during the daytime hours at their earliest convenience. Early results were not promising; there was low uptake among Hispanics, notwithstanding their eligibility. One interpretation of these findings was their collective reluctance or hesitancy, which became part of a broader narrative on the mistrust exhibited by underrepresented communities of health systems. While there is a legacy of discrimination and bias toward underrepresented patients and team members, those factors were not determinative in explaining the trends that we observed in our communities.

Belonging is required to establish trust, and it is often a byproduct of efforts to collaborate, understand barriers to care, exhibit empathy, and foster collective efficacy. In our initial design, we did not engage external stakeholders or community leaders, and while we clearly understood the disproportionate impact of COVID-19 on underrepresented communities, we less clearly understood the barriers to care. These oversights precluded us from exhibiting empathy or creating an opportunity for collective empathy, as we could not even reach our populations of interest.

Our analysis of data highlighted multiple gaps in our initial approach. Many underrepresented patients who were eligible for vaccine did not have email addresses on file. Without phone outreach, which was implemented in subsequent phases, those individuals may not have received an invitation. Some individuals also worked shifts that did not allow for them to go to our facilities during the allotted hours of operation, and finally, some individuals simply did not have sufficient means of transportation outside of their communities.

In response, a team led by a nurse, who was engaged with the local Hispanic community and served in a leadership role, served as a liaison between our system and local community organizations. She identified the existent barriers to care, and her team helped devise a potential solution that would address the gaps in uptake: set up a vaccine clinic on the weekend (Fig. 6.1) in the community, meet communities where they are, and proactively partner with community organizations to reach out to eligible individuals.

This collaboration gave us the opportunity to reconnect with our empathy toward this population and truly serve. And the collective efficacy became readily apparent in the results that followed. By the end of the weekend, there was 100% vaccine uptake without a single dose wasted. One recipient was a 96-year-old gentleman who captured the spirit of the moment as he held up his vaccine card (Fig. 6.2), reminding us that we were truly in this together.

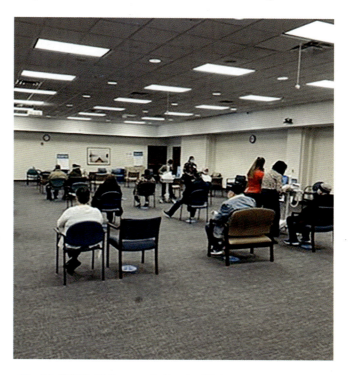

• **Fig. 6.1** COVID-19 Community Vaccine Clinic.

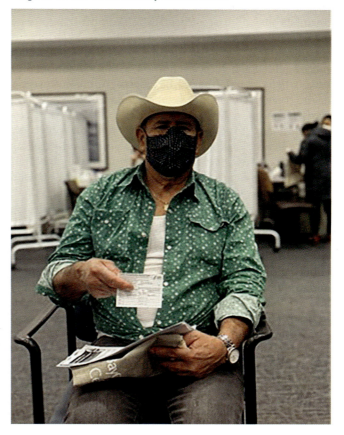

• **Fig. 6.2** A 96-Year-Old Vaccine Recipient.

References

1. Centers for Disease Control and Prevention (CDC). *People With Certain Medical Conditions*; 2022. Available at https://www.cdc.gov/coronavirus/2019-ncov/need-extra-precautions/people-with-medical-conditions.html.

2. Centers for Disease Control and Prevention (CDC). *Risk for COVID-19 Infection, Hospitalization, and Death by Age Group*; 2022. Available at https://www.cdc.gov/coronavirus/2019-ncov/covid-data/investigations-discovery/hospitalization-death-by-age.html.

3. University of Wisconsin Center for Health Disparities Research. *About the Neighborhood Atlas*; 2022. Available at https://www.neighborhoodatlas.medicine.wisc.edu/.

4. Centers for Disease Control and Prevention. *CDC/ATSDR SVI Fact Sheet*; 2021. Available at https://www.atsdr.cdc.gov/placeand-health/svi/fact_sheet/fact_sheet.html.

PART 3

Breast Cancer Treatment in the Community

7

Contemporary Surgical Approaches to Breast Cancer

ASHLEY MARUMOTO, ARMANDO E. GIULIANO, AMEER GOMBERAWALLA, NICOLE M. ZAREMBA, AND HARRY NAYAR

BIOPSY TECHNIQUES

Key Points

- Biopsy of suspicious breast lesions is necessary prior to considering operation.

Historical Context

Historically, biopsy of suspicious breast lesions required surgical excision. Lesions were sampled and sent for frozen section prior to performing a radical or modified radical mastectomy.[1] It was not until the 1970s that percutaneous biopsy was introduced as an alternative. Image-guided biopsy was first described by Roberts et al. in 1975.[2] However, it wasn't widely utilized until 1993 following the success of ultrasound (US)-guided core needle biopsy (CNB).[2–4]

Shorter recovery times, reduced cost, fewer complications, and smaller scars make percutaneous biopsy more favorable than surgical biopsy. Furthermore, the use of a minimally invasive biopsy technique to establish a breast cancer diagnosis before any surgical procedure is a Breast Quality Measure by the American Society of Breast Surgeons (ASBrS).[5,6] For these reasons, image-guided percutaneous biopsies are preferable and commonly performed.

Indications

The Breast Imaging and Reporting Data Systems (BI-RADS) lexicon for mammography was established in 1993. BI-RADS describes key imaging findings and classifies breast lesions into different categories, which provides direction for management and follow-up. Lesions that are BI-RADS 4 or 5 on mammography require further evaluation with biopsy. US and magnetic resonance imaging (MRI) are other modalities with their own criteria to identify abnormal breast lesions requiring biopsy.

Fine Needle Aspiration Versus Core Needle Biopsy

For breast lesions, CNB is preferred over fine needle aspiration (FNA). CNB provides evaluation of tissue histology, while FNA only provides cytologic evaluation and cannot distinguish invasive from noninvasive cancer. Additionally, biomarker status is a crucial component of the breast cancer diagnosis and is difficult with FNA.[5] FNA is associated with higher rates of insufficient samples and higher false-negative rates.[5,7] However FNA is often able to provide a diagnosis when axillary lymph nodes are being sampled near a large vessel or when cystic lesions require evaluation.[8]

Types of Needles and Devices

Both spring-loaded and vacuum-assisted devices are available. Vacuum-assisted devices have the advantage of allowing for a single insertion as well as larger tissue and broader tissue sampling secondary to a rotating device. Needle sizes typically range from 7 to 14 gauge and vary depending on the device type and by imaging modality. The number of samples obtained also vary by needle size, with smaller needles requiring more samples for increased accuracy.

Palpable Lesions Versus Nonpalpable Lesions

Breast lesions may be palpable or nonpalpable. If a lesion is palpable, image guidance with US is recommended.[5] For lesions that are not palpable, stereotactic imaging, US, or MRI are necessary to identify and biopsy the lesion. The choice of modality depends on the ability to visualize the lesion as well as technical convenience. For instance, if a lesion is seen on both mammogram and US, US would be the preferred method of biopsy owing to ease and technical simplicity compared with stereotactic biopsy. For lesions demonstrated across multiple modalities, the radiologist must ensure that the lesions and targets are concordant between the images.

Considerations

As with all procedures, written informed consent is necessary prior to performing breast biopsy. Patients should be informed that biopsy may yield benign, malignant or nondiagnostic results. Pathologic results must be correlated with clinical findings and interpreted as concordant or discordant. Risks of the procedure include bleeding, infection, and missed lesions, and should be discussed. Anticoagulation is a relative contraindication to performing breast biopsy. For patients taking anticoagulant medications, it is usually recommended that patients hold their anticoagulation periprocedurally. Additionally, patients should be informed that a clip will be placed to mark the location of the biopsy. Regardless of the modality used or if the lesion is palpable or not, a clip should be placed at the biopsy site. In the event that biopsy results necessitate surgical intervention, the clip marks the site for surgery. If biopsy results are benign and concordant, the presence of a clip allows for continued surveillance and denotes that the lesion has been previously sampled.

Stereotactic Biopsy

Stereotactic biopsy is the preferred modality for lesions that are mammographically detected without a sonographic correlate and can be performed via two-dimensional or three-dimensional mammographic guidance. Patients may be positioned prone or upright with advantages and disadvantages to each.[9] In the prone position, the breast is placed through an opening in the table (Fig. 7.1). It may be difficult for some patients to maneuver onto the table. In the upright position, the breast is compressed between two plates similar to the usual technique for mammography (Fig. 7.2). In this

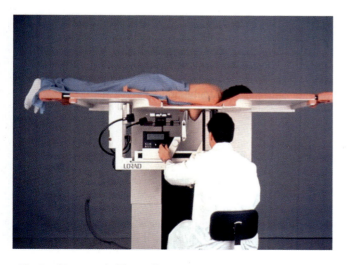

• **Fig. 7.1** Stereotactic Biopsy Prone.

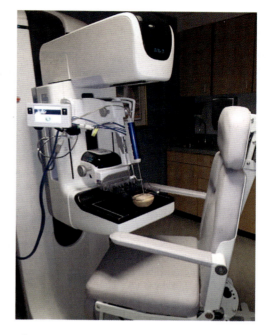

• **Fig. 7.2** Stereotactic Biopsy Upright. (From Bahl M, Maunglay M, D'Alessandro HA, Lehman CD. Comparison of upright digital breast tomosynthesis-guided versus prone stereotactic vacuum-assisted breast biopsy. *Radiology*. 2019;290(2):298-304.)

position, the patient may experience vasovagal responses or move in response to seeing the needle. Upright tomosynthesis-guided vacuum-assisted breast biopsy has a higher rate of successful biopsy than prone and can be performed in a shorter amount of time with one-fourth of the exposure.[10]

The breast is compressed and the target area positioned through the window in the paddle. A scout view is obtained. Prior to biopsy, it is necessary to ensure that there is adequate distance from the skin to the lesion so that the biopsy is within the breast tissue and not too superficial. Biopsies that are too superficial may excise skin as well as breast tissue. Local anesthetic is injected, biopsy performed, and a marking clip is placed. The number of samples depends on the size of the needle. For 10–11-gauge needles, typically 12 samples are obtained, while for 7–9-gauge needles, 4 samples are typical. A specimen radiograph is necessary to verify that the targeted lesion was biopsied. Manual compression is provided and the skin incision is reapproximated with steri-strip or surgical glue. A postprocedural mammogram is obtained to document accurate tissue sampling as well as to document marker placement. Biopsy clips have been known to migrate due to hematoma formation or upon release of breast compression, known as the accordion effect. Given its implications for future localization and surgical planning, clip migration must be documented in the biopsy report.[9]

Ultrasound Biopsy

For sonographically detected lesions, US-guided biopsy is preferable to stereotactic biopsy (Fig. 7.3). US-guided biopsy does not require breast compression, does not utilize

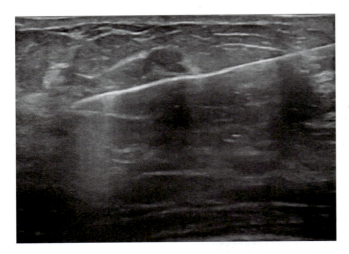

• **Fig. 7.3** Ultrasound Biopsy. (From Park VY, Kim EK, Moon HJ, Yoon JH, Kim MJ. Evaluating imaging-pathology concordance and discordance after ultrasound-guided breast biopsy. *Ultrasonography*. 2018;37(2):107-120.)

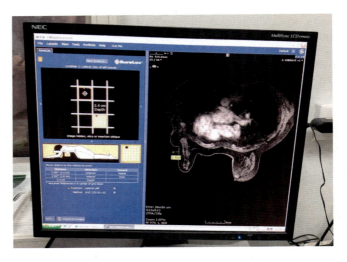

• **Fig. 7.4** Magnetic Resonance Image Biopsy. (From Gao P, Kong X, Song Y, et al. Recent progress for the techniques of MRI-guided breast interventions and their applications on surgical strategy. *J Cancer*. 2020;11(16):4671-4682.)

ionizing radiation, and provides real-time visualization of the needle with shorter procedure times, lower costs, improved patient comfort, and is technically less challenging.[9]

Typically, US is used for masses but can be utilized for calcifications. When calcifications or nonmass lesions are biopsied under US guidance, vacuum-assisted biopsy has been found to be more accurate than 14-gauge CNB.[11] Furthermore, when calcifications are biopsied under US guidance, it is imperative to obtain postprocedural imaging. For US-guided biopsies, patients are positioned supine but may be bolstered in the lateral decubitus position if needed depending on the location of the lesion in the breast. Sometimes the ipsilateral arm is positioned overhead to facilitate biopsy. The US probe is held either by the radiologist or the technologist and is used to identify the lesion. After injection of local anesthetic, the skin is entered approximately 1–2 cm from the edge of the transducer and the needle is visualized throughout the entire procedure to ensure adequate tissue sampling and to avoid inadvertent injury. This is most easily achieved when the needle runs parallel to the transducer. An image is obtained as the needle traverses the lesion. As with stereotactic biopsy, a biopsy clip is placed followed by postprocedural imaging. Clip migration is less common with US-guided biopsies compared with stereotactic biopsies.[9]

Magnetic Resonance Biopsy

Magnetic resonance (MR)-guided biopsies are indicated for lesions detected with MR but without mammographic or US correlates. MR-guided biopsy is technically challenging, expensive, and time consuming. The patient is positioned prone with the breast positioned through an opening in the table with biopsy grid used to localize the lesion (Fig. 7.4). Light compression maintains breast position while permitting vascular perfusion with contrast. Fluctuations in a patient's hormones causing changes in tissue enhancement or breast compression occluding inflow of contrast material may result in lesion nonvisualization.[12] If this occurs, short-term follow-up is recommended to ensure stability of lesions that are not visualized at the time of biopsy. If the lesion is identified, the needle is positioned using a grid and fired. Four to six samples from a 7–9-gauge needle are typically obtained. As with other modalities, a clip is routinely placed at the biopsy site.

Postbiopsy Considerations and Concordance

Following the procedure, a report is written describing the modality used, the lesion location and laterality, the number of tissue specimens obtained, clip placement, any associated complications, and results from the post-biopsy mammogram, including clip location. The procedure report is addended to reflect the pathology results and whether or not they are concordant with the clinical and imaging findings. Imaging-pathologic concordance must take into consideration several factors. Appropriate targeting of the lesion is essential. Stereotactic biopsy can be more easily monitored by postprocedural mammogram, while US-guided biopsies rely on real-time needle visualization. The biopsy specimen must also be adequate and requires sampling of the most suspicious area of the lesion.[2]

Imaging-pathologic concordance is imperative to determine next steps for biopsied lesions. Benign concordant results should be followed in 6 months with the same modality used for biopsy in order to determine lesion stability. Suspicious lesions with benign pathology are considered discordant and require further intervention. Discordant results may either be rebiopsied or surgically excised.[5]

SURGICAL OPTIONS

Key Points

- Trials have demonstrated the safety of surgical de-escalation for selected patients with breast cancer.
- It is necessary to consider patient age, clinical and imaging findings, and biomarker status when discussing surgical timing and options for patients with breast cancer.
- Treatment recommendations for breast cancer operations continue to evolve rapidly.

Historical Context

Breast cancer once relied on invasive, disfiguring operations for treatment. Today, a woman can often be cured with breast-conserving surgery and adjuvant therapies. Dr. Halsted pioneered the radical mastectomy in the late 1800s during which the entire breast, pectoralis major and minor muscles, and axillary lymph nodes were removed. It was believed that the tumor spread in a contiguous manner until the 1960s, when research demonstrated that breast cancer was often a systemic disease.[13] Concurrent improvements in systemic therapy permitted a shift toward consideration of surgical de-escalation.

In the 1960s, the National Surgical Adjuvant Breast and Bowel Project (NSABP) was created by Dr. Bernard Fisher in order to collaborate on research and determine the best treatment for breast cancer.[14] Two of the most influential studies from NSABP as they relate to breast cancer surgery include NSABP B-04 and NSABP B-06.[15–21]

Between 1971 and 1974, NSABP B-04 randomized women with clinically node-negative disease to radical mastectomy, total mastectomy with radiation, or total mastectomy without radiation, and women with clinically node-positive disease to radical mastectomy or total mastectomy with radiation.[15] Early results demonstrated no significant difference in disease-free survival, distant disease–free survival, and overall survival, and even after 25 years of follow-up no survival benefit was seen in any group. Interestingly, there was a statistically significant difference in locoregional recurrence among clinically node-negative women favoring those that underwent total mastectomy with radiation.[20,21]

In NSABP B-06, patients were randomized to undergo modified radical mastectomy, lumpectomy with axillary dissection, or lumpectomy with axillary dissection plus whole-breast radiation.[16,17] Once again, no difference in survival could be seen.[16,17] However differences in local control were identified. Among women who underwent lumpectomy, the lowest ipsilateral breast tumor recurrence (IBTR) was seen in those who were treated with radiation.[20,21]

These studies paved the way for further de-escalation of locoregional therapy. Between 1999 and 2004, NSABP B-32 demonstrated that sentinel node biopsy for clinically node-negative patients was as effective as standard axillary dissection with fewer side effects.[22] Around the same time, the Alliance for Clinical Trials in Oncology Z0011 trial (ACOSOG Z0011) examined whether axillary dissection could be omitted for clinically node-negative women with axillary metastases identified by sentinel node biopsy undergoing lumpectomy and whole-breast radiation. Women in whom sentinel node biopsy identified one to two positive lymph nodes were randomized to undergo axillary dissection or no further surgery. No significant differences in disease-free survival, overall survival, or local or regional recurrences were seen between groups.[23,24] ACOSOG Z0011 demonstrated that it was safe to omit axillary dissection in women with limited axillary disease treated with breast conservation. The study was criticized for closing early due to enrolling only 891 of the anticipated 1900 patients, as well as a lower than anticipated event rate. Study results stood the test of time and long-term follow-up continued to demonstrate no significant differences in outcomes.[25,26]

Other studies including IBCSG 23-01 and the AMAROS trials also demonstrated no advantage to routine axillary dissection for women with minimal axillary disease.[27–29] As a result, many clinically node-negative women with early-stage breast cancer can now be spared the morbidity of axillary dissection. Results from Z0011 were practice changing and led to changes in national guidelines.[30–33]

Surgical Localization of the Biopsied Lesion

Following breast or axillary needle biopsy, it is imperative that a clip be placed in order to mark the location for future surgical excision. For women with nonpalpable lesions undergoing breast-conserving surgery, localization of the lesion is necessary. In the event that mastectomy is performed, localization is often not necessary, but may be considered for very superficial, deep, or lateral lesions. Localization can be performed via a number of different modalities.

Wire localization of breast lesions has been utilized since the 1970s (Fig. 7.5). During wire localization, the radiologist, or surgeon, will place a wire into or adjacent to the breast lesion under image guidance. This may be performed with either stereotactic, US or MR guidance. This procedure is often performed on the day of operation, as a wire protruding from the skin can be uncomfortable for the patient and is at risk of dislodgement. The surgeon uses the wire as a guide to locate and remove the lesion and the previously placed clip.

Seed localization utilizing a detectable seed instead of a wire was developed as an alternative to wire localization (Fig. 7.6). Multiple seed localization technologies exist. Radioactive seeds containing iodine-125 were the first on the market[34] and additional technologies followed. In 2014, SAVI SCOUT radar localization from Cianna Medical Inc., and in 2016 Magseed by Endomagnetics Inc., were approved by the US Food and Drug Administration for preoperative breast localization.[35,36] Most recently in 2017, the LOCalizer by Hologic Inc. was approved by the Food and Drug Administration and uses radiofrequency identification. Axillary lymph nodes may be localized by wire or seed placement in order to perform targeted axillary dissection (TAD).[37] Studies have shown that outcomes favor seed technology and do not significantly differ between the various seed technologies.[34,38,39]

Seed localization is usually performed by the radiologist preoperatively and identified by the surgeon intraoperatively with various probes. Advantages and disadvantages for each type of seed technology exist. The major advantage to seed technology is the ability to place the seed prior to the day of surgery. Additional advantages include improved patient and clinician satisfaction as well as decreased operative times. Disadvantages are specific to the seed technologies themselves. Radioactive seeds are governed by state regulations and facilities require trained personnel and licensing to oversee the program. While radioactive seeds are titanium-encapsulated, the capsule can be transected resulting in the release of radioactive material. Radar seeds can be deactivated by direct contact with electrocautery. While magnetic seeds do not deactivate with electrocautery, metal instruments interfere with detection.

Regardless of device used, review of the preoperative images by the operating team is necessary in order to create a surgical plan. Intraoperative specimen imaging is necessary to ensure seed removal.

Breast Conservation

The decision to proceed with breast conservation depends on patient desire and candidacy for breast conservation. As previously discussed, multiple randomized controlled trials have demonstrated that there is no difference in overall survival when comparing breast conservation to mastectomy. As such, it is vital that patients who are candidates for breast conservation understand that choice of surgery will not impact their survival, but small differences in local recurrence exist.

Absolute contraindications to breast conservation include pregnancy, diffuse malignant or indeterminate calcifications, inflammatory breast cancer, or persistently positive margins. Relative contraindications include multicentric tumors, large tumors relative to the breast volume, or inability to be treated with radiation (i.e., due to genetic mutation, prior radiation, collagen-vascular disease, noncompliance, or absence of a radiation center).

Breast-conserving surgery is also known as segmental mastectomy, partial mastectomy, or lumpectomy. However, segmental or partial mastectomy is the preferred

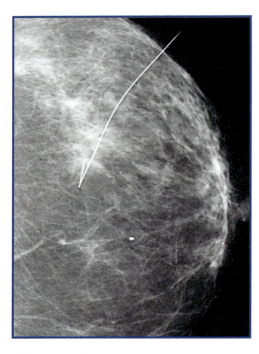

• **Fig. 7.5** Wire Localization.

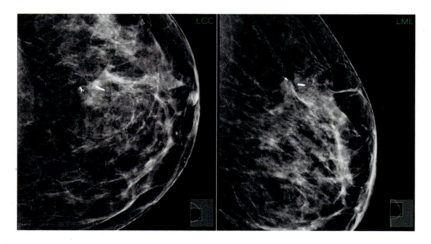

• **Fig. 7.6** Seed Localization. (From Ross FA, Elgammal S, Reid J, et al. Magseed localisation of non-palpable breast lesions: experience from a single centre. *Clin Radiol.* 2022;77(4):291-298.)

nomenclature, as the lesion of interest is often occult and not a "lump." As with all procedures, informed consent is obtained prior to the operation. Nonpalpable lesions are localized preoperatively. Preoperative films are reviewed by the surgical team in order to ensure that the correct lesion was localized and to develop an operative plan. Either a periareolar incision or incision over the lesion of interest can be made. The lesion and a small rim of surrounding tissue are removed.

The surgeon may choose to mark the specimen with sutures to denote surgical margins. Alternatively, many centers routinely perform shave margins of the lumpectomy cavity. A single-center randomized controlled trial evaluating shave margins demonstrated a reduced positive margin rate and reduced re-excision rate when cavity shave margins were obtained.[40] Findings were later validated in a multicenter randomized trial.[41] Retrospective evaluation demonstrated the lowest recurrence when both the lumpectomy specimen and cavity shave margins were negative.[42] Interestingly, the highest recurrence rate was seen when the lumpectomy specimen was negative and the shave margins positive.[42] This can be explained by the phenomenon that tumors may not necessarily grow contiguously.

A specimen radiograph is obtained to verify that the lesion, wire or seed, and clip are obtained (Fig. 7.7). The specimen is then sent to pathology for evaluation. The lumpectomy cavity may be closed in multiple layers to occlude the dead space or allow for a seroma to fill the cavity, which can help preserve the normal breast contour. Pathology results are reviewed at the postoperative appointment.

At times, the clip is not obtained in the lumpectomy specimen. Residual clips can contribute to increased patient and surgeon anxiety. When this occurs, it is important to have a discussion with the patient. Excision of the lesion, and not the clip, is the goal of the operation. Postoperative mammography can evaluate for clip dislodgement within the lumpectomy bed or if the clip was lost at the time of surgery. If the lesion of interest was not removed or positive margins remain, re-excision is necessary and the clip can be removed at that time. If the lesion was obtained with negative margins, clip removal is not necessary.

Margins Following Breast-Conserving Surgery

At the postoperative visit, the surgeon reviews the pathology report with the patient, specifically discussing tumor biology and margin status. The Society of Surgical Oncology and American Society for Radiation Oncology have published margin guidelines for breast-conserving surgery for both invasive and in situ disease.[43] For invasive disease, no ink on tumor is considered a negative margin.[44] However for ductal carcinoma in situ (DCIS) a 2-mm margin is recommended.[43] For lesions with both invasive disease and DCIS, invasive margin guidelines should be followed and no ink on tumor is considered sufficient, even when an extensive intraductal component (EIC) is present.[44] However for patients with tumors with EIC, postoperative mammography should be considered to assist in identifying residual calcifications. DCIS with microinvasion should be treated as DCIS with 2-mm margins. When positive margins occur, re-excision is often indicated as positive margins result in at least double the rate of recurrence. However, sometimes re-excision is not possible. These circumstances warrant a discussion with the multidisciplinary team.

Mastectomy

The decision to undergo mastectomy is a highly personal one. A woman may decide to undergo mastectomy for personal reasons or she may not be a candidate for breast conservation. Historically, men with breast cancer were treated with mastectomy; however National Comprehensive Cancer Network guidelines recommend considering breast conservation versus mastectomy in men based on criteria used for women.[31] There are no absolute contraindications to mastectomy aside from inability to tolerate the operation. Women who undergo mastectomy should be offered consultation for reconstruction with a plastic surgeon.[45]

The Women's Health and Cancer Rights Act was signed into law on October 21, 1998 and mandates that insurance covers all reconstructive operations related to mastectomy, as well as surgery to the contralateral breast for symmetry. Alternatively, women may choose to remain flat following total mastectomy. The "going flat" movement is gaining popularity.[46] For women who desire reconstruction, skin-sparing mastectomy or nipple-sparing techniques may be considered. The nipple-areolar complex is removed in the skin-sparing technique while it is preserved in the nipple-sparing technique. Women are considered candidates for nipple preservation provided the lesion is a sufficient distance away from the nipple. Traditionally this distance was considered 2 cm; however patients may be eligible for nipple-sparing mastectomy even when this distance is less than 2 cm.[47] Women with a prior history of breast surgery,

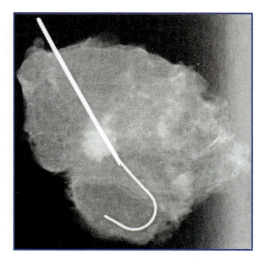

• **Fig. 7.7** Specimen Radiograph.

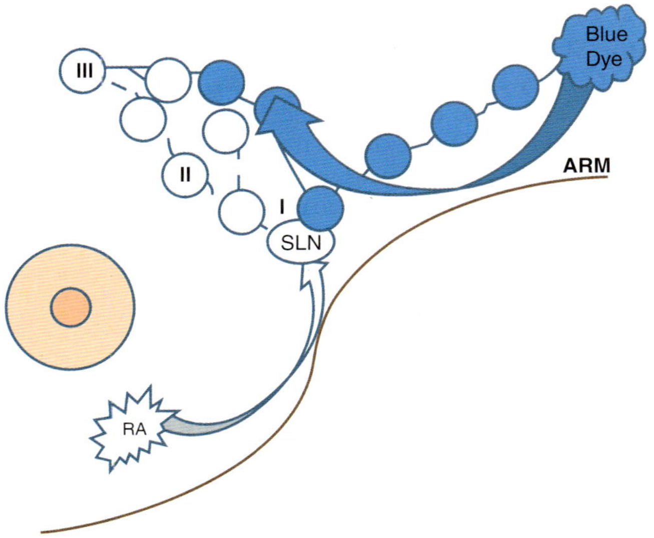

• **Fig. 7.12** Axillary Reverse Mapping (ARM). Variations of ARM lymphatics may place them within operative field of dissection of level I or II lymph nodes or in juxtaposition to the sentinel lymph node. *RA*, Radioactive; *SLN*, sentinel lymph node.

nodes and had 100% seed placement and removal.[144] Miller et al. found similar success with magnetic seed for lymph node localization.[145] With reliable SLNB after NAC, aggressive axillary surgery can be avoided.

Axillary Reverse Mapping

Axillary reverse mapping (ARM) is a technique used to distinguish the lymphatic drainage of the arm from that of the breast. It identifies upper-extremity (UE) lymphatics coursing through the axilla to minimize unnecessary disruption of the arm lymphatics while performing lymph node surgery.[146–148] ARM entails mapping UE lymphatics with blue dye at the time of SLNB mapping in the breast with technetium-99, allowing for differentiation of lymphatics draining the breast (hot) and the UE (blue). Variations in UE lymphatic drainage patterns exist and may coalesce or cross over with those draining the breast (Fig. 7.12).

There are three factors to consider with ARM: feasibility, prevention of BCRL, and oncologic safety. A large phase II single-arm trial with 654 patients evaluated the feasibility of ARM. They reported identification of blue UE lymphatics in 29% of SLNB patients and 72% of ALND patients.[149–157] Boneti et al. identified blue in 39% of those patients having SLNB and in 81% of patients having ALND.[151] Wijaya et al. performed a review and meta-analysis of 29 studies with 4954 patients combined. They found the feasibility to be 37% in SLNB and 82% in ALND.[158] The larger percent of identification in ALND is due to the larger operative field and greater area of dissection, aiding in visibility.

In terms of prevention of BCRL, Tummel et al. prospectively reported on patients in a single-arm study. They found the rate of BCRL after SLNB with ARM was 0.8% and ALND with ARM was 6.5% after 26 months follow-up.[157]

In the meta-analysis by Wijaya et al., they found the BCRL rate was 2% in those with SLNB and ARM and 14% with ALND and ARM.[158]

In an analysis of five randomized controlled trials evaluating ALND versus ALND with ARM, all five studies favor ALND plus ARM for lower BCRL rates.[259]

In a small fraction of patients, the ARM (blue) node will also be the SLN. This can call into question the oncologic safety. Tummel et al.[152] found that crossover SLN (hot) and blue was seen in 3.8% of SLNB procedures. Crossover happened in 5.6% of those undergoing ALND. In the subset of patients in which an identified blue lymphatic was transected, there was an overall lymphedema rate of 18.7% when not reanastomosed compared with 0% when reanastomosed at 14 months of follow-up.[157] Of note, the axillary recurrence rate was 0.2% in those with SLNB and 1.4% in those with ALND.

Future work includes the Alliance trial A221702, a randomized prospective phase III trial that studies how well ARM works in preventing lymphedema in patients with breast cancer undergoing ALND. Patients will be randomized to ARM versus no ARM. This randomized trial will help establish change in practice as needed, based on the evidence found.

Lymphatic Microsurgical Preventive Healing Approach

A logical progression from ARM is the lymphatic microsurgical preventive healing approach (LyMPHA) procedure. LyMPHA provides a preventive lymphavenous anastomosis. In those patients where the malignant node is found to be draining the arm, a lymphovascular anastomosis can prevent secondary lymphedema (Fig. 7.13). Boccardo et al. described the technique in the *Annals of Surgical Oncology*.[160–162] in a randomized study in 2011, Boccardo et al. compared LyMPHA in 46 patients undergoing complete ALND. At 6 months of follow-up, he showed that one (4.34%) patient with LyMPHA developed lymphedema versus seven (30.43%) control patients.[161] Long-term follow-up at 4 years showed no sign of lymphedema in 71 of 74 (96%) of patients who underwent LyMPHA.[160] Feldman et al. found the lymphedema rate was three of 24 (12.5%) in successfully completed and four of eight (50%) in unsuccessfully treated patients. They found LyMPHA to be feasible, safe, and effective for the primary prevention of BCRL.[163]

Ozmen et al.[164] evaluated the simplified lymphatic microsurgical preventing healing approach (S-LyMPHA). S-LyMPHA is a slightly modified and simplified version of LyMPHA. It is performed by the operating surgeon performing the ALND. During the ALND, transected blue lymphatic channels are identified and at the completion of the dissection, those channels are carefully dissected and invaginated using a sleeve technique into the cut end of a neighboring vein with two 7–0 nonabsorbable stitches. The microscope is not used in any part of this surgery.[164] They evaluated 380 patients who underwent ALND and found a

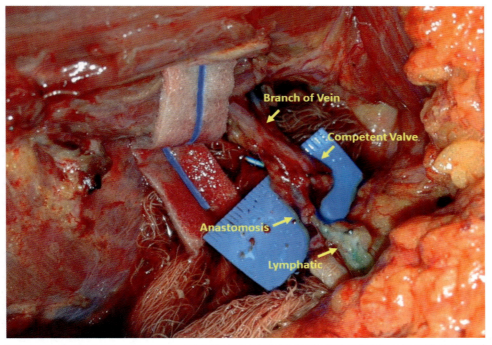
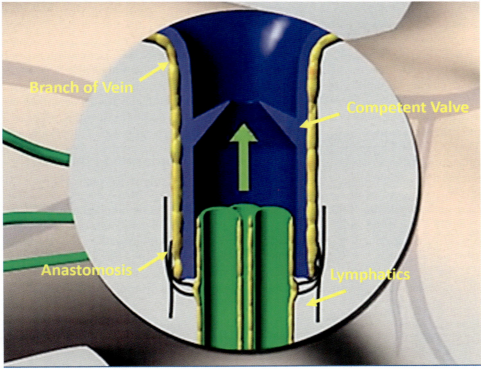

• **Fig. 7.13** LyMPHA Schematic and LyMPHA Operative View.

significantly lower rate of lymphedema in both univariate and multivariate analysis (3% vs. 19%.)

Johnson et al. recently described the benefits of LyMPHA in those patients undergoing ALND and nodal radiation. They performed a literature review and included 19 studies. The pooled cumulative incidence of lymphedema was 33.4% in those undergoing ALND and RLNR versus 10.3% in those undergoing ALND, RLNR, and LyMPHA (P = .004).[165]

ARM and LyMPHA help prevent BCRL by identifying nodes draining the arm, as well as establishing a reconnection for the disrupted lymphatics. Further randomized multicenter trials would need to be conducted to establish more long-term data.

Less Radiation to Prevent Lymphedema

Partial Breast Irradiation

For patients who undergo lumpectomy, radiation therapy is usually recommended. Traditionally whole-breast radiation is recommended; however there is data to show that in patients with early-stage, favorable breast cancer, partial breast irradiation (PBI) is safe and effective. PBI can be delivered as external beam radiation therapy (EBRT), as targeted intraoperative radiation (TARGIT-IORT), balloon catheter, or interstitial catheter brachytherapy (Fig. 7.14). Intraoperative radiation can be given as low-energy x-rays or as intraoperative electron radiotherapy. There have been two large, prospective randomized trials comparing whole-breast radiation to both forms of IORT, electron and 50 kV photons, showing low local recurrence rates and excellent overall survival outcomes.[166,167]

There are now long-term survival and local control outcomes from the TARGIT-A trial. Vaidya et al.[168] randomized patients to a one-time dose of external beam of whole-breast radiotherapy or TARGIT-IORT immediately after lumpectomy in the operating room. With a median follow-up of 8.6 years and maximum follow-up of 18.90 years, no statistical difference was found for local recurrence-free survival, mastectomy-free survival, distant disease-free survival, overall survival, and breast cancer mortality. Of note, mortality from other causes was significantly lower in the TARGIT-IORT group. This group has previously published on radiation-related quality-of-life parameters after TARGIT-IORT.[169] They found that patients receiving IORT alone reported less general pain and arm symptoms as well as better role functioning than those in the EBRT group. Most common issues were pain in the arm or shoulder and difficulty moving or raising the arm sideways. The frequencies of moderate or severe breast and arm symptoms reported by patients in each group for swelling in the arm versus hand were 8% versus 4% with TARGIT-IORT compared with 9% versus 7% with EBRT. The TARGIT-A trial has not yet reported specifically on BCRL. We hypothesize that since RLNR is avoided with TARGIT-IORT, the BCRL rate will likely be lower compared with EBRT. A review of the radiation fields used in the ACOSOG Z0011 trial found that in approximately half of patients in both study arms, the radiation fields were within 2 cm of the humeral head, possibly causing substantial incidental axillary irradiation.[270] Lymphedema rates from TARGIT-A would be valuable data to be able to identify ways to prevent lymphedema with more directed radiotherapy.

The ELIOT study had a similar design to TARGIT-A, but used electron technology. It randomized 1305 women between whole-breast radiation and single-dose intraoperative electron radiotherapy. Median follow-up was 5.8 years and there was no difference in overall survival or breast cancer recurrence.[167]

Obi et al.[171] reported outcomes and acute toxicities from a single institution with intraoperative radiation. They analyzed 201 patients with a median follow-up of 23 months and found the rate of arm lymphedema was 0.5% ($n = 1$) in their group.

Warren et al.[117] conducted a prospective cohort study of 1476 breast cancer patients using volume measurements with a perometer to assess the impact of various radiation techniques on rates of BCRL. At a median follow-up of 25.4 months, the 2-year cumulative incidence of BCRL was 6.8%. Cumulative incidence by radiation therapy type was as follows: 3.0% no radiation; 3.1% breast or chest wall alone; 21.9% supraclavicular; and 21.1% with supraclavicular and posterior axillary boost. Of interest they treated 6% of patients with PBI. In a univariate analysis for factors with risk of lymphedema, those who received PBI only had a hazard ratio of 0.38; however this was not statistically significant given the low number of patients. This highlights the potential benefit of PBI in avoiding RLNR and decreasing the risk of BCRL from radiation. This has been suggested in other studies as well.[172]

Omit Radiation in the Elderly and Neoadjuvant Responders

CALGB 9343 randomized women older than 70 years with T1N0M0 ER-positive breast cancer who received lumpectomy without any axillary surgery at all to either tamoxifen plus radiation therapy or tamoxifen alone. While the tamoxifen plus radiation therapy group experienced greater locoregional control—98% versus 90% in the tamoxifen

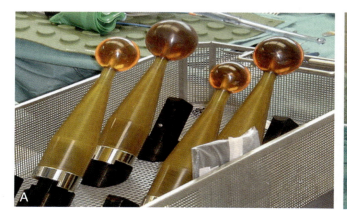
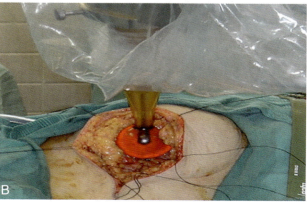

• **Fig. 7.14** Intraoperative Radiation. (Used with permission from Kuerer HM. Surgical consideration for accelerated partial breast irradiation. In: Wazer DE, Arthur DW, Vicini FA, eds. *Accelerated Partial Breast Irradiation-Techniques and Clinical Implementation.* Springer Nature; 2006.)

only group—there were no differences in cancer-specific survival, overall survival, or breast-preservation rates.[132] They concluded that women over the age of 70 years with favorable, small, estrogen-responsive tumors could avoid radiation if they commit to taking endocrine therapy.

Future work in this realm includes the NSABP B-51/RTOG 1304 trial, a randomized phase III trial evaluating the role of radiation therapy for patients who have positive lymph nodes prior to NAC who convert to pathologically negative nodes after NAC. We look forward to the results of this trial to help us to continue to improve our goal of reducing rates of BCRL.

Post Lymphedema Treatment

Nonsurgical Management of Arm Lymphedema

For patients in which lymphedema has been established, there are both nonoperative and operative management options. The mainstay of nonoperative treatment is complex decongestive therapy. There are two phases consisting of reduction and maintenance. The reduction phase includes manual lymph drainage, sequential gradient pump, exercises, low-stretch bandages, and skin care. The maintenance phase consists of compression garment, exercises, and skin care.

There has not been one strategy identified as the most beneficial. A randomized controlled trial tested complex decongestive therapy over standard compressive therapy. There was no significant difference in the percent volume reduction of the arm at 6 weeks and 52 weeks. In addition, reports of quality of life did not differ.[173] Compression garments have been shown to prevent progression in subclinical BCRL as well as reduce arm volume.[14,124,217,218] Manual lymphatic drainage is important for volume reduction. It has been shown to be beneficial to patients with mild-to-moderate BCRL in conjunction with compression bandaging.[176]

Physical therapy by lymphedema-trained therapists has been shown to be more beneficial than just patient education and physical therapy alone.[121,220] Aerobic and resistance exercise does not incite or exacerbate BCRL.[178–182] The data suggests that monitored management with trained physical therapists is better than self-directed treatment.[183]

Two randomized controlled trials looked at the role of early detection and intervention. A study from Madrid enrolled 120 patients without BCRL who had ALND. They were randomized to a program of manual lymphatic drainage, massage, and exercise or BCRL education alone. At 1-year follow-up, 25% of patients randomized to education alone developed BCRL compared with 7% in the other group.[78] Another study randomized 65 women without BCRL who had ALND to prospective monitoring and treatment with physiotherapy or surveillance alone. They found at 2 years the incidence of BCRL was 11% in the early intervention group compared with 30% in those with surveillance alone.[177] This data supports the recommendation that early detection and monitored treatment are beneficial at preventing progression.

Surgical Treatment of Arm Lymphedema

Surgical management is another option, particularly for patients who do not respond to noninvasive treatment. There are two main surgical strategies: ablative and physiologic procedures.

Ablative procedures reduce limb volume by surgically removing edematous tissue. Liposuction or suction-assisted protein lipectomy are used as volume-reduction treatments because they are less invasive than older debulking procedures and do not require skin grafting. Liposuction/suction-assisted protein lipectomy has been shown to have significant volume reductions.[184–186] However, compression garments must be worn continuously to maintain the decreased volume.[185,186]

Physiologic procedures treat the etiology of BCRL by re-establishing and/or redirecting axillary lymphatic flow. Reapproximation or rerouting of lymphatic drainage pathways can be achieved by establishing unobstructed connections with distal healthy tissue or proximal venous tissues.

Procedures utilizing distal tissues generally involve lymphatic grafts or vascularized flaps containing lymphatic soft tissue. The lymphaticolymphatic bypass procedure involves an anastomosis between healthy lymphatic tissue of the lower extremity to the affected arm's axillary lymphatics and supraclavicular lymphatics. This has been shown to produce long-term patency and reduce UE volume.[187,188]

Another major surgical treatment involves vascularized lymph node transfer. A lymph node flap is harvested with its vascular supply from a donor site and introduced into the affected extremity. Blood supply is achieved through an anastomosis from the lymph node flap's blood vessels to the native axillary blood vessels.[189,190] There has been reduction in limb volume following this procedure, circumference differentiation of 7.3%, and reduction rate of 40.4% at a mean follow-up of 39.1 months. Furthermore by mapping the lymphatic drainage of the donor site, selective removal of lymph nodes can be achieved to decrease the risk of lymphedema in the donor site (Fig. 7.15).[191]

Lastly, lymphatic venous anastomosis uses proximal tissue instead of grafts to re-establish lymphatic drainage. Multiple lymphatic vessels are anastomosed to venules, allowing lymphatic drainage into the venous system. Chang et al. performed 89 lymphatic venous anastomoses in women with UE lymphedema. Symptom improvement was reported in 96% of patients, and mean volume reduction was 42% overall.[192,193] There are no randomized clinical trials as of yet to fully compare and evaluate the benefits of these surgical procedures.

Section Summary

BCRL is a challenging consequence of breast cancer treatment. It is imperative for the contemporary practitioner to evolve as new methods, treatment algorithms, and techniques become available. Various methods of surveillance, early detection, avoidance of practices, and treatment adjustments can improve outcomes for our patients, as we continue to improve the level of care available.

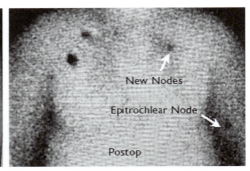

• **Fig. 7.15** Vascularized Lymph Node Transfer. (Chapter 16 by Mark L. Smith and Joseph H. Dayan. Microsurgical Procedures: Vascularized Lymph Node Transfer from the Thoracodorsal Axis, 132–143. In *Principles and Practice of Lymphedema Surgery*, Second edition, Ming-Huei Cheng, David W Chang, Ketan M Patel, 2018, Elsevier Inc.)

DCIS, LOBULAR CARCINOMA IN SITU, AND OTHER HIGH-RISK LESIONS

Key Points

- The management of DCIS is similar to invasive cancer with surgery and radiation as the mainstay of treatment.
- Ongoing clinical trials are exploring the potential role of de-escalated treatment of DCIS.
- Most high-risk lesions require surgical excision to establish a diagnosis and determine the best course of treatment.

Epidemiology

The incidence of DCIS has increased since population-based breast cancer screening recommendations began in the 1970s. The incidence of DCIS increased more than 11-fold from 7 cases per 100,000 in 1980 to 83 cases per 100,000 in 2008. However, a small decline in the rate of DCIS of 2.1% per year was noted from 2012 to 2016.[194] Furthermore, the incidence of advanced breast cancer has not significantly decreased, suggesting that screening has resulted in overdiagnosis and possibly treatment.[195] Currently, DCIS represents approximately 20–25% of breast cancers.

Diagnosis

DCIS is considered stage 0 cancer by the 8th Edition of the American Joint Committee on Cancer.[196] Due to the advent of screening recommendations, most patients are diagnosed with nonpalpable, clinically occult lesions. Only 10% of DCIS cases are detected as masses or nipple discharge. Given its association with calcifications, DCIS is most commonly diagnosed by mammography. However up to 25% of DCIS lesions do not contain calcifications. DCIS may be associated with a mass lesion or architectural distortion.[197] The sensitivity of MRI for detecting DCIS may be superior to mammography but has less specificity. The presence of DCIS alone is not an indication for further evaluation with breast MRI.

Natural History

It is believed that DCIS progresses slowly, if at all. While DCIS is a direct precursor to invasive breast cancer, it is not necessarily an obligate precursor. It is estimated that less than 1% of patients with DCIS will progress to invasive disease annually.[198] However the risk of progression depends on many factors. Research attempting to stratify patients and determine who will progress to invasive disease has to date been unsuccessful. Hormone-replacement therapy has not been shown to significantly increase the risk of developing DCIS.[199] Fortunately the prognosis of DCIS is excellent, with only a 1–3% 20-year breast cancer–specific mortality rate.

Pathology

Ductal atypia represents a heterogeneous group of lesions on a continuum.[200] DCIS is one such lesion in which a proliferation of atypical epithelial cells is contained within the lumen of the breast ducts. Architectural, cytologic, and nuclear features, as well as size, distinguish DCIS from atypical ductal hyperplasia. Grading of DCIS is based on cytonuclear features including morphology, cytoplasmic features, degree of nuclear pleomorphism, and degree of mitotic activity resulting in low (1), intermediate (2), or high (3) grade histology. Among pathologists, there is interobserver variability for atypical proliferative lesions. Hormone receptor status is routinely evaluated, as the results may help guide adjuvant therapy recommendations, while HER2 status is not routinely performed for DCIS.[201] DCIS lesions diagnosed with core biopsy may be upstaged to invasive disease following pathologic evaluation of the entire specimen. Upstage rates depend on a number of factors including size, mass lesion, and grade. Rates of upstaging and can be as high as 43%.[202,203]

Treatment

There is no single treatment approach that is suitable for all patients with DCIS. As such, there is concern that DCIS is being overtreated in many cases. While some patients may benefit from aggressive treatment, others may be able to be treated conservatively. Historically, DCIS was treated with mastectomy. Now, the decision for mastectomy versus breast conservation depends upon patient preference as well as clinical factors. If a patient is a candidate for breast conservation, lumpectomy with consideration for postoperative radiotherapy with or without chemoprevention is a reasonable option. Chemoprevention without operation is being considered for patients whose DCIS is hormone receptor-positive.

A sentinel node biopsy is recommended for patients undergoing mastectomy for DCIS and may be offered to patients undergoing lumpectomy who have tumors with higher risk features.[204]

Recommendations regarding margin width for DCIS have evolved. Previously, a 1-cm margin was recommended. However, recent guidelines now recommend a 2-mm margin for DCIS. For lesions with both invasive disease and DCIS, no ink on tumor is considered sufficient, even with an EIC. On the other hand, margins for DCIS with microinvasion should be treated as DCIS.[31,43,44]

Recurrence

The most common failure following lumpectomy for DCIS is IBTR. Approximately half of all recurrences will be invasive.[205] No randomized trial has directly compared mastectomy to breast-conserving surgery for the treatment of DCIS. Multiple trials have evaluated the effect of adjuvant radiotherapy on recurrence, with some trials also evaluating the role of tamoxifen. Five randomized trials have demonstrated the efficacy of treating DCIS with adjuvant radiotherapy following breast-conserving surgery, with two including the addition of tamoxifen.[205–211] Radiotherapy reduced IBTR for DCIS treated with lumpectomy in all studies and reduced the risk of local recurrence by up to 50%, with durable results even with long-term follow-up.[205,209,211] Tamoxifen reduces IBTR by about one-third.[205,209] In NSABP B-17 and B-24, about 20% of patients treated with lumpectomy without radiation experienced an invasive recurrence at 15 years compared with 8.5% of patients who received lumpectomy, radiation, and tamoxifen therapy.[205] Despite the impact on recurrence, studies have found no difference in overall survival with radiation.[204] It is important to counsel patients on these details and to weigh the risks and benefits when considering surgery and adjuvant therapies. A multidisciplinary team can aid in these discussions and decisions.

Prognostic Scores

A number of prognostic indices and nomograms exist for DCIS. The first nomogram developed for DCIS was the Van Nuys Prognostic Index (VNPI), which was first introduced in 1996.[212] It was developed to aid in treatment decision-making and to predict the risk of recurrence for patients with DCIS. The VNPI initially stratified patients into risk groups based on tumor size, margin width, and

pathologic classification, and has been updated to include patient age.[213] The Memorial Sloan Kettering Cancer Center DCIS (MSKCC DCIS) calculator is another nomogram that incorporates ten clinicopathologic as well as treatment factors.[214]

Commercially available calculators also exist to predict the chance of recurrence and benefit of radiotherapy for patients with DCIS. Oncotype DX Breast DCIS Score developed by Exact Sciences uses 12 genes (7 cancer-related genes and 5 reference genes) to predict the risk of ipsilateral recurrence.[215,216] However only 29.4% of patients were treated with tamoxifen in the validation study.[215] DCISionRT from PreludeDx, Inc. is another score used to identify the benefit of radiotherapy.[217]

Despite their availability, nomogram and calculator use varies among practitioners and is not routinely performed. Studies have demonstrated conflicting results regarding concordance among the various tests. A study comparing the VNPI, MSKCC DCIS Nomogram, and Oncotype DX® DCIS Score found varying risk estimates among the predictive tools.[218] However, there may be concordance between the MSKCC DCIS nomogram and the commercially available Oncotype DX® DCIS Score for women over 50 years.[214] Treatment decisions for patients with DCIS require a thorough discussion between clinician and patient.

Future Perspectives

Given the concern for overdiagnosis and treatment, prospective studies are evaluating the role of surgery in the treatment of DCIS in the hopes of identifying a patient population in whom treatment can be de-escalated. Currently, the LORD trial in Europe, LORIS in the United Kingdom, LORETTA trial in Japan, and COMET trial in the United States are evaluating the role of active surveillance versus standard treatment in patients with DCIS.[219] The results from these trials will hopefully better elucidate a group of patients for whom nonoperative treatment would be beneficial.

Other High-Risk Lesions

Atypical hyperplasia and lobular carcinoma in situ (LCIS) are benign breast lesions without the potential for disease progression. LCIS was removed from the 8th edition of the American Joint Committee on Cancer Breast Cancer Staging System.[196] Rather these high-risk lesions relate to a patient's breast cancer risk, which can be four- to tenfold higher than the general population. LCIS confers an increased risk of invasive disease in either breast of 1–2% per year.[220]

While high risk lesions are noninvasive precursors, they require thoughtful attention and consideration for further treatment. High-risk lesions may be upstaged to invasive disease following surgical excision. Atypical ductal hyperplasia contains similar histologic features to DCIS. As such, core biopsied lesions showing atypical ductal hyperplasia should be surgically excised for definitive diagnosis.[220] Surgical excision of LCIS and atypical lobular hyperplasia, on the other hand, is more controversial. If there is clinical, imaging, and pathologic concordance, these lesions can be managed without excision.[221] Patients with LCIS should undergo high-risk surveillance and be referred for consideration of chemoprevention. Pleiomorphic LCIS (PLCIS), on the other hand, is distinct from classic LCIS. It is a rare, more aggressive lesion with no consensus for treatment; however it is generally recommended that PLCIS be treated similar to DCIS.[222]

Other high-risk lesions include papillary lesions, complex sclerosing lesions, columnar cell lesions, and flat epithelial atypia, among others. Rates of upstage to cancer after core biopsy vary among the different lesions and the decision to excise should be based on clinical, imaging, and pathologic concordance. Patients with high-risk lesions on CNB require consideration of clinical, imaging, and pathologic factors to determine the best course of action.

BREAST RECONSTRUCTION

Key Points

- Coverage must be provided for all stages of breast reconstruction.
- Breast reconstruction should be considered for all breast cancer surgery; i.e., mastectomy and breast conservation with oncoplastic reconstruction to repair the defect.

Introduction to Breast Reconstruction

Breast reconstruction is a standard of care in the treatment of breast cancer and an integral part of the overall multidisciplinary approach to breast cancer treatment. It is often addressed with breast cancer patients during the initial surgical consultation. In 1998 the Women's Health and Cancer Rights Act was signed into law.[223] It provides protections to patients who choose to have breast reconstruction in connection with a mastectomy or partial mastectomy. It states that coverage must be provided for all stages of reconstruction of the breast on which the mastectomy (or partial mastectomy) has been performed; surgery and reconstruction of the other breast to produce a symmetrical appearance; and prostheses and treatment of physical complications of all stages of the mastectomy, including lymphedema (Centers for Medicare & Medicaid Services). In this section, we will address breast reconstruction with breast-conservation surgery, or oncoplastic breast reconstruction.

ONCOPLASTIC BREAST RECONSTRUCTION

Key Points

- Definition
- Volume displacement versus volume replacement
- Classification
- Benefits

Oncoplastic breast surgery is the combination of surgical oncologic principals with plastic surgery techniques. The ASBrS developed a consensus definition of oncoplastic surgery as a form of "Breast conservation surgery incorporating an oncologic partial mastectomy with ipsilateral defect repair using volume displacement or volume replacement techniques with contralateral symmetry surgery as appropriate." Volume displacement is defined as closing the lumpectomy defect and redistributing the resection volume over the preserved breast. Volume displacement is divided into two levels: level 1 (<20% resection volume) and level 2 (20–50% resection volume).[224] Volume replacement includes those situations when volume is added using flaps or implants to correct the partial mastectomy defect.[225] The primary goal of oncoplastic breast surgery is complete excision of the malignancy with appropriate histologic margins with a secondary goal of maintaining or improving cosmesis and contour of the breast. There are several benefits to the oncoplastic approach. Oncoplastic breast conservation is more likely to achieve negative margins and has demonstrated decreased rates of re-excision[226,227]; review of patient-reported outcomes (PROs) data show superior aesthetic and psychosocial outcomes with oncoplastic breast conservation when comparted with mastectomy and immediate reconstruction[228]; and oncoplastic breast conservation is cost effective and often complete in one operation.[229,230]

PREOPERATIVE CONSIDERATIONS

Key Points

- History and physical exam
- Imaging
- Pedicles
- Informed consent

Goals of oncoplastic breast surgery include complete removal of the tumor with clear margins and good-to-excellent cosmetic results in a single operation. To achieve these goals, thorough preoperative planning is required. This starts with a systematic physical exam to determine breast size, tumor size, and the tumor-to-breast size ratio as well as the baseline grade of ptosis. Attention is placed on noting any previous scars, quality of the skin, and breast composition: fatty versus dense. Equally important is knowledge of the patient's medical history, comorbidities, and medications with special consideration to those with diabetes, vascular disease, pulmonary disease, steroid use, and smoking status among others. These can affect wound healing and may contribute to the choice of surgical procedure (Fig. 7.16).

Along with the history and physical exam, an equally in-depth review of imaging studies is necessary. The surgeon must assess the imaging abnormality, focality, and satellite lesions, as well as distance from the nipple-areolar complex to determine which oncoplastic procedure is appropriate.

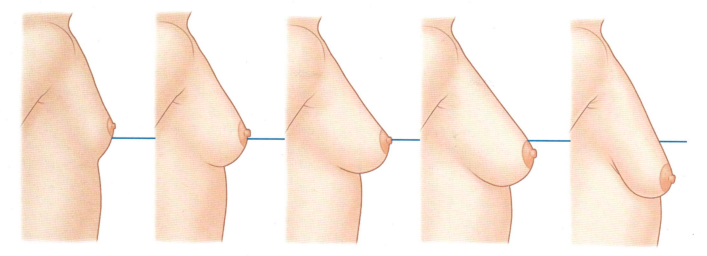

• **Fig. 7.16** Regnault Classification of Ptosis. (From Hartmann EC, Spring MA, Stevens WG. One- and two-stage considerations for augmentation mastopexy. In: *Plastic Surgery,* Vol 5: *Breast.* 7th Ed. Amsterdam: Elsevier; 108-123.e2.)

MRI of the breasts is often helpful for preoperative planning in oncoplastic breast reconstruction.

Keeping in mind all of these points, consideration is then given to which pedicle is best to maintain vascular supply to the nipple-areolar complex or if the patient requires a nipple delay or a free nipple graft. There are five main options for vascular pedicles: central, lateral, superior, superior medial, and inferior. A pedicle that is remote from the area to be excised is best to avoid complications such as loss of sensation, necrosis, flattening, and/or possible nipple loss (Figs. 7.17A–B, and 7.18).

Many basic, level 1, oncoplastic approaches and procedures are performed by the breast surgeon performing the partial mastectomy. However, more advanced, level 2, oncoplastic breast reconstruction is often performed in conjunction with or by a plastic surgeon. The breast surgeon and plastic surgeon work closely together to plan a procedure that achieves the aforementioned goals. Setting expectations with the patient is important. There must be a clear understanding that this is first an oncologic procedure, and clear margins remain the priority above all else. With this comes a discussion of patient expectations regarding postoperative breast size and what is feasible considering the tumor-to-breast volume ratio. In addition the surgeon should ensure the patient understands their own baseline asymmetries and the risk for further asymmetries post-treatment, as well as have a discussion about changes that continue to occur with and after radiation therapy, which is often necessary to complete their cancer treatment. Like with any other surgical procedure, detailed informed consent includes details of risks specific to oncoplastic reconstruction, including but not limited to altered or loss of sensation to a portion of the breast and/or nipple-areolar complex, loss of nipple projection, erectile function, pigmentation, possible nipple loss, scarring, and asymmetry.

BASIC ONCOPLASTIC APPROACH

Key Points

- Mobilizing
- Closing the defect

To achieve the best possible cosmetic result and rounded contour of the breast, the lumpectomy defect must be repaired. All level 1 oncoplastic breast surgery involves closing the lumpectomy cavity with glandular flaps created by dual-plane undermining of the mastectomy plane and the retromammary plane with reapproximation of the mobilized surrounding breast tissue. Mobilizing the surrounding breast tissue off the overlying skin is performed by dissecting in the plane of loose areolar tissue that separates the subcutaneous fat from the underlying breast tissue. This mobilization can be performed for an area up to two-thirds of the breast tissue. However skin undermining should be limited in very fatty breast tissue to reduce the risk for postoperative fat necrosis. Closing the partial mastectomy defect also often includes mobilizing the same breast parenchyma off the pectoralis fascia in the retromammary plane to allow for additional tissue mobility.

Most oncoplastic procedures include resection of skin. This is beneficial for a variety of reasons: skin overlying the tumor can be included in the partial mastectomy, reducing the risk of a close or positive anterior margin; and reducing the skin envelope of the breast can allow for a better contour postoperatively by reducing the size of a postoperative seroma. However with little to no postoperative seroma, which is traditionally used for radiation planning and boost, it is imperative that all six margins of the lumpectomy cavity are marked prior to any tissue rearrangement for future radiation planning. This can also be helpful in the setting

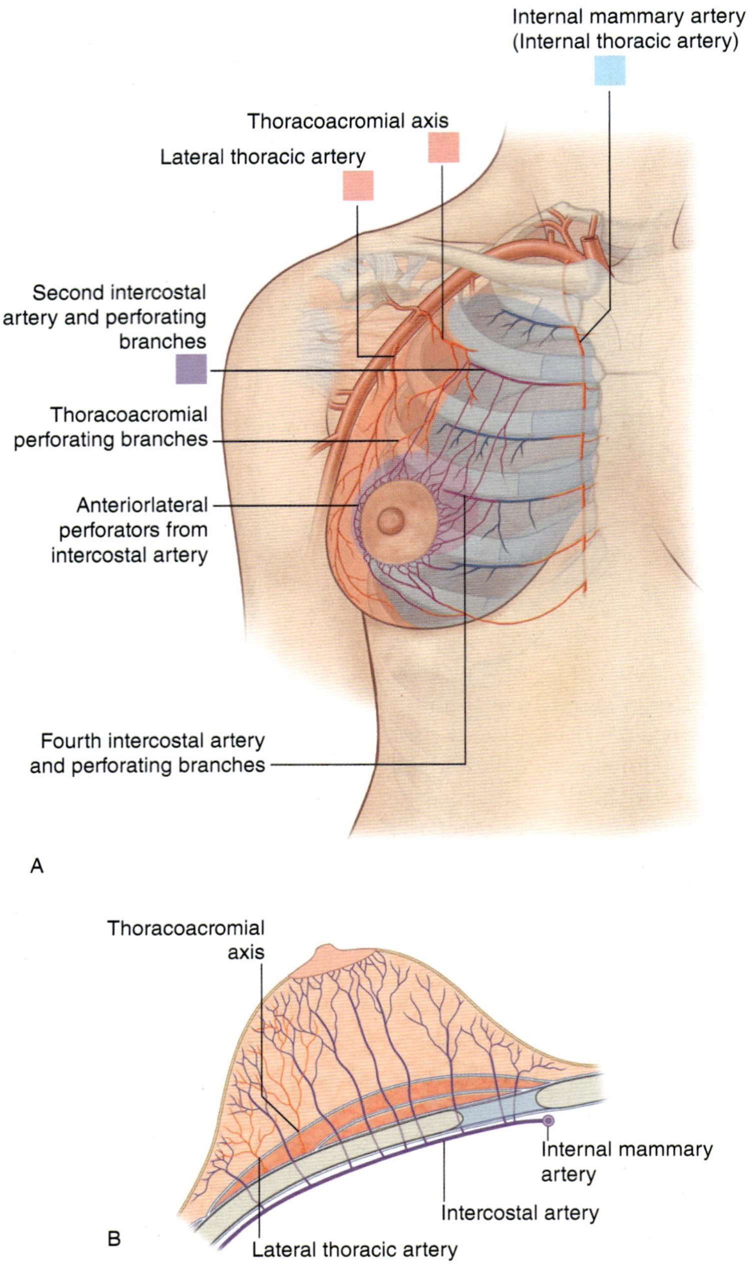

66 PART 3 **Breast Cancer Treatment in the Community**

• **Fig. 7.17** (A and B) Vascular anatomy of the breast. (From Hartmann EC, Spring MA, Stevens WG. One- and two-stage considerations for augmentation mastopexy. In: *Plastic Surgery,* Vol 5: *Breast.* 7th Ed. Amsterdam: Elsevier; 108-123.e2.)

of close or positive margins requiring additional surgery to help with targeted re-excision.

LEVEL 1 ONCOPLASTIC PROCEDURES

Key Points

• Ellipse
Level 1 oncoplastic surgery is best for smaller to moderate-sized breasts with minimal ptosis and tumors that require resection of less than 20% of the breast tissue.

The simplest and most basic oncoplastic incision is the ellipse or parallelogram, in which two parallel incisions of equal length are joined at each end in a tight "V". It can be used to access a tumor in any location of the breast. Incisions can be placed along the anterior axillary line or inframammary crease to allow for a hidden scar. If the tumor is not accessible through these locations, a radially placed incision with judicious skin removal is best to avoid displacement of the nipple areolar complex. With this approach, often a contralateral procedure for symmetry can be avoided as the nipple remains in place. A radial ellipse can remove skin overlying the tumor, increasing the likelihood of a clear

CHAPTER 7 Contemporary Surgical Approaches to Breast Cancer 67

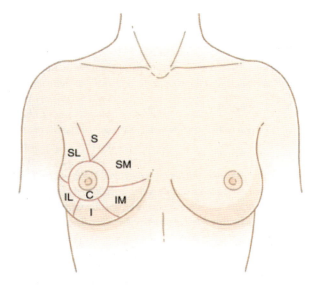

• **Fig. 7.18** Vascular Pedicles of the Breast. *C*: Central; *I*: inferior; *IL*: inferior lateral; *IM*: inferior medial; *S*: superior; *SL*: superior lateral; *SM*: superior medial. (From Venturi M. Reduction mammaplasty techniques for oncoplastic surgery. In: *Oncoplastic Surgery of the Breast*. Amsterdam: Elsevier; 8, 50-56.)

anterior margin. As with all oncoplastic procedures, taking skin does decrease the size of the skin envelope of the breast, allowing for a better postoperative contour and minimal seroma assuming the lumpectomy cavity is appropriately repaired.

UPPER POLE

Key Points

- Crescent mastopexy
- Batwing and hemi-batwing mastopexy
- Circumareolar (donut) mastopexy

Basic oncoplastic approaches to breast tumors located in the upper poles include crescent, batwing or hemi-batwing excisions, in addition to the approaches described later that allow access to any quadrant of the breast (Fig. 7.19). The upper pole includes tumors located between 8:00 and 4:00 going clockwise.

Crescent Mastopexy

A crescent mastopexy allows excision of a tumor from the upper pole while lifting the nipple-areolar complex (Fig. 7.20). It is best for breasts with minimal, grade 1, ptosis that requires minimal reshaping. This approach does lift the nipple-areolar complex, so it is best accompanied by a contralateral mastopexy for symmetry or can be used to correct baseline breast asymmetry.

(Hemi)Batwing Mastopexy

The batwing and hemi-batwing mastopexy combine the radial ellipse with the crescent mastopexy (Fig. 7.21). It achieves dual goals of lifting the nipple-areolar complex while also excising a medial and/or lateral segment of the breast. It is still best for breasts with mild-to-moderate grade 1–2 ptosis. While the incisions and scars are not hidden, it does carry less risk of wound-healing complications compared with some of the more complex level 2 oncoplastic approaches. This approach can easily be performed under local anesthesia with or without sedation. It is therefore quite useful in higher risk patients, patients who prefer to avoid general anesthesia, or those who prefer a shorter, simpler breast-conserving operation but still require resection of significant breast volume that would otherwise leave a postoperative contour deformity.

Circumareolar (Donut) Mastopexy

A circumareolar or donut mastopexy allows excision of a tumor from any location in the breast (Fig. 7.22). With this approach, the nipple-areolar complex is typically left in place but the skin envelope of the breast is reduced, allowing for a more rounded aesthetic outcome and a lifted appearance to the breast. In this approach, an incision is made around the areolar border and a second circular incision is made no more than 2 cm outside of the first. The skin between the two incisions is de-epithelialized, and the tumor is accessed by deepening the incision into the breast parenchyma in the quadrant of the tumor. Ideally, the deep incision is no more than 50% of the outer incision to preserve blood supply to the nipple-areolar complex. The defect is closed similar to the other oncoplastic procedures with a combination of undermining and advancement of the adjacent tissues. The incisions are then closed by approximating the two circumareolar incisions with permanent suture to avoid stretching of the nipple areaolar complex (Fig. 7.22).

Lower Pole

Basic oncoplastic approaches to breast tumors located in the lower poles include the triangle and inframammary excisions, in addition to the radial ellipse, donut mastopexy, and level 2 approaches described later that allow access to any quadrant of the breast. The lower pole includes tumors located between 3:00 and 9:00 going clockwise (Fig. 7.23).

This approach removes an isosceles triangular-shaped wedge of tissue from the lower breast hemisphere. It is ideal for patients with tumors in the 5:00, 6:00, or 7:00 position who do not want the nipple-areola complex elevated as it would be with a standard reduction. It leaves a cosmetic inverted T-shaped scar at the inframammary crease and 6:00. Closure is accomplished by extending the inframammary incision toward the medial and lateral edges of the

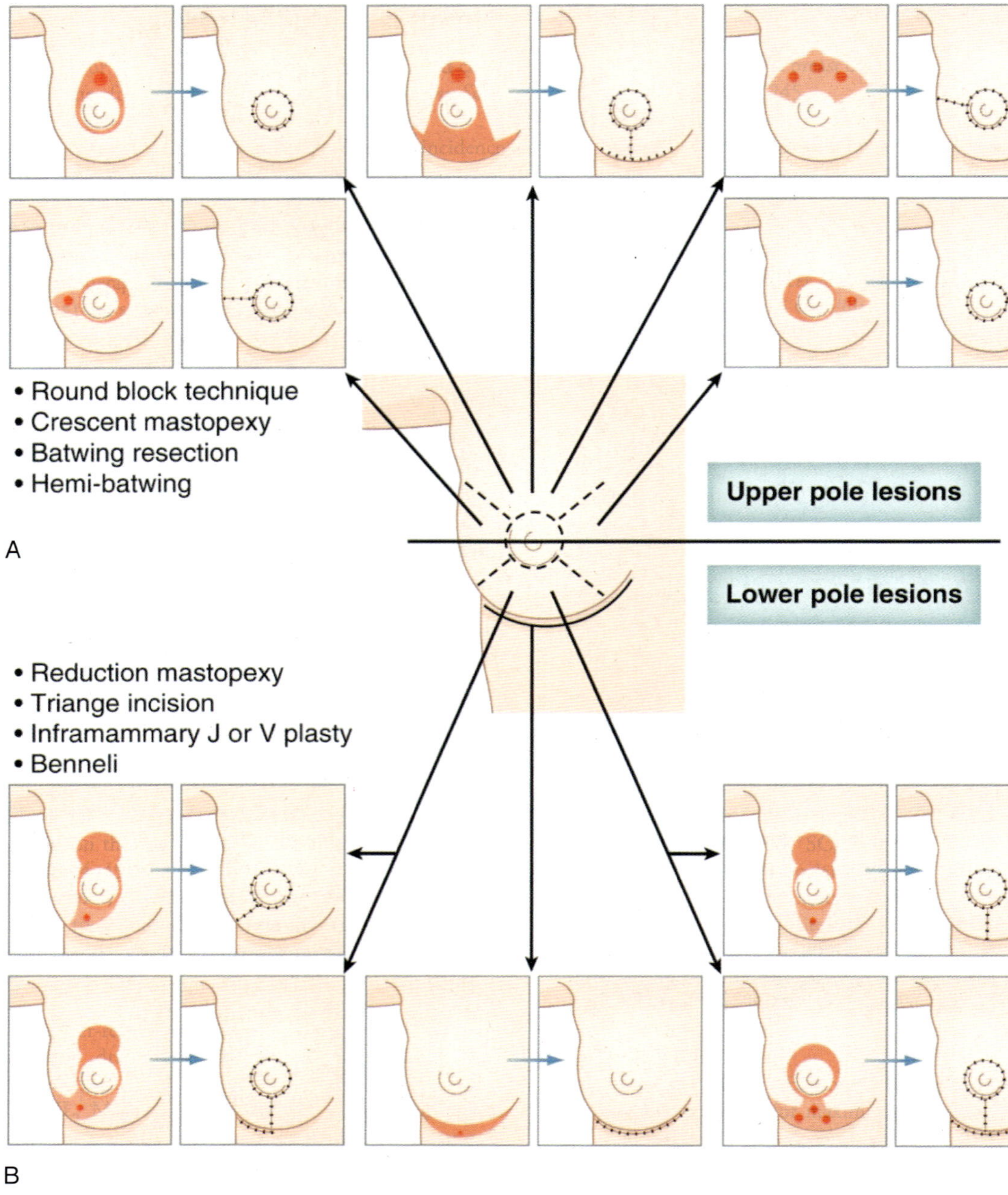

• **Fig. 7.19** Oncoplastic Incisions by Tumor Location. (Adapted from Fitoussi A, Berry MG, Couturaud B, et al. *Oncoplastic and reconstructive surgery for breast cancer: The Institut Curie Experience*. Paris: Springer; 2009. https://doi.org/10.1007/978-3-642-00144-4.)

breast to mobilize dermoglandular flaps towards the center of the breast and re-approximate in layers (Fig. 7.24).

This excision accesses the breast through a crescent incision using the inframammary crease as the superior portion, and the inferior portion of the crescent is 1 cm inferior to this. The horizontal incision length can utilize the majority of the inframammary crease, usually 12 cm or larger, depending on breast size. Only a partial-thickness incision to the dermis is made for the central 6 cm to preserve vascular supply to the dermal parenchymal flap. Skin within the incision is de-epithelialized for advancement to fill the lumpectomy defect. The breast is accessed by deepening the superior portion of the de-epithelialized skin, about 2 mm from the edge of the incision. Once the partial mastectomy is complete, the medial and lateral portions of the de-epithelialized inframammary breast/abdominal tissue are incised down to and mobilized off the underlying chest wall musculature, including the fascia, leaving the central 6 cm attached to the dermis and fascia to maintain vascular supply. The mobilized de-epithelized dermis is transposed into the lumpectomy defect and sutured into place (Fig. 7.25).

CHAPTER 7 Contemporary Surgical Approaches to Breast Cancer 69

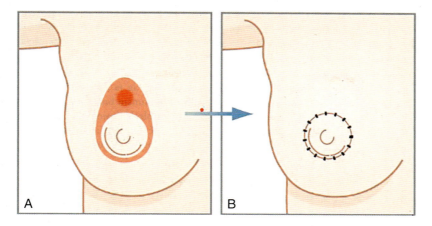

• **Fig. 7.20** Crescent Mastopexy. (Adapted from Fitoussi A, Berry MG, Couturaud B, et al. *Oncoplastic and reconstructive surgery for breast cancer: The Institut Curie Experience*. Paris: Springer; 2008.)

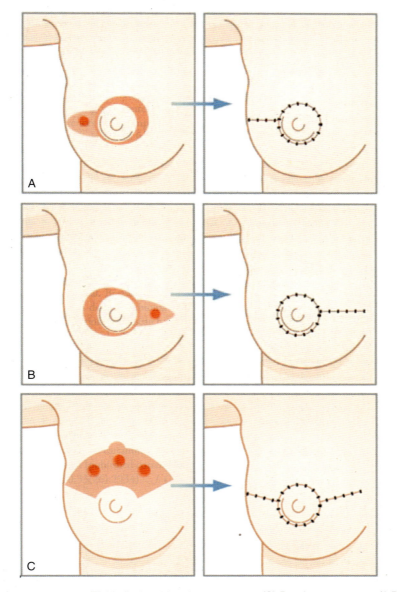

• **Fig. 7.21** (A) Lateral hemi-batwing mastopexy. (B) Medial hemi-batwing mastopexy (C) Batwing mastopexy. (A,B,C, Adapted from Fitoussi A, Berry MG, Couturaud B, et al. *Oncoplastic and reconstructive surgery for breast cancer: The Institut Curie Experience*. Paris: Springer; 2009. https://doi.org/10.1007/978-3-642-00144-4.)

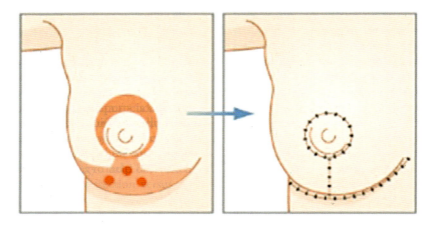

• **Fig. 7.22** Circumareolar (Donut/Benelli/Round Block) Mastopexy. Illustration of a local tissue rearrangement performed after an upper lumpectomy without neoadjuvant chemotherapy resection and reconstruction with local glandular flaps and round block technique. (A) Preoperative design with incision located on the upper quadrant of the left breast and including the total periareolar area. (B) Breast defect after the upper lumpectomy. (C) Glandular flap advancement and final result (D) following primary closure through round block technique. (From Mendonça Munhoz A. Partial breast reconstruction with local tissue rearrangements. In: *Atlas of Reconstructive Breast Surgery.* Amsterdam: Elsevier. 16, 189-203; Yang JD, Lee JW, Cho YK, et al. Surgical techniques for personalized oncoplastic surgery in breast cancer patients with small- to moderate-sized breasts (part 1): volume displacement. *J Breast Cancer.* 2012;15(1):1-6.)

• **Fig. 7.23** Triangle Mastopexy. (Adapted from Fitoussi A, Berry MG, Couturaud B, et al. *Oncoplastic and reconstructive surgery for breast cancer: The Institut Curie Experience*. Paris: Springer; 2009. https://doi.org/10.1007/978-3-642-00144-4.)

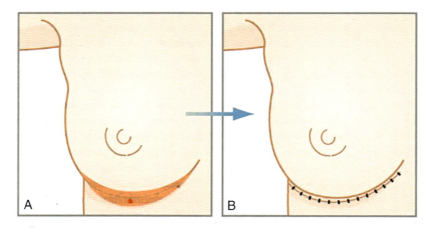

• **Fig. 7.24** Inframammary Excision. The various incisions for tumors located in different parts of the breast. (A) Upper pole lesions can be served by a variety of techniques, including round block, crescent mastopexy, and batwing or hemi-batwing. (B) Lower pole lesions may use techniques that require a mastopexy based on a superior pedicle flap. Including reduction mastopexy, triangle incision, J or V plasty, and Benneli. (Adapted from Fitoussi A, Berry MG, Couturaud B, et al. *Oncoplastic and reconstructive surgery for breast cancer: The Institut Curie Experience*. Paris: Springer; 2009. https://doi.org/10.1007/978-3-642-00144-4.)

CHAPTER 7 Contemporary Surgical Approaches to Breast Cancer

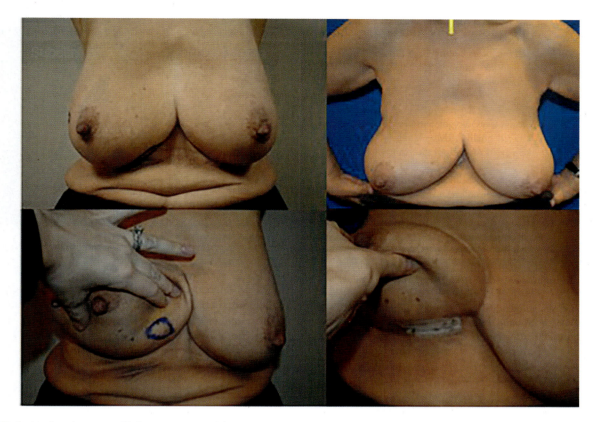

• **Fig. 7.25** A step-by-step case of inframammary excision.

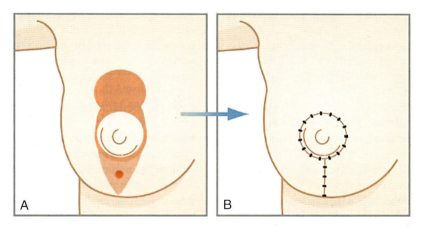

• **Fig. 7.26** Vertical Mastopexy. (Adapted from Fitoussi A, Berry MG, Couturaud B, et al. *Oncoplastic and reconstructive surgery for breast cancer: The Institut Curie Experience.* Paris: Springer; 2009. https://doi.org/10.1007/978-3-642-00144-4.)

Level 2 and Extreme Oncoplastic Procedures

Level 2 oncoplastic surgery is best for moderate- to larger-sized breasts with ptosis and tumors that require resection of 20–50% of the breast tissue. These procedures allow access to any quadrant of the breast for resection of a tumor and can be modified to include skin if the anterior margin approaches skin. The two major level 2 oncoplastic approaches are the vertical mastopexy and the reduction mammoplasty. Both approaches require additional planning for a pedicle that is remote from the tumor and allow for mobilization of the nipple-areolar complex with adequate vascular supply.

Vertical Mastopexy

The vertical mastopexy uses a circumareolar incision with a vertical circular or elliptical extension at 6:00. It is best for smaller to moderate-sized breasts with grade 1 or 2 ptosis (Figs. 7.26–7.28).

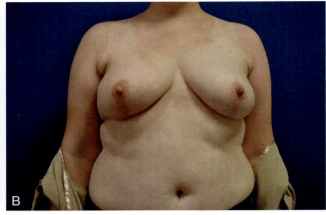

• Fig. 7.27 Before (A) and after (B) radiation photos of vertical mastopexy oncoplastic reconstruction. Post photo is 1 year post completion of adjuvant radiation.

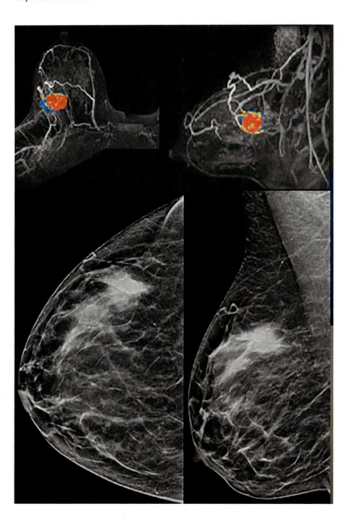

• Fig. 7.28 Preoperative magnetic resonance image and mammogram of the patient in Fig. 7.22.

Wise Pattern Reduction Mammoplasty

The wise pattern reduction mammoplasty is the workhorse of oncoplastic surgery. It can access any quadrant of the breast and be used for moderate- to large-sized breasts, including those with macromastia and grade 3 ptosis. Depending on nipple distance from sternal notch and tumor location, a free nipple graft is sometimes necessary with this approach (Figs. 7.29–7.32).

Split Wise Pattern Reduction Mammoplasty

For more complex cases requiring upper pole skin for an anterior margin, the traditional wise pattern can be split to allow for this, still achieving optimal oncologic and cosmetic results.[105] These approaches, termed extreme oncoplasty, have allowed for breast conservation in patients that would traditionally have required a mastectomy to achieve negative margins (Figs. 7.33 and 7.34).

Conclusion

Oncoplastic breast-conservation surgery incorporates an oncologic partial mastectomy with repair of the defect using volume-displacement or volume-replacement techniques with or without contralateral symmetry surgery as appropriate. These procedures vary in complexity and can be performed by any general or breast surgeon with or without a plastic surgeon. It is cost effective and results in superior aesthetic and psychosocial outcomes regardless of index tumor location. An oncoplastic approach should be considered for most patients who are otherwise candidates for breast conservation.

BREAST RECONSTRUCTION

Key Points

- Breast reconstruction after mastectomy is a preference-sensitive condition and surgeons should embrace a shared decision-making model.
- Foregoing breast reconstruction, or "going flat," should be discussed.

CHAPTER 7 Contemporary Surgical Approaches to Breast Cancer

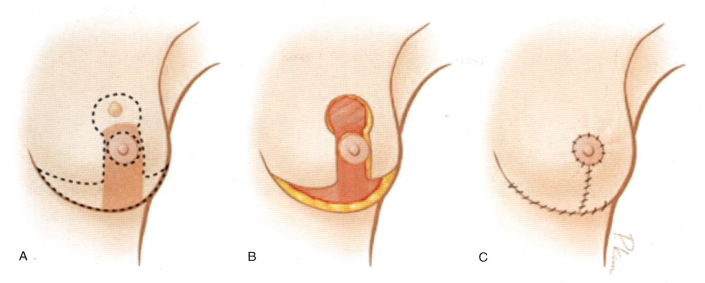

• **Fig. 7.29** Wise Pattern with Inferior Pedicle for Upper Pole Tumor. Illustration of a local tissue rearrangement performed with local glandular flaps. (A) Preoperative design with parallelogram incision located on the upper-lateral quadrant of the left breast. (B) Breast defect after the upper-lateral lumpectomy. (C) Glandular flaps advancement and final result following primary closure. (Adapted from Yang JD, et al. Surgical techniques for personalized oncoplastic surgery in breast cancer patients with small- to moderate-sized breasts (part 1): volume displacement. *J Breast Cancer*. 2012;15(1):1–6.)

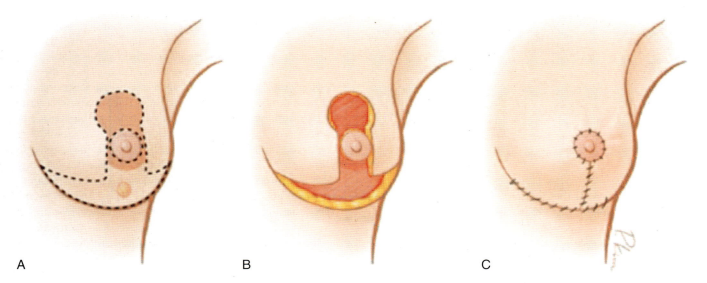

• **Fig. 7.30** Wise Pattern with Superior Pedicle for Lower Pole Tumor. Illustration of a local tissue rearrangement performed with local glandular flaps. (A) Preoperative design with parallelogram incision located on the upper-lateral quadrant of the left breast. (B) Breast defect after the upper-lateral lumpectomy. (C) Glandular flaps advancement and final result following primary closure. (Adapted from Yang JD, et al. Surgical techniques for personalized oncoplastic surgery in breast cancer patients with small- to moderate-sized breasts (part 1): volume displacement. *J Breast Cancer*. 2012;15(1):1–6.)

- Postmastectomy reconstruction can be classified by timing (immediate vs. delayed) and method (implant- and tissue-based).

Introduction

After completing this chapter, the reader should be able to describe various options for reconstruction following mastectomy.

Breast reconstruction following mastectomy is a federally mandated benefit. However while breast reconstruction is a vitally important aspect in the rehabilitation process for most breast cancer patients, the option of foregoing reconstruction should always be presented. Breast reconstruction can either be achieved through the use of implants (e.g., alloplastic reconstruction) or by the use of one's own tissues (e.g., autogenous reconstruction); hybrid techniques that combine both are also described. Despite

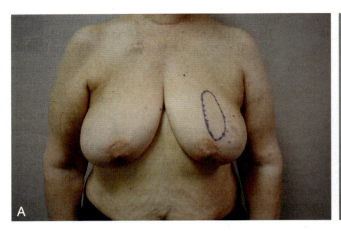 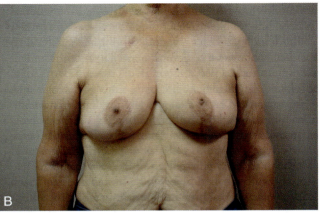

- **Fig. 7.31** (A) Before and (B) after radiation photos of vertical mastopexy oncoplastic reconstruction. The post photo is 1 year post completion of adjuvant radiation.

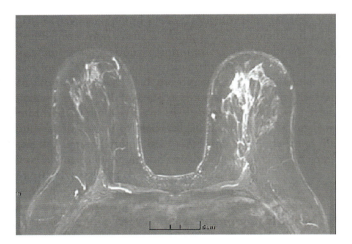

- **Fig. 7.32** Preoperative magnetic resonance image of the patient in Fig. 7.32.

the method chosen, the goal remains the same: to create symmetric breast mounds that look normal in clothing.

Patient Selection

Breast reconstruction is a preference-sensitive treatment. As such counseling should be patient-centered, with priority given to the patient's goals and values. Several important patient- and diagnosis-specific factors should be considered (Table 7.1).

A thorough history and physical examination are requisite, and the surgeon should strive to understand the patient's expectations while reviewing and recommending reconstructive options.[232]

Implant-Based Reconstruction, Technical Aspects

The patient should be marked preoperatively. Important landmarks include the midline, breast meridian, inferior mammary fold, and upper and lateral boundaries of the breast footprint. The incision plan should be developed collaboratively with the oncologic surgeon to allow for adequate and safe ablation of the malignancy while also preserving perfusion of the mastectomy skin flaps and cosmesis. Incision choices for nipple-sparing mastectomy include periareolar, with various extensions, and inferior mammary fold (Fig. 7.35).

In the immediate setting, a tissue expander is placed in the breast pocket at the time of the mastectomy, either in the retropectoral, prepectoral, or hybrid plane (Table 7.2). Regardless of where the tissue expander is placed, the goal remains the same: to re-establish the breast footprint and create symmetry. This tissue expander is inflated over a series of clinic appointments until the desired size and symmetry is achieved. In a second operation, the tissue expander is removed and a breast implant, typically silicone, is placed, with or without adjunct procedures, such as fat grafting. The breast implant constitutes the definitive reconstruction. In a certain subset of patients, it may be possible to forego the tissue-expansion phase and place a breast implant at the time of mastectomy, so called direct-to-implant breast reconstruction. However patients should still be counseled that direct-to-implant reconstruction should be considered a multistep process and revisions are common.

Complications

In addition to conventional surgical risk, counseling should also entail specific prosthetic-related complications. Infection/exposure is perhaps the most common early complication. Salvage may be attempted with hospital admission, aggressive aspiration of fluid if present, and intravenous antibiotics, operative exploration, and explanation of the cause is considered definitive management. Late complications include asymmetry, wrinkling/rippling, rupture, and capsular contracture (Table 7.3 and Fig. 7.36).[232,233]

The use of textured devices has been associated with the development of breast implant-associated anaplastic large-cell

CHAPTER 7 Contemporary Surgical Approaches to Breast Cancer   75

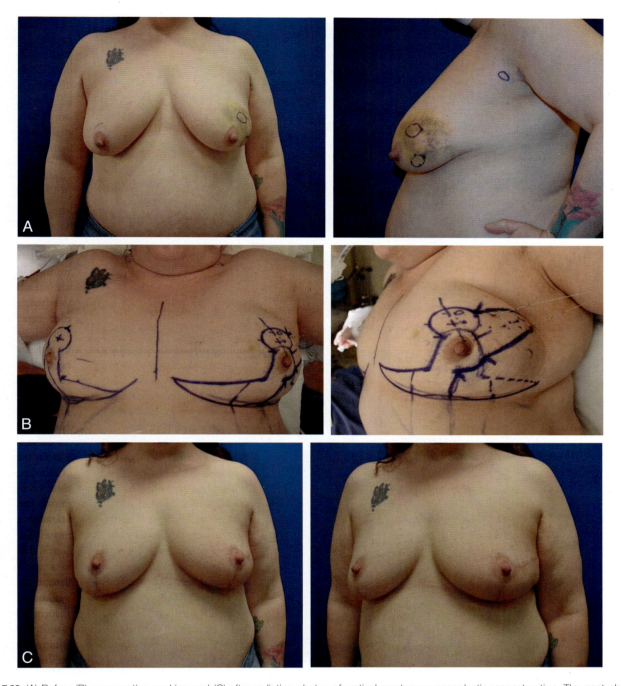

• **Fig. 7.33** (A) Before (B) preoperative marking and (C) after radiation photos of vertical mastopexy oncoplastic reconstruction. The post photo is 4 months post completion of adjuvant radiation.

lymphoma. There is also recent evidence of aggressive squamous cell cancers developing around breast implants. A complete review of this entity is beyond the scope of this chapter; readers may be directed to breastcancer.org for more information.

Tissue-Based Reconstruction

Patient Selection

Tissue-based reconstruction, or autogenous reconstruction, utilizes tissue from a remote area of the body to recreate a breast mound.[234–236] Most women are candidates for either alloplastic or autogenous reconstruction. It is vitally important to present all options to the patient and find the one that is most congruent with their preferences, goals, and values. The breast cancer treatment plan, including the possibility of adjuvant chemotherapy, postmastectomy radiation treatment, and contralateral prophylactic mastectomy should be reviewed.[232] Once these factors are determined, possible donor tissue locations are considered (Table 7.4).

Abdominally based tissue is by far the most common donor site for microvascular breast reconstruction today.

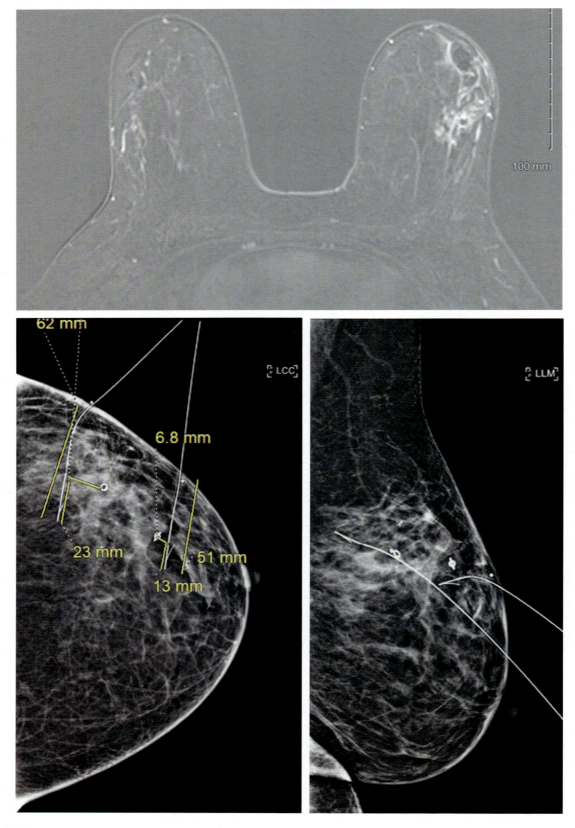

• Fig. 7.34 (A) Preoperative magnetic resonance image and (B) mammogram of the patient in Fig. 7.33.

CHAPTER 7 Contemporary Surgical Approaches to Breast Cancer

TABLE 7.1	Factors to Consider when Evaluating Patients for Breast Reconstruction
Diagnosis-Specific Factors	**Patient Factors**
Neoadjuvant chemotherapy	Age
Postmastectomy radiation	BMI
Skin involvement	Smoking status
Mastectomy type (nipple-sparing vs. skin-sparing)	Cup size
Unilateral vs. bilaterality	Previous operations

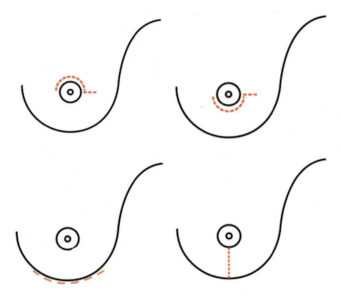

• Fig. 7.35 Nipple Delay Incision Pattern. *Top left:* supra-areolar; *top right:* infra-areolar; *bottom left:* inframammary fold; *bottom right:* vertical. (From Miles OJ, Wiffen JL, Grinsell DG. Nipple delay prior to nipple-sparing mastectomy: the protective effect on nipple-areola complex ischaemia. *J Plastic Reconstr Aesthet Surg.* 2022:75(7);2229–2235.)

TABLE 7.2	Technical Considerations in Alloplastic Breast Reconstruction
Implant location	Retropectoral vs. prepectoral
Use of scaffold	Bioresorbable vs. acellular dermal matrix
Implant size	Volume, projection
Implant type	Silicone vs. saline; textured vs. smooth

TABLE 7.3	Baker Classification Capsular Contracture
Stage 1	Soft breast
Stage 2	Firm breast
Stage 3	Deformed breast
Stage 4	Painful breast

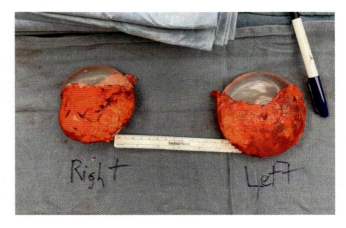

• Fig. 7.36 Example of capsular contracture *(left)* demonstrating a thickened, fibrotic capsule following explantation and capsulectomy.

TABLE 7.4	Tissue-Based Breast Reconstruction Techniques
Abdominally based tissue	e.g., Free TRAM, msfTRAM, DIEP, SIEA
Thigh based	Gracilis, PAP flap
Gluteal based	SGAP, IGAP
Posterior trunk	Latissimus, TDAP

DIEP, Deep inferior epigastric artery perforator; *IGAP,* inferior gluteal artery perforator flap; *msfTRAM,* muscle sparing free-transverse rectus abdominis muscle; *PAP,* profunda artery perforator flap, *SGAP,* superior gluteal artery perforator flap, *SIEA,* superficial inferior epigastric artery; *TDAP,* thoracodorsal artery perforator flap, *TRAM,* transverse rectus abdominis muscle.

The deep inferior epigastric artery perforator flap, or DIEP flap, utilizes only the skin and fat of the lower abdomen, which is both available and expendable in many women (Fig. 7.37).

Technique

The patient is marked in both the standing and beach chair positions. Important abdominal landmarks include the midline, bilateral anterior superior iliac spines, and the umbilicus. In contrast to the transverse rectus abdominis muscle flap, the DIEP flap spares all of the abdominal musculature and fascia, thus preserving core strength (Fig. 7.38).

The operation proceeds in the following sequence:
1. Identification and selection of perforators
2. Subfascial dissection of pedicle
3. Flap harvest
4. Exposure and dissection of recipient vessels
5. Microvascular anastomosis
6. Flap inset
7. Closure of the donor site.

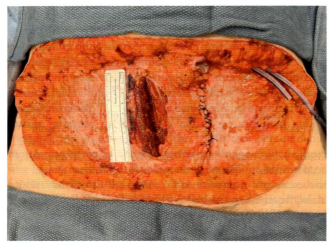

• **Fig. 7.37** Preoperative *(left)* and Postoperative *(right)* photos of bilateral nipple-sparing mastectomy with autologous reconstruction following nipple delay. (From Miles OJ, Wiffen JL, Grinsell DG. Nipple delay prior to nipple-sparing mastectomy: the protective effect on nipple-areola complex ischaemia. *J Plastic Reconstr Aesthet Surg*. 2022;75(7):2229–2235.)

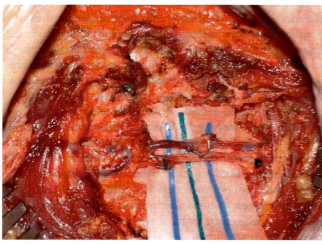

• **Fig. 7.38** *(Top)* Donor site appearance following harvest of bilateral deep inferior epigastric artery perforator flaps. *(Bottom)* Internal mammary recipient vessels dissected and prepared for microvascular anastomosis.

Complications

Complications associated with tissue-based reconstruction include flap loss, fat necrosis, donor site complications (e.g., hernia/bulge, weakness, wound-healing delay), and DVT/PE.[230] Most microvascular complications occur within the first 24–48 hours, thus necessitating an early flap-monitoring protocol. Examples of monitoring technique include clinical examination, Doppler checks, and transcutaneous oximetry. The rates of complications are variable depending on numerous patient and technical factors.

Conclusion

Like most other areas in the multidisciplinary management of breast cancer, surgical treatment continues to evolve. The management of disease on the chest wall has become less radical as we have gained better understanding of the pathophysiology of the disease and of combined modality treatment. Management of the lymphatics have opened new methods for the diagnosis, prevention, and treatment of lymphedema. Newer techniques in oncoplastic procedures and breast reconstruction whether by using implants, tissue transfer or microvascular anastomoses for free tissue flaps have demonstrated excellent cosmetic appearance of the post treatment breast. Continued research in this area will allow further improvement in and refinement of surgical techniques and reconstruction for breast cancer patients.

References

1. Gonzalez E, Grafton WD, Morris DM, Barr LH. Diagnosing breast cancer using frozen sections from Tru-cut needle biopsies. Six-year experience with 162 biopsies, with emphasis on outpatient diagnosis of breast carcinoma. *Ann Surg*. 1985;202(6):696–701.

2. Park VY, Kim EK, Moon HJ, Yoon JH, Kim MJ. Evaluating imaging-pathology concordance and discordance after ultrasound-guided breast biopsy. *Ultrasonography*. 2018;37(2):107–120.

3. Parker SH, Jobe WE, Dennis MA, et al. US-guided automated large-core breast biopsy. *Radiology*. 1993;187(2):507–511.

4. Vandromme MJ, Umphrey H, Krontiras H. Image-guided methods for biopsy of suspicious breast lesions. *J Surg Oncol*. 2011;103(4):299–305.

5. American Society of Breast Surgeons. Consensus guideline on image-guided percutaneous biopsy of palpable and nonpalpable breast lesions. https://www.breastsurgeons.org/docs/statements/Consensus-Guideline-on-Image-Guided-Percutaneous-Biopsy-of-Palpable-and-Nonpalpable-Breast-Lesions.pdf. Accessed September 25, 2023.

6. American Society of Breast Surgeons. Preoperative diagnosis of breast cancer quality measure. https://www.breastsurgeons.org/statements/QM/A SBrS_Preoperative_diagnosis_of_breast_cancer.pdf Accessed September 24, 2021.

7. Wang M, He X, Chang Y, Sun G, Thabane L. A sensitivity and specificity comparison of fine needle aspiration cytology and core needle biopsy in evaluation of suspicious breast lesions: a systematic review and meta-analysis. *Breast*. 2017;31: 157–166.

8. Lukasiewicz E, Ziemiecka A, Jakubowski W, Vojinovic J, Bogucevska M, Dobruch-Sobczak K. Fine-needle versus core-needle biopsy - which one to choose in preoperative assessment of focal lesions in the breasts? Literature review. *J Ultrason*. 2017;17(71):267–274.

9. Mahoney MC, Newell MS. Breast intervention: how I do it. *Radiology*. 2013;268(1):12–24.

10. Bahl M, Maunglay M, D'Alessandro HA, Lehman CD. Comparison of upright digital breast tomosynthesis-guided versus prone stereotactic vacuum-assisted breast biopsy. *Radiology*. 2019;290(2):298–304.

11. Bae S, Yoon JH, Moon HJ, Kim MJ, Kim EK. Breast microcalcifications: diagnostic outcomes according to image-guided biopsy method. *Korean J Radiol*. 2015;16(5):996–1005.

12. Gao P, Kong X, Song Y, et al. Recent progress for the techniques of MRI-guided breast interventions and their applications on surgical strategy. *J Cancer*. 2020;11(16):4671–4682. Published 2020 May 20.

13. Fisher B, Redmond C, Fisher ER. The contribution of recent NSABP clinical trials of primary breast cancer therapy to an understanding of tumor biology--an overview of findings. *Cancer*. 1980;46(4 Suppl):1009–1025.

14. Wickerham DL, O'Connell MJ, Costantino JP, et al. The half century of clinical trials of the National Surgical Adjuvant Breast And Bowel Project. *Semin Oncol*. 2008;35(5):522–529.

15. Fisher B, Montague E, Redmond C, et al. Comparison of radical mastectomy with alternative treatments for primary breast cancer. A first report of results from a prospective randomized clinical trial. *Cancer*. 1977;39(6 Suppl):2827–2839.

16. Fisher B, Redmond C, Fisher ER, et al. Ten-year results of a randomized clinical trial comparing radical mastectomy and total mastectomy with or without radiation. *N Engl J Med*. 1985;312(11):674–681.

17. Fisher B, Bauer M, Margolese R, et al. Five-year results of a randomized clinical trial comparing total mastectomy and segmental mastectomy with or without radiation in the treatment of breast cancer. *N Engl J Med*. 1985;312:665–673.

18. Fisher B, Redmond C, Poisson R, et al. Eight-year results of a randomized clinical trial comparing total mastectomy and lumpectomy with or without irradiation in the treatment of breast cancer. *N Engl J Med*. 1989;320:822–828.

19. Fisher B, Anderson S, Redmond CK, et al. Reanalysis and results after 12 years of follow-up in a randomized clinical trial comparing total mastectomy with lumpectomy with or without irradiation in the treatment of breast cancer. *N Engl J Med*. 1995;333:1456–1461.

20. Fisher B, Jeong JH, Anderson S, Bryant J, Fisher ER, Wolmark N. Twenty-five-year follow-up of a randomized trial comparing radical mastectomy, total mastectomy, and total mastectomy followed by irradiation. *N Engl J Med*. 2002;347(8):567–575.

21. Fisher B, Anderson S, Bryant J, et al. Twenty-year follow-up of a randomized trial comparing total mastectomy, lumpectomy, and lumpectomy plus irradiation for the treatment of invasive breast cancer. *N Engl J Med*. 2002;347:1233–1241.

22. Krag DN, Anderson SJ, Julian TB, et al. Sentinel-lymph-node resection compared with conventional axillary-lymph-node dissection in clinically node-negative patients with breast cancer: overall survival findings from the NSABP B-32 randomised phase 3 trial. *Lancet Oncol*. 2010;11:927–933.

23. Giuliano AE, McCall L, Beitsch P, et al. Locoregional recurrence after sentinel lymph node dissection with or without axillary dissection in patients with sentinel lymph node metastases: the American College of Surgeons Oncology Group Z0011 randomized trial. *Ann Surg*. 2010;252:426–432.

24. Giuliano AE, Hunt KK, Ballman KV, et al. Axillary dissection vs no axillary dissection in women with invasive breast cancer and sentinel node metastasis: a randomized clinical trial. *JAMA*. 2011;305:569–575.

25. Giuliano AE, Ballman K, McCall L, et al. Locoregional recurrence after sentinel lymph node dissection with or without axillary dissection in patients with sentinel lymph node metastases: long-term follow-up from the·American College of Surgeons Oncology Group (Alliance) ACOSOG Z0011 randomized trial. *Ann Surg*. 2016;264(3):413–420.

26. Giuliano AE, Ballman KV, McCall L, et al. Effect of axillary dissection vs no axillary dissection on 10-year overall survival among women with invasive breast cancer and sentinel node metastasis: the ACOSOG Z0011 (Alliance) randomized clinical trial. *JAMA*. 2017;318(10):918–926.

27. Galimberti VCB, Zurrida S, Viale G, et al. International Breast Cancer Study Group Trial 23- 01 Investigators. Update of International Breast Cancer Study Group Trial 23-01 to compare axillary dissection versus no axillary dissection in patients with clinically node negative breast cancer and micrometastases in the sentinel node. *Cancer Res*. 2011;71:102s.

28. Galimberti V, Cole BF, Viale G, et al. Axillary dissection versus no axillary dissection in patients with breast cancer and sentinel-node micrometastases (IBCSG 23-01): 10-year follow-up of a randomised, controlled phase 3 trial. *Lancet Oncol*. 2018;19(10):1385–1393.

29. Donker M, van Tienhoven G, Straver ME, et al. Radiotherapy or surgery of the axilla after a positive sentinel node in breast cancer (EORTC 10981-22023 AMAROS): a randomised, multicentre, open-label, phase 3 non-inferiority trial. *Lancet Oncol*. 2014;15(12):1303–1310.

30. American Society of Breast Surgeons Consensus Guidelines: Performance and Practice Guidelines for Sentinel Lymph Node Biopsy in Breast Cancer Patients. https://www.breastsurgeons.org/docs/statements/Performance-and-Practice-Guidelines-for-Sentinel-Lymph-Node-Biopsy-in-Breast-Cancer-Patients.pdf Accessed 10/3/2021

31. National Comprehensive Cancer Network Guidelines (NCCN). nccn.org.

32. Tseng J, Alban RF, Siegel E, Chung A, Giuliano AE, Amersi FF. Changes in utilization of axillary dissection in women with invasive breast cancer and sentinel node metastasis after the ACOSOG Z0011 trial. *Breast J.* 2021;27(3):216–221.

33. Howard DH, Soulos PR, Chagpar AB, Mougalian S, Killelea B, Gross CP. contrary to conventional wisdom, physicians abandoned a breast cancer treatment after a trial concluded it was ineffective. *Health Aff (Millwood).* 2016;35(7):1309–1315.

34. Jeffries DO, Dossett LA, Jorns JM. Localization for breast surgery: the next generation. *Arch Pathol Lab Med.* 2017;141(10):1324–1329.

35. SCOUT Report: News and Views on Surgical Guidance and Breast Tumor Localization: https://www.merit.com/wp-content/uploads/2020/09/201609-SCOUTReport-ExtendedFlexibilityReflectorPlacementSupportsImprovedPatientAndHospitalScheduling.pdf. Accessed 10/3/2021.

36. Endomagnetics Inc. Magseed. 2016: https://www.endomag.com/indications-for-use/ Accessed 10/3/2021.

37. Food and Drug Administration. Hologic. https://www.accessdata.fda.gov/cdrh_docs/pdf18/K181692.pdf, Accessed 7/10/2023.

38. Srour MK, Kim S, Amersi F, Giuliano AE, Chung A. Comparison of wire localization, radioactive seed, and Savi scout® radar for management of surgical breast disease. *Breast J.* 2020;26(3):406–413.

39. Srour MK, Kim S, Amersi F, Giuliano AE, Chung A. Comparison of multiple wire, radioactive seed, and Savi Scout® radar localizations for management of surgical breast disease. *Ann Surg Oncol.* 2021;28(4):2212–2218.

40. Chagpar AB, Killelea BK, Tsangaris TN, et al. A randomized, controlled trial of cavity shave margins in breast cancer. *N Engl J Med.* 2015 Aug 6;373(6):503–510.

41. Dupont E, Tsangaris T, Garcia-Cantu C, et al. Resection of cavity shave margins in stage 0-III breast cancer patients undergoing breast conserving surgery: a prospective multicenter randomized controlled trial. *Ann Surg.* 2021 May 1;273(5):876–881.

42. Abdelsattar JM, Afridi FG, Dai Z, et al. The effect of lumpectomy and cavity shave margin status on recurrence and survival in breast-conserving surgery. *Am Surg.* 2023;89(3):424–443.

43. Morrow M, Van Zee KJ, Solin LJ, et al. Society of Surgical Oncology-American Society for Radiation Oncology-American Society of Clinical Oncology Consensus Guideline on margins for breast-conserving surgery with whole-breast irradiation in ductal carcinoma in situ. *J Clin Oncol.* 2016;34(33):4040–4046.

44. Moran MS, Schnitt SJ, Giuliano AE, et al. Society of Surgical Oncology-American Society for Radiation Oncology consensus guideline on margins for breast-conserving surgery with whole-breast irradiation in stages I and II invasive breast cancer. *Int J Radiat Oncol Biol Phys.* 2014;88(3):553–564.

45. BIN V-J. Accessed 10/5/2021 (male breast cancer)

46. Baker JL, Dizon DS, Wenziger CM, et al. "Going flat" after mastectomy: patient-reported outcomes by online survey. *Ann Surg Oncol.* 2021;28(5):2493–2505.

47. Balci FL, Kara H, Dulgeroglu O, Uras C. Oncologic safety of nipple-sparing mastectomy in patients with short tumor-nipple distance. *Breast J.* 2019;25(4):612–618.

48. Jensen JA, Lin JH, Kapoor N, Giuliano AE. Surgical delay of the nipple-areolar complex: a powerful technique to maximize nipple viability following nipple-sparing mastectomy. *Ann Surg Oncol.* 2012;19(10):3171–3176.

49. Giannotti DG, Hanna SA, Cerri GG, Barbosa Bevilacqua JL. analysis of skin flap thickness and residual breast tissue after mastectomy. *Int J Radiat Oncol Biol Phys.* 2018;102(1):82–91.

50. Jogerst K, Thomas O, Kosiorek HE, et al. Same-day discharge after mastectomy: breast cancer surgery in the era of ERAS®. *Ann Surg Oncol.* 2020;27(9):3436–3445.

51. Morton DL, Wen DR, Wong JH, et al. Technical details of intraoperative lymphatic mapping for early stage melanoma. *Arch Surg.* 1992;127(4):392–399.

52. Giuliano AE, Kirgan DM, Guenther JM, Morton DL. Lymphatic mapping and sentinel lymphadenectomy for breast cancer. *Ann Surg.* 1994 Sep;220(3):391–398. discussion 398-401.

53. Society of Surgical Oncology: Five Things Physicians and Patients Should Question (Updated 2021): https://www.choosingwisely.org/societies/society-of-surgical-oncology/ Accessed 10/3/2021

54. Jakub JW, Murphy BL, Gonzalez AB, et al. A validated nomogram to predict upstaging of ductal carcinoma in situ to invasive disease. *Ann Surg Oncol.* 2017;24(10):2915–2924.

55. Thompson JF, Niewind P, Uren RF, Bosch CM, Howman-Giles R, Vrouenraets BC. Single-dose isotope injection for both preoperative lymphoscintigraphy and intraoperative sentinel lymph node identification in melanoma patients. *Melanoma Res.* 1997 Dec;7(6):500–506.

56. BINV-D. Accessed 10/2/2021 (axillary staging)

57. Vitug AF, Newman LA. Complications in breast surgery. *Surg Clin North Am.* 2007;87(2):431-x.

58. Boughey JC, Suman VJ, Mittendorf EA, et al. Sentinel lymph node surgery after neoadjuvant chemotherapy in patients with node-positive breast cancer: the ACOSOG Z1071 (Alliance) clinical trial. *JAMA.* 2013;310(14):1455–1461.

59. American Society of Breast Surgeons. Position Statement on Management of the Axilla In Patients with Invasive Breast Cancer. 2019 www.breastsurgeons.org. Accessed 10/2/2021.

60. Caudle AS, Yang WT, Krishnamurthy S, et al. Improved axillary evaluation following neoadjuvant therapy for patients with node-positive breast cancer using selective evaluation of clipped nodes: implementation of targeted axillary dissection. *J Clin Oncol.* 2016;34(10):1072–1078.

61. NSABP B-51. Standard or comprehensive radiation therapy in treating patients with early-stage breast cancer previously treated with chemotherapy and surgery. clinicaltrials.gov Accessed 10/2/2021

62. Moo TA, Edelweiss M, Hajiyeva S, et al. is low-volume disease in the sentinel node after neoadjuvant chemotherapy an indication for axillary dissection? [published correction appears in *Ann Surg Oncol.* 2020 Dec;27(Suppl 3):966]. *Ann Surg Oncol.* 2018;25(6):1488–1494.

63. Alliance for Clinical Trials in Oncology. Comparison of axillary lymph node dissection with axillary radiation for patients with node-positive breast cancer treated with chemotherapy. clinicaltrials.gov Accessed 10/2/2021

64. Samiei S, van Nijnatten TJA, de Munck L, et al. Correlation between pathologic complete response in the breast and absence of axillary lymph node metastases after neoadjuvant systemic therapy. *Ann Surg.* 2020;271(3):574–580.

65. Tadros AB, Yang WT, Krishnamurthy S, et al. Identification of patients with documented pathologic complete response in the breast after neoadjuvant chemotherapy for omission of axillary surgery [published correction appears in *JAMA Surg.* 2017 Jul 1;152(7):708]. *JAMA Surg.* 2017;152(7):665–670.

66. van la Parra RF, Kuerer HM. Selective elimination of breast cancer surgery in exceptional responders: historical perspective and current trials. *Breast Cancer Res.* 2016;18(1):28 Published 2016 Mar 8.

67. Clinical Trials. Eliminating surgery or radiotherapy after systemic therapy in treating patients with HER2 positive or triple negative breast cancer. https://clinicaltrials.gov/ct2/show/NCT02945579 Accessed 10/3/2021

68. Pasket E, Dean J, Oliveri J, Harrop J. Cancer-related lymphedema risk factors, diagnosis, treatment, and impact. *Journal of Clinical Oncology.* 2012;30(30):3726–3733.

69. Yah-Chen T, Ying Xu J, Cormier S, et al. Incidence, treatment costs, and complications of lymphedema after breast cancer among women of working age: a 2-year follow-up study. *Journal of Clinical Oncology.* 2009;27:2007–2014.

70. Hespe GE NM, Mehrara BJ. *Pathophysiology of lymphedema. Lymphadema Presentation. Diagnosis and Treatment.* Springer; 2015.

71. McLaughlin SA, Wright MJ, Morris KT, et al. Prevalence of lymphedema in women with breast cancer 5 years after sentinel lymph node biopsy or axillary dissection: objective measurements. *J Clin Oncol.* 2008;26(32):5213–5219.

72. Shah C, Arthur D, Riutta J, Whitworth P, Vicini FA. Breast-cancer related lymphedema: a review of procedure-specific incidence rates, clinical assessment AIDS, treatment paradigms, and risk reduction. *Breast J.* 2012;18(4):357–361.

73. Leidenius M, Leivonen M, Vironen J, von Smitten K. The consequences of long-time arm morbidity in node-negative breast cancer patients with sentinel node biopsy or axillary clearance. *J Surg Oncol.* 2005;92(1):23–31.

74. Blanchard DK, Donohue JH, Reynolds C, Grant CS. Relapse and morbidity in patients undergoing sentinel lymph node biopsy alone or with axillary dissection for breast cancer. *Arch Surg.* 2003;138(5):482–487.

75. Ashikaga T, Krag DN, Land SR, et al. Morbidity results from the NSABP B-32 trial comparing sentinel lymph node dissection versus axillary dissection. *J Surg Oncol.* 2010;102(2):111–118.

76. Paskett ED, Dean JA, Oliveri JM, Harrop JP. Cancer-related lymphedema risk factors, diagnosis, treatment, and impact: a review. *J Clin Oncol.* 2012;30(30):3726–3733.

77. Mansel RE, Fallowfield L, Kissin M, et al. Randomized multicenter trial of sentinel node biopsy versus standard axillary treatment in operable breast cancer: the ALMANAC trial. *J Natl Cancer Inst.* 2006;98(9):599–609.

78. Soran A, Ozmen T, McGuire KP, et al. The importance of detection of subclinical lymphedema for the prevention of breast cancer-related clinical lymphedema after axillary lymph node dissection; a prospective observational study. *Lymphat Res Biol.* 2014;12(4):289–294.

79. Laidley A B, Anglin B. The impact of L-Dex((R)) measurements in assessing breast cancer-related lymphedema as part of routine clinical practice. *Front Oncol.* 2016;6:192.

80. Torres Lacomba M, Yuste Sánchez MJ, Zapico Goñi A, et al. Effectiveness of early physiotherapy to prevent lymphoedema after surgery for breast cancer: randomised, single blinded, clinical trial. *BMJ.* 2010;340:b5396.

81. Stout Gergich NL, Pfalzer LA, McGarvey C, Springer B, Gerber LH, Soballe P. Preoperative assessment enables the early diagnosis and successful treatment of lymphedema. *Cancer.* 2008;112(12):2809–2819.

82. Executive C. The diagnosis and treatment of peripheral lymphedema: 2016 consensus document of the International Society of Lymphology. *Lymphology.* 2016;49(4):170–184.

83. Armer JM, Hulett JM, Bernas M, Ostby P, Stewart BR, Cormier JN. Best practice guidelines in assessment, risk reduction, management, and surveillance for post-breast cancer lymphedema. *Curr Breast Cancer Rep.* 2013;5(2):134–144.

84. Ostby PL, Armer JM, Dale PS, Van Loo MJ, Wilbanks CL, Stewart BR. Surveillance recommendations in reducing risk of and optimally managing breast cancer-related lymphedema. *J Pers Med.* 2014;4(3):424–447.

85. Harrington S, Gilchrist L, Sander A. Breast Cancer EDGE Task Force Outcomes: clinical measures of pain. *Rehabil Oncol.* 2014;32(1):13–21.

86. Supplement to the NLN position breast cancer screening: screening and early detection of breast cancer-related lymphedema. 2012.

87. McLaughlin SA, Staley AC, Vicini F, et al. Considerations for clinicians in the diagnosis, prevention, and treatment of breast cancer-related lymphedema: recommendations from a multidisciplinary expert ASBrS panel: Part 1: definitions, assessments, education, and future directions. *Ann Surg Oncol.* 2017;24(10):2818–2826.

88. Armer JM, Stewart BR. Post-breast cancer lymphedema: incidence increases from 12 to 30 to 60 months. *Lymphology.* 2010;43(3):118–127.

89. McLaughlin SA, DeSnyder SM, Klimberg S, et al. Considerations for clinicians in the diagnosis, prevention, and treatment of breast cancer-related lymphedema, recommendations from an expert panel: Part 2: preventive and therapeutic options. *Ann Surg Oncol.* 2017;24(10):2827–2835.

90. Lopez Penha TR, Slangen JJ, Heuts EM, Voogd AC, Von Meyenfeldt MF. Prevalence of lymphoedema more than five years after breast cancer treatment. *Eur J Surg Oncol.* 2011;37(12):1059–1063.

91. National Comprehensive Cancer Network. Breast Cancer. 2016.

92. National lymphedema network. Available from: http://www.nationallymphedemanetwork.org.

93. Tierney S, Aslam M, Rennie K, Grace P. Infrared optoelectronic volumetry, the ideal way to measure limb volume. *Eur J Vasc Endovasc Surg.* 1996;12(4):412–417.

94. Sun F, Hall A, Tighe MP, et al. Perometry versus simulated circumferential tape measurement for the detection of breast cancer-related lymphedema. *Breast Cancer Res Treat.* 2018;172(1):83–91.

95. Sharkey AR, King SW, Kuo RY, Bickerton SB, Ramsden AJ, Furniss D. Measuring limb volume: accuracy and reliability of tape measurement versus perometer measurement. *Lymphat Res Biol.* 2018;16(2):182–186.

96. Sander AP, Hajer NM, Hemenway K, Miller AC. Upper-extremity volume measurements in women with lymphedema: a comparison of measurements obtained via water displacement with geometrically determined volume. *Phys Ther.* 2002;82(12):1201–1212.

97. Cornish BH, Chapman M, Hirst C, et al. Early diagnosis of lymphedema using multiple frequency bioimpedance. *Lymphology.* 2001;34(1):2–11.

98. Bundred NJ, Stockton C, Keeley V, et al. Comparison of multi-frequency bioimpedance with perometry for the early detection and intervention of lymphoedema after axillary node clearance for breast cancer. *Breast Cancer Res Treat.* 2015;151(1):121–129.

99. Fu MR, Cleland CM, Guth AA, et al. L-dex ratio in detecting breast cancer-related lymphedema: reliability, sensitivity, and specificity. *Lymphology*. 2013;46(2):85–96.

100. Gaw R, Box R, Cornish B. Bioimpedance in the assessment of unilateral lymphedema of a limb: the optimal frequency. *Lymphat Res Biol*. 2011;9(2):93–99.

101. Shah C. Bioimpedance spectroscopy in the detection of breast cancer-related lymphedema: an ounce of prevention. *Breast J*. 2019;25(6):1323–1325.

102. Vicini F, Shah C, Lyden M, Whitworth P. Bioelectrical impedance for detecting and monitoring patients for the development of upper limb lymphedema in the clinic. *Clin Breast Cancer*. 2012;12(2):133–137.

103. Whitworth PW, Shah C, Vicini F, Cooper A. Preventing breast cancer-related lymphedema in high-risk patients: the impact of a structured surveillance protocol using bioimpedance spectroscopy. *Front Oncol*. 2018;8:197.

104. Whitworth PW, Cooper A. Reducing chronic breast cancer-related lymphedema utilizing a program of prospective surveillance with bioimpedance spectroscopy. *Breast J*. 2018;24(1):62–65.

105. Bulley C, Gaal S, Coutts F, et al. Comparison of breast cancer-related lymphedema (upper limb swelling) prevalence estimated using objective and subjective criteria and relationship with quality of life. *Biomed Res Int*. 2013;2013:807569.

106. Ridner SH, Dietrich MS. Development and validation of the Lymphedema Symptom and Intensity Survey-Arm. *Support Care Cancer*. 2015;23(10):3103–3112.

107. Bulley C, Coutts F, Blyth C, et al. A morbidity screening tool for identifying fatigue, pain, upper limb dysfunction and lymphedema after breast cancer treatment: a validity study. *Eur J Oncol Nurs*. 2014;18(2):218–227.

108. Fu MR, Axelrod D, Cleland CM, et al. Symptom report in detecting breast cancer-related lymphedema. *Breast Cancer (Dove Med Press)*. 2015;7:345–352.

109. Gartner R, Jensen MB, Kronborg L, Ewertz M, Kehlet H, Kroman N. Self-reported arm-lymphedema and functional impairment after breast cancer treatment--a nationwide study of prevalence and associated factors. *Breast*. 2010;19(6):506–515.

110. DiSipio T, Rye S, Newman B, Hayes S. Incidence of unilateral arm lymphoedema after breast cancer: a systematic review and meta-analysis. *Lancet Oncol*. 2013;14(6):500–515.

111. Tsai RJ, Dennis LK, Lynch CF, Snetselaar LG, Zamba GK, Scott-Conner C. The risk of developing arm lymphedema among breast cancer survivors: a meta-analysis of treatment factors. *Ann Surg Oncol*. 2009;16(7):1959–1972.

112. Asdourian MS, Skolny MN, Brunelle C, Seward CE, Salama L, Taghian AG. Precautions for breast cancer-related lymphoedema: risk from air travel, ipsilateral arm blood pressure measurements, skin puncture, extreme temperatures, and cellulitis. *Lancet Oncol*. 2016;17(9):e392–e405.

113. Ferguson CM, Swaroop MN, Horick N, et al. Impact of ipsilateral blood draws, injections, blood pressure measurements, and air travel on the risk of lymphedema for patients treated for breast cancer. *J Clin Oncol*. 2016;34(7):691–698.

114. McLaughlin SA, Wright MJ, Morris KT, et al. Prevalence of lymphedema in women with breast cancer 5 years after sentinel lymph node biopsy or axillary dissection: patient perceptions and precautionary behaviors. *J Clin Oncol*. 2008;26(32):5220–5226.

115. Shaitelman SF, Chiang YJ, Griffin KD, et al. Radiation therapy targets and the risk of breast cancer-related lymphedema: a systematic review and network meta-analysis. *Breast Cancer Res Treat*. 2017;162(2):201–215.

116. Kilbreath SL, Refshauge KM, Beith JM, et al. Risk factors for lymphoedema in women with breast cancer: a large prospective cohort. *Breast*. 2016;28:29–36.

117. Warren LE, Miller CL, Horick N, et al. The impact of radiation therapy on the risk of lymphedema after treatment for breast cancer: a prospective cohort study. *Int J Radiat Oncol Biol Phys*. 2014;88(3):565–571.

118. Zou L, Liu FH, Shen PP, et al. The incidence and risk factors of related lymphedema for breast cancer survivors post-operation: a 2-year follow-up prospective cohort study. *Breast Cancer*. 2018;25(3):309–314.

119. Norman SA, Localio AR, Kallan MJ, et al. Risk factors for lymphedema after breast cancer treatment. *Cancer Epidemiol Biomarkers Prev*. 2010;19(11):2734–2746.

120. Helyer LK, Varnic M, Le LW, Leong W. Obesity is a risk factor for developing postoperative lymphedema in breast cancer patients. *Breast J*. 2010;16(1):48–54.

121. Specht MC, Miller CL, Russell TA, et al. Defining a threshold for intervention in breast cancer-related lymphedema: what level of arm volume increase predicts progression? *Breast Cancer Res Treat*. 2013;140(3):485–494.

122. Sayegh HE, Asdourian MS, Swaroop MN, et al. Diagnostic methods, risk factors, prevention, and management of breast cancer-related lymphedema: past, present, and future directions. *Curr Breast Cancer Rep*. 2017;9(2):111–121.

123. Showalter SL, Brown JC, Cheville AL, Fisher CS, Sataloff D, Schmitz KH. Lifestyle risk factors associated with arm swelling among women with breast cancer. *Ann Surg Oncol*. 2013;20(3):842–849.

124. McLaughlin SA, Bagaria S, Gibson T, et al. Trends in risk reduction practices for the prevention of lymphedema in the first 12 months after breast cancer surgery. *J Am Coll Surg*. 2013;216(3):380–389. quiz 511-3.

125. Executive Committee. The Diagnosis and Treatment of Peripheral Lymphedema: 2016 Consensus Document of the International Society of Lymphology. *Lymphology*. 2016 Dec;49(4):170–184. PMID: 29908550.

126. Fisher B, Slack NH. Number of lymph nodes examined and the prognosis of breast carcinoma. *Surg Gynecol Obstet*. 1970;131(1):79–88.

127. Fisher B, Fisher ER, Redmond C. Ten-year results from the National Surgical Adjuvant Breast and Bowel Project (NSABP) clinical trial evaluating the use of L-phenylalanine mustard (L-PAM) in the management of primary breast cancer. *J Clin Oncol*. 1986;4(6):929–941.

128. Schwartz, G.F., Giuliano A.E., Veronesi U.; Consensus Conference Committee. Proceedings of the consensus conference on the role of sentinel lymph node biopsy in carcinoma of the breast, April 19–22, 2001, Philadelphia, Pennsylvania. Cancer, 2002. 94(10): p. 2542-51.

129. Giuliano AE, Ballman KV, McCall L, et al. Effect of axillary dissection vs no axillary dissection on 10-year overall survival among women with invasive breast cancer and sentinel node metastasis: the ACOSOG Z0011 (Alliance) Randomized clinical trial. *JAMA*. 2017;318(10):918–926.

130. Donker M, et al. Radiotherapy or surgery of the axilla after a positive sentinel node in breast cancer (EORTC 10981-22023

131. AMAROS): a randomised, multicentre, open-label, phase 3 non-inferiority trial. *Lancet Oncol.* 2014;15(12):1303–1310.

131. ASBrS, Choosing Wisely.

132. Hughes KS, van Tienhoven G, Straver ME, et al. Lumpectomy plus tamoxifen with or without irradiation in women 70 years of age or older with early breast cancer. *N Engl J Med.* 2004;351(10):971–977.

133. Martelli G, Miceli R, Daidone MG, et al. Axillary dissection versus no axillary dissection in elderly patients with breast cancer and no palpable axillary nodes: results after 15 years of follow-up. *Ann Surg Oncol.* 2011;18(1):125–133.

134. Hung P, Wang SY, Killelea BK, et al. Long-term outcomes of sentinel lymph node biopsy for ductal carcinoma in situ. *JNCI Cancer Spectr.* 2019;3(4):pkz052.

135. Van Roozendaal LM, Goorts B, Klinkert M, et al. Sentinel lymph node biopsy can be omitted in DCIS patients treated with breast conserving therapy. *Breast Cancer Res Treat.* 2016;156(3):517–525.

136. Karakatsanis A, Hersi AF, Pistiolis L, et al. Effect of preoperative injection of superparamagnetic iron oxide particles on rates of sentinel lymph node dissection in women undergoing surgery for ductal carcinoma in situ (SentiNot study). *Br J Surg.* 2019;106(6):720–728.

137. Boughey JC, Suman VJ, Mittendorf EA, et al. Sentinel lymph node surgery after neoadjuvant chemotherapy in patients with node-positive breast cancer: the ACOSOG Z1071 (Alliance) clinical trial. *JAMA.* 2013;310(14):1455–1461.

138. Kuehn T, Bauerfeind I, Fehm T, et al. Sentinel-lymph-node biopsy in patients with breast cancer before and after neoadjuvant chemotherapy (SENTINA): a prospective, multicentre cohort study. *Lancet Oncol.* 2013;14(7):609–618.

139. Boileau JF, Poirier B, Basik M, et al. Sentinel node biopsy after neoadjuvant chemotherapy in biopsy-proven node-positive breast cancer: the SN FNAC study. *J Clin Oncol.* 2015;33(3):258–264.

140. Classe JM, Loaec C, Gimbergues P, et al. Sentinel lymph node biopsy without axillary lymphadenectomy after neoadjuvant chemotherapy is accurate and safe for selected patients: the GANEA 2 study. *Breast Cancer Res Treat.* 2019;173(2):343–352.

141. Caudle AS, Yang WT, Mittendorf EA, et al. Selective surgical localization of axillary lymph nodes containing metastases in patients with breast cancer: a prospective feasibility trial. *JAMA Surg.* 2015;150(2):137–143.

142. Allweis TM, Menes T, Rotbart N, et al. Ultrasound guided tattooing of axillary lymph nodes in breast cancer patients prior to neoadjuvant therapy, and identification of tattooed nodes at the time of surgery. *Eur J Surg Oncol.* 2020;46(6):1041–1045.

143. Yuan L, Qi X, Zhang Y, et al. Comparison of sentinel lymph node detection performances using blue dye in conjunction with indocyanine green or radioisotope in breast cancer patients: a prospective single-center randomized study. *Cancer Biol Med.* 2018;15(4):452–460.

144. Simons JM, Scoggins ME, Kuerer HM, et al. Prospective registry trial assessing the use of magnetic seeds to locate clipped nodes after neoadjuvant chemotherapy for breast cancer patients. *Ann Surg Oncol.* 2021

145. Miller ME, Patil N, Li P, et al. Hospital system adoption of magnetic seeds for wireless breast and lymph node localization. *Ann Surg Oncol.* 2021;28(6):3223–3229.

146. Klimberg VS. A new concept toward the prevention of lymphedema: axillary reverse mapping. *J Surg Oncol.* 2008;97(7):563–564.

147. Thompson M, Korourian S, Henry-Tillman R, et al. Axillary reverse mapping (ARM): a new concept to identify and enhance lymphatic preservation. *Ann Surg Oncol.* 2007;14(6):1890–1895.

148. Boneti C, Korourian S, Bland K, et al. Axillary reverse mapping: mapping and preserving arm lymphatics may be important in preventing lymphedema during sentinel lymph node biopsy. *J Am Coll Surg.* 2008;206(5):1038–1042. discussion 1042-4.

149. Ahmed M, Rubio IT, Kovacs T, Klimberg VS, Douek M. Systematic review of axillary reverse mapping in breast cancer. *Br J Surg.* 2016;103(3):170–178.

150. Beek MA, Gobardhan PD, Schoenmaeckers EJ, et al. Axillary reverse mapping in axillary surgery for breast cancer: an update of the current status. *Breast Cancer Res Treat.* 2016;158(3):421–432.

151. Boneti C, Badgwell B, Robertson Y, Korourian S, Adkins L, Klimberg V. Axillary reverse mapping (ARM): initial results of phase II trial in preventing lymphedema after lymphadenectomy. *Minerva Ginecol.* 2012;64(5):421–430.

152. Boneti C, Korourian S, Diaz Z, et al. Scientific Impact Award: Axillary reverse mapping (ARM) to identify and protect lymphatics draining the arm during axillary lymphadenectomy. *Am J Surg.* 2009;198(4):482–487.

153. Gebruers N, Tjalma WA. Clinical feasibility of axillary reverse mapping and its influence on breast cancer related lymphedema: a systematic review. *Eur J Obstet Gynecol Reprod Biol.* 2016;200:117–122.

154. Han C, Yang B, Zuo WS, Zheng G, Yang L, Zheng MZ. The feasibility and oncological safety of axillary reverse mapping in patients with breast cancer: a systematic review and meta-analysis of prospective studies. *PLOS ONE.* 2016;11(2):e0150285.

155. Noguchi M, Noguchi M, Ohno Y, et al. Feasibility study of axillary reverse mapping for patients with clinically node-negative breast cancer. *Eur J Surg Oncol.* 2016;42(5):650–656.

156. Ochoa D, Korourian S, Boneti C, Adkins L, Badgwell B, Klimberg VS. Axillary reverse mapping: five-year experience. *Surgery.* 2014;156(5):1261–1268.

157. Tummel E, Ochoa D, Korourian S, et al. Does axillary reverse mapping prevent lymphedema after lymphadenectomy? *Ann Surg.* 2017;265(5):987–992.

158. Wijaya WA, Peng J, He Y, Chen J, Cen Y. Clinical application of axillary reverse mapping in patients with breast cancer: a systematic review and meta-analysis. *Breast.* 2020;53:189–200.

159. Guo X, Jiao D, Zhu J, et al. The effectiveness of axillary reverse mapping in preventing breast cancer-related lymphedema: a meta-analysis based on randomized controlled trials. *Gland Surg.* 2021;10(4):1447–1459.

160. Boccardo F, Casabona F, De Cian F, et al. Lymphatic microsurgical preventing healing approach (LYMPHA) for primary surgical prevention of breast cancer-related lymphedema: over 4 years follow-up. *Microsurgery.* 2014;34(6):421–424.

161. Boccardo FM, Casabona F, Friedman D, et al. Surgical prevention of arm lymphedema after breast cancer treatment. *Ann Surg Oncol.* 2011;18(9):2500–2505.

162. Boccardo F, Casabona F, De Cian F, et al. Lymphedema microsurgical preventive healing approach: a new technique for primary prevention of arm lymphedema after mastectomy. *Ann Surg Oncol.* 2009;16(3):703–708.

163. Feldman S, Bansil H, Ascherman J, et al. Single institution experience with lymphatic microsurgical preventive healing approach (LYMPHA) for the primary prevention of lymphedema. *Ann Surg Oncol.* 2015;22(10):3296–3301.

164. Ozmen T, Layton C, Friedman-Eldar O, et al. Evaluation of simplified lymphatic microsurgical preventing healing approach (S-LYMPHA) for the prevention of breast cancer-related clinical lymphedema after axillary lymph node dissection. *Ann Surg.* 2019;270(6):1156–1160.

165. Johnson AR, Kimball S, Epstein S, et al. Lymphedema incidence after axillary lymph node dissection: quantifying the impact of radiation and the lymphatic microsurgical preventive healing approach. *Ann Plast Surg.* 2019;82(4S Suppl 3):S234–S241.

166. Vaidya JS, Wenz F, Bulsara M, et al. Risk-adapted targeted intraoperative radiotherapy versus whole-breast radiotherapy for breast cancer: 5-year results for local control and overall survival from the TARGIT-A randomised trial. *Lancet.* 2014;383(9917):603–613.

167. Veronesi U, Orecchia R, Maisonneuve P, et al. Intraoperative radiotherapy versus external radiotherapy for early breast cancer (ELIOT): a randomised controlled equivalence trial. *Lancet Oncol.* 2013;14(13):1269–1277.

168. Vaidya JS, Bulsara M, Baum M, et al. Long term survival and local control outcomes from single dose targeted intraoperative radiotherapy during lumpectomy (TARGIT-IORT) for early breast cancer: TARGIT-A randomised clinical trial. *BMJ.* 2020;370:m2836.

169. Welzel G, Boch A, Sperk E, et al. Radiation-related quality of life parameters after targeted intraoperative radiotherapy versus whole breast radiotherapy in patients with breast cancer: results from the randomized phase III trial TARGIT-A. *Radiat Oncol.* 2013;8:9.

170. Jagsi R, Chadha M, Moni J, et al. Radiation field design in the ACOSOG Z0011 (Alliance) trial. *J Clin Oncol.* 2014;32(32):3600–3606.

171. Obi E, Tom MC, Manyam BV, et al. Outcomes with intraoperative radiation therapy for early-stage breast cancer. *Breast J.* 2020;26(3):454–457.

172. Shah C, Vicini F, Beitsch P, et al. The use of bioimpedance spectroscopy to monitor therapeutic intervention in patients treated for breast cancer related lymphedema. *Lymphology.* 2013;46(4):184–192.

173. Andersen L, Højris I, Erlandsen M, Andersen J. Treatment of breast-cancer-related lymphedema with or without manual lymphatic drainage--a randomized study. *Acta Oncol.* 2000;39(3):399–405.

174. McNeely ML, Magee DJ, Lees AW, et al. The addition of manual lymph drainage to compression therapy for breast cancer related lymphedema: a randomized controlled trial. *Breast Cancer Res Treat.* 2004;86(2):95–106.

175. Dayes IS, Whelan TJ, Julian JA, et al. Randomized trial of decongestive lymphatic therapy for the treatment of lymphedema in women with breast cancer. *J Clin Oncol.* 2013;31(30):3758–3763.

176. Ezzo J, Manheimer E, McNeely ML, et al. Manual lymphatic drainage for lymphedema following breast cancer treatment. *Cochrane Database Syst Rev.* 2015;5p. CD003475.

177. Box RC, Reul-Hirche HM, Bullock-Saxton JE, Furnival CM. Physiotherapy after breast cancer surgery: results of a randomised controlled study to minimise lymphoedema. *Breast Cancer Res Treat.* 2002;75(1):51–64.

178. Sagen A, Karesen R, Risberg MA. Physical activity for the affected limb and arm lymphedema after breast cancer surgery. A prospective, randomized controlled trial with two years follow-up. *Acta Oncol.* 2009;48(8):1102–1110.

179. Schmitz KH, Ahmed RL, Troxel A, et al. Weight lifting in women with breast-cancer-related lymphedema. *N Engl J Med.* 2009;361(7):664–673.

180. Schmitz KH, Troxel AB, Cheville A, et al. Physical Activity and Lymphedema (the PAL trial): assessing the safety of progressive strength training in breast cancer survivors. *Contemp Clin Trials.* 2009;30(3):233–245.

181. Ahmed RL, Thomas W, Yee D, Schmitz KH. Randomized controlled trial of weight training and lymphedema in breast cancer survivors. *J Clin Oncol.* 2006;24(18):2765–2772.

182. Rogan S, Taeymans J, Luginbuehl H, Aebi M, Mahnig S, Gebruers N. Therapy modalities to reduce lymphoedema in female breast cancer patients: a systematic review and meta-analysis. *Breast Cancer Res Treat.* 2016;159(1):1–14.

183. Moseley AL, Carati CJ, Piller NB. A systematic review of common conservative therapies for arm lymphoedema secondary to breast cancer treatment. *Ann Oncol.* 2007;18(4):639–646.

184. Granzow JW, Soderberg JM, Kaji AH, Dauphine C. An effective system of surgical treatment of lymphedema. *Ann Surg Oncol.* 2014;21(4):1189–1194.

185. Greene AK, Maclellan RA. Operative treatment of lymphedema using suction-assisted lipectomy. *Ann Plast Surg.* 2016;77(3):337–340.

186. Boyages J, Kastanias K, Koelmeyer LA, et al. Liposuction for advanced lymphedema: a multidisciplinary approach for complete reduction of arm and leg swelling. *Ann Surg Oncol.* 2015;22(Suppl 3):S1263–S1270.

187. Baumeister RG, Siuda S, Bohmert H, Moser E. A microsurgical method for reconstruction of interrupted lymphatic pathways: autologous lymph-vessel transplantation for treatment of lymphedemas. *Scand J Plast Reconstr Surg.* 1986;20(1):141–146.

188. Baumeister RG, Mayo W, Notohamiprodjo M, Wallmichrath J, Springer S, Frick A. Microsurgical lymphatic vessel transplantation. *J Reconstr Microsurg.* 2016;32(1):34–41.

189. Cheng MH, Chen SC, Henry SL, Tan BK, Chia-Yu Lin M, Huang JJ. Vascularized groin lymph node flap transfer for postmastectomy upper limb lymphedema: flap anatomy, recipient sites, and outcomes. *Plast Reconstr Surg.* 2013;131(6):1286–1298.

190. Cheng MH, Huang JJ, Wu CW, et al. The mechanism of vascularized lymph node transfer for lymphedema: natural lymphaticovenous drainage. *Plast Reconstr Surg.* 2014;133(2):192e–198e.

191. Dayan JH, Dayan E, Smith ML. Reverse lymphatic mapping: a new technique for maximizing safety in vascularized lymph node transfer. *Plast Reconstr Surg.* 2015;135(1):277–285.

192. Poumellec MA, Foissac R, Cegarra-Escolano M, Barranger E, Ihrai T. Surgical treatment of secondary lymphedema of the upper limb by stepped microsurgical lymphaticovenous anastomoses. *Breast Cancer Res Treat.* 2017;162(2):219–224.

193. Chang DW, Suami H, Skoracki R. A prospective analysis of 100 consecutive lymphovenous bypass cases for treatment of extremity lymphedema. *Plast Reconstr Surg.* 2013;132(5):1305–1314.

194. Breast Cancer Facts and Figures 2019-2020. https://www.cancer.org/content/dam/cancer-org/research/cancer-facts-and-statistics/breast-cancer-facts-and-figures/breast-cancer-facts-and-figures-2019-2020.pdf. Accessed 10/4/2021

195. Bleyer A, Welch HG. Effect of three decades of screening mammography on breast-cancer incidence. *N Engl J Med.* 2012;367(21):1998–2005.

196. Giuliano AE, Edge SB, Hortobagyi GN. Eighth Edition of the AJCC Cancer Staging Manual: breast cancer. *Ann Surg Oncol.* 2018;25(7):1783–1785.

197. Tajima CC, de Sousa LLC, Venys GL, Guatelli CS, Bitencourt AGV, Marques EF. Magnetic resonance imaging of the breast:

role in the evaluation of ductal carcinoma in situ. *Radiol Bras*. 2019;52(1):43–47.

198. Groen EJ, Elshof LE, Visser LL, et al. Finding the balance between over- and under-treatment of ductal carcinoma in situ (DCIS). *Breast*. 2017;31:274–283.

199. Chlebowski RT, Hendrix SL, Langer RD, et al. Influence of estrogen plus progestin on breast cancer and mammography in healthy postmenopausal women: the Women's Health Initiative Randomized Trial. *JAMA*. 2003;289(24):3243–3253.

200. Silverstein MJ. Ductal carcinoma in situ of the breast. *BMJ*. 1998;317(7160):734–739.

201. Gorringe KL, Fox SB. Ductal carcinoma in situ biology, biomarkers, and diagnosis. *Front Oncol*. 2017;7:248 Published 2017 Oct 23.

202. Kim S, Kim J, Park HS, et al. An updated nomogram for predicting invasiveness in preoperative ductal carcinoma in situ of the breast. *Yonsei Med J*. 2019;60(11):1028–1035.

203. Park HS, Park S, Cho J, Park JM, Kim SI, Park BW. Risk predictors of underestimation and the need for sentinel node biopsy in patients diagnosed with ductal carcinoma in situ by preoperative needle biopsy. *J Surg Oncol*. 2013;107(4):388–392.

204. Trialists Early Breast Cancer. Collaborative Group (EBCTCG); Correa C, McGale P, Taylor C, et al. Overview of the randomized trials of radiotherapy in ductal carcinoma in situ of the breast. *J Natl Cancer Inst Monogr*. 2010;2010(41):162–177.

205. Wapnir IL, Dignam JJ, Fisher B, et al. Long-term outcomes of invasive ipsilateral breast tumor recurrences after lumpectomy in NSABP B-17 and B-24 randomized clinical trials for DCIS. *J Natl Cancer Inst*. 2011;103(6):478–488.

206. Emdin SO, Granstrand B, Ringberg A, et al. SweDCIS: Radiotherapy after sector resection for ductal carcinoma in situ of the breast. Results of a randomised trial in a population offered mammography screening. *Acta Oncol*. 2006;45(5):536–543.

207. Wärnberg F, Garmo H, Emdin S, et al. Effect of radiotherapy after breast-conserving surgery for ductal carcinoma in situ: 20 years follow-up in the randomized SweDCIS Trial. *J Clin Oncol*. 2014;32(32):3613–3618.

208. EORTC Breast Cancer Cooperative Group; EORTC Radiotherapy Group; Bijker N, Meijnen P, Peterse JL, et al. Breast-conserving treatment with or without radiotherapy in ductal carcinoma-in-situ: ten-year results of European Organisation for Research and Treatment of Cancer randomized phase III trial 10853--a study by the EORTC Breast Cancer Cooperative Group and EORTC Radiotherapy Group. J Clin Oncol. 2006;24(21):3381-3387.

209. Cuzick J, Sestak I, Pinder SE, et al. Effect of tamoxifen and radiotherapy in women with locally excised ductal carcinoma in situ: long-term results from the UK/ANZ DCIS trial. *Lancet Oncol*. 2011;12(1):21–29.

210. McCormick B, Winter K, Hudis C, et al. RTOG 9804: a prospective randomized trial for good-risk ductal carcinoma in situ comparing radiotherapy with observation [published correction appears in *J Clin Oncol*. 2015 Sep 10;33(26):2934]. . *J Clin Oncol*. 2015;33(7):709–715.

211. McCormick B, Winter KA, Woodward W, et al. Randomized phase III trial evaluating radiation following surgical excision for good-risk ductal carcinoma in situ: long-term report from NRG Oncology/RTOG 9804. *J Clin Oncol*. 2021;39(32):3574–3582.

212. Silverstein MJ, Lagios MD, Craig PH, et al. A prognostic index for ductal carcinoma in situ of the breast. *Cancer*. 1996;77(11):2267–2274.

213. Silverstein MJ. The University of Southern California/Van Nuys prognostic index for ductal carcinoma in situ of the breast. *Am J Surg*. 2003;186(4):337–343.

214. Van Zee KJ, Zabor EC, Di Donato R, et al. Comparison of local recurrence risk estimates after breast-conserving surgery for DCIS: DCIS nomogram versus refined oncotype DX breast DCIS score. *Ann Surg Oncol*. 2019;26(10):3282–3288.

215. Solin LJ, Gray R, Baehner FL, et al. A multigene expression assay to predict local recurrence risk for ductal carcinoma in situ of the breast. *J Natl Cancer Inst*. 2013;105(10):701–710.

216. Oncotype D.X. Breast D.C.I.S. https://www.oncotypeiq.com/en-US/breast-cancer/healthcare-professionals/oncotype-dx-breast-dcis-score/clinical-evidence. Access 10/4/2021

217. The Science of Our Name. DCISionRT. https://preludedx.com/dcisionrt/#validation. Accessed 10/4/2021

218. Lei RY, Carter DL, Antell AG, et al. A comparison of predicted ipsilateral tumor recurrence risks in patients with ductal carcinoma in situ of the breast after breast-conserving surgery by breast radiation oncologists, the Van Nuys Prognostic Index, the Memorial Sloan Kettering Cancer Center DCIS Nomogram, and the 12-Gene DCIS Score Assay. *Adv Radiat Oncol*. 2020;6(2):100607 Published 2020 Nov 1.

219. Kanbayashi C, Thompson AM, Hwang ES, et al. (2019). The international collaboration of active surveillance trials for low-risk DCIS (LORIS, LORD, COMET, LORETTA). *Journal of Clinical Oncology*. 2019;37(15 Suppl.):TPS603-TPS603.

220. Thomas PS. Diagnosis and management of high-risk breast lesions. *J Natl Compr Canc Netw*. 2018;16(11):1391–1396.

221. Lewin AA, Mercado CL. Atypical ductal hyperplasia and lobular neoplasia: update and easing of guidelines. *AJR Am J Roentgenol*. 2020;214(2):265–275.

222. Calle C, Kuba MG, Brogi E. Non-invasive lobular neoplasia of the breast: morphologic features, clinical presentation, and management dilemmas. *Breast J*. 2020;26(6):1148–1155.

223. Women's Health and Cancer Rights Act (WHCRA). https://www.cms.gov/CCIIO/Programs-and-Initiatives/Other-Insurance-Protections/whcra_factsheet. Accessed 02/28/2022

224. Patel K, Bloom J, Nardello S, Cohen S, Reiland J, Chatterjee A. An oncoplastic surgery primer: common indications, techniques, and complications in level 1 and 2 volume displacement oncoplastic surgery. *Ann Surg Oncol*. 2019 Oct;26(10):3063–3070.

225. Chatterjee A, Gass J, Patel K, et al. A consensus definition and classification system of oncoplastic surgery developed by the American Society of Breast Surgeons. *Ann Surg Oncol*. 2019 Oct;26(11):3436–3444.

226. De La Cruz L, Blankenship S, Chatterjee A, et al. Outcomes after oncoplastic breast-conserving surgery in breast cancer patients: a systematic literature review. *Ann Surg Oncol*. 2016;23(10):3247–3258.

227. Losken A, Dugal C, Styblo T, Carlson G. A meta-analysis comparing breast conservation therapy alone to the oncoplastic technique. *Ann Plast Surg*. 2014;72(2):145–149.

228. Kelsall J, McCulley S, Brock L, Akerlund M, Macmillan R. Comparing oncoplastic breast conserving surgery with mastectomy and immediate breast reconstruction: case-matched patient reported outcomes. *J Plast Reconstr Aesthet Surg*. 2017;70(10):1377–1385.

229. Chatterjee A, Offodile II AC, Asban A, et al. A cost-utility analysis comparing oncoplastic breast surgery to standard lumpectomy in large breasted women. *Adv Breast Cancer Res*. 2018;7(2):14.

230. Asban A, Homsy C, Chen L, Fisher C, Losken A, Chatterjee A. A cost-utility analysis comparing large volume displacement oncoplastic surgery to mastectomy with single stage implant reconstruction in the treatment of breast cancer. *Breast*. 2018;41:159–164.

231. Silverstein MJ, Savalia N, Khan S, Ryan J. Extreme oncoplasty: breast conservation for patients who need mastectomy. *Breast J.* 2015 Jan-Feb;21(1):52–59.

232. Chung K. *Grabb and Smith's Plastic Surgery.* Lippincott Williams & Wilkins; 2019.

233. Lennox PA, Bovill ES, Macadam SA. Evidence-based medicine: alloplastic breast reconstruction. *Plastic and reconstructive surgery.* 2017;140(1):94e–108e.

234. Chang EI. Latest advancements in autologous breast reconstruction. *Plastic and reconstructive surgery.* 2021;147(1):111e–122e.

235. Farhadi J, Hofer SOP, Masia J. Contemporary indications in breast reconstruction. *Clinics in plastic surgery.* 2018;45(1):i.

236. Macadam SA, Bovill ES, Buchel EW, Lennox PA. Evidence-based medicine: autologous breast reconstruction. *Plastic and reconstructive surgery.* 2017;139(1):204e–229e.

8

Radiation Therapy

KENNETH T. BASTIN, ELLEN L. ZIAJA, GREG KAUFFMANN, DONALD ALLEN GOER, JAY K. HARNESS, AND JULIANN REILAND

Radiation therapy is frequently employed in treating breast cancer and is thus available in virtually all radiation centers. Given the commonality of breast cancer across the world, management of this disease occupies a large volume of patient care in a radiation oncology clinic. As science advances and innovative approaches are validated in the literature, breast cancer management in the modern era has become more complex and specialized. A multidisciplinary approach employing input from a diverse group of specialties bringing their knowledge base to the table contributes to an elevated standard of care.

In our institution, multidisciplinary care is practiced in two main forums: (1) multidisciplinary cancer conferences in which new cancer cases are presented in a prospective fashion seeking input on management across disciplines, and (2) multidisciplinary clinics in which a newly diagnosed patient meets with their cancer team of physicians and healthcare extenders in a single setting to provide a streamlined recommendation. Both approaches work to provide the patient with a personalized care plan and a consensus recommendation. In both settings, the current breast cancer management guidelines from the National Comprehensive Cancer Network are discussed as validation for the treatment plan and patients are screened for potential eligibility into available clinical research trials, which may also provide an alternative treatment pathway. We also have standardized treatment pathways among our group to ensure that we are providing consistent care to patients across our 11 sites of care, and accommodate innovation with rapid introduction across our system.

Radiation Therapy Background

Radiation is a natural phenomenon present throughout the universe in the form of electromagnetic radiation and particles emitted from radioactive decay. Naturally occurring radiation was first described by Becquerel in 1896.[1] The first described human-made radiation was announced by William Roentgen in 1895.[2] Marie and Pierre Curie, co-discovering both radium and polonium as natural radioactive elements,[3] shared the 1903 Nobel Prize with Henri Becquerel. Radioactivity measurements have been described using the Becquerel and Curie in their honor. In 1920, the Curie Institute in Paris was formed for medical research. Ironically Curie died in 1934 at the age of 66 of probable aplastic anemia, likely a side effect of chronic radiation exposure. Roentgen, who initially discovered high-energy electromagnetic energy emanating from an electrified vacuum tube, coined the discovery as "X-rays" and won the Nobel Prize in physics in 1901. Roentgen is considered the father of radiology (Fig. 8.1).

In the mid-1900s, cobalt-60 was used as a human-made radioactive source for delivery of radiation. However the penetrating energy of the cobalt-60 gamma rays was relatively low, thus limiting effective and safe radiation doses for deep-seated tumors in the chest, abdomen, and pelvis.

Brothers Russell and Sigurd Varian invented the linear accelerator in Palo Alto, California, which delivered higher penetrating radiation than cobalt therapy. Linear accelerators (LINACs) are used in virtually all cancer centers for treatment today and Varian remains an international leader in this technology. One current Varian model, the TrueBeam, has multiple features including beam shaping, arc and rotational radiation delivery, and built-in computed tomography (CT)-based imaging for radiation delivery (Fig. 8.2). The system also allows for radiation delivery timed with respiratory gating, which is especially relevant to cancer treatment in the chest, breast, and abdominal areas.

Proton therapy has expanded in its use across the United States based on the physical feature that protons (positively charged particles) will deliver radiation treatment to a defined depth in tissue based on the selected beam energy (the Bragg Peak). Protons require significantly greater financial start-up investment, and for most nonpediatric applications have not proven clearly superior to high-energy photon (X-ray) treatment. Ongoing clinical trials will better define the role of proton therapy for more common cancers such as breast and prostate cancer.

Clinical radiation treatment requires the accurate measurement and delivery of radiation doses, which is defined by the term *Gray* (Gy) or *centigray* (cGy). Radiation delivery from an external body source is referred to as tele-therapy, whereas radiation delivery from an internalized source (using radioactive seeds, interstitial needles, or balloon) is referred to as brachytherapy.

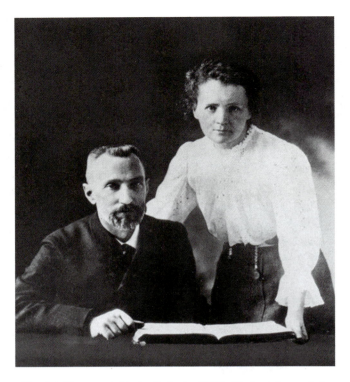

• **Fig. 8.1** Pierre and Marie Curie in 1903. Modern-day radiation treatment is virtually completely machine produced, including the production of high-energy X-rays (photons), electrons, protons, beams from cyclotrons, or (rarely) neutron therapy. Radium-226 occurring as a natural element is no longer used in medical care. Commonly used radioisotopes, including iodine-125, iridium 192, and cobalt-60, are created using industrial production methods.

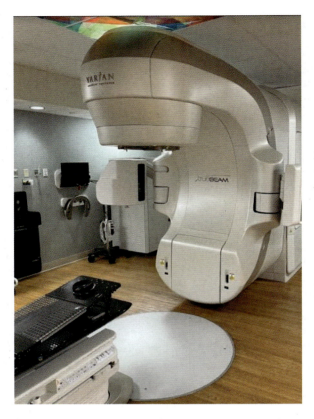

• **Fig. 8.2** A Varian TrueBeam LINAC with a built-in computed tomography scanner, multi-energy photon options, electron beam energies, and multipositional table. (Photo by author.)

It is the radiation oncologist who defines anatomical targets and avoidance tissue, typically from CT-based imaging, then defines fractional and total doses. A clinical dosimetrist is trained to incorporate the physician's anatomic contouring into a treatment plan, and subsequently the medical physicist, specializing in radiation therapy, will review and approve the technical aspects of the plan. The radiation oncologist is ultimately responsible for supervising the patient's treatment. The team approach for radiation delivery involves coordination and strict quality assurance.

Radiation Therapy Definitions

Radiation therapy energy produced by a linear accelerator will determine its effective penetration into tissue. Modern-day LINAC units typically deliver a maximum photon energy ranging between 6 and 20 million electron volts (MeV). In contrast, diagnostic X-ray imaging typically uses 50–150 kV energies, with this much lower energy range taking advantage of differences in X-ray interaction based on tissue density (i.e., bone versus soft tissue) by virtue of the photoelectric effect. LINAC treatment systems typically have a range of energies available for treatment, chosen during the treatment planning phase.

Modern LINACs shape the radiation field using either stationary multiple beams or dynamic moving beams, all preplanned using dedicated computer and software technology. Intensity-modulated radiation therapy (IMRT) refers to the shaping of radiation fields using dynamic field-shaping technology and requires greater planning and quality assurance but may deliver better avoidance of normal tissue with treatment. Three-dimensional radiation therapy uses stationary and well-defined radiation field shapes, may be most appropriate for palliative cases, and dosimetry may equal IMRT involving large field treatment.

Imaging on the linear accelerator is always incorporated during a treatment course, as it confirms setup accuracy and may include daily or weekly CT/kV/MV depending upon clinical indications. The imaging is not for diagnostic purposes but rather to confirm set up immediately prior to radiation treatment.

A radiation simulation is a setup session that precedes any radiation delivery and allows for the planning. Simulation typically occurs up to 1 week before treatment and may incorporate a CT scan for baseline imaging. In many clinical situations, a pre-existing positron emission tomography (PET) scan or magnetic resonance image (MRI) can be fused digitally with CT imaging to allow the radiation oncologist better definition of the treatment target and avoidance of normal tissue (Fig. 8.3).

The radiation treatment course is defined not only by the target and avoidance of normal tissues but by the treatment dose per fraction of delivery and the total number of

CHAPTER 8 Radiation Therapy 89

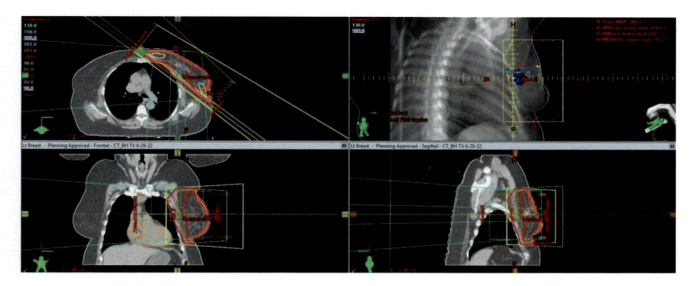

• **Fig. 8.3** Dosimetry of a left-breast radiation setup, axial/coronal/sagittal views.

EBRT Isodose & Treatment Plan Documentation

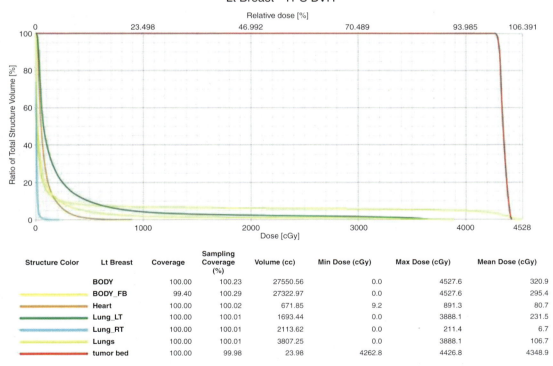

• **Fig. 8.4** Dose volume histogram showing low doses to critical structures (heart/lungs) while meeting prescription dosing to the target.

fractions (Fig. 8.4). Both are important from a biological perspective and are defined by palliative versus curative, and preoperative or postoperative clinical situations. For example breast cancer treatment may be delivered using a 5 day per week 6-week course to a total maximum dose of 5000–6000 cGy. Alternatively, some courses can be completed in 16 fractions over just 3 weeks for a total dose of 4256 cGy. In some clinical situations the surgical bed requires additional radiation, possibly adding five more fractions to a dose of 1000 cGy. The radiation prescription is personalized to the patient's situation, treatment intent, pathology, and according to the clinical trial protocol if enrolled.

Radiation Biology

The recognized target of radiation is the DNA within cells. Radiation can cause direct double-stranded breaks in DNA, resulting in eventual cell death. Alternatively, free radical formation (indirect effect) can produce permanent DNA damage and death. Free radical formation is enhanced by the presence of oxygen, meaning that hypoxic tumors are less effectively treated with radiation. Approximately 70% of radiation tumor kill is from the indirect effect.[4]

Competent DNA repair is retained in most normal tissue but reduced in tumor cells, thus allowing for preferred tumor killing with radiation treatment. Radiation therapy tumor kill can be enhanced using concurrent chemotherapy as radiation sensitizers, and is commonly used in treating rectal cancer, lung cancer, and head neck cancer. Radiation sensitizers, however, are not typically used for treating breast cancer.

Different human tissues have different tolerances to radiation treatment. Rapidly growing tissue in the gastrointestinal system and head and neck mucosal surfaces respond briskly to radiation, whereas musculoskeletal tissue has minimal immediate effect. In addition, the total radiation dose to an organ is defined based on complication risks. Clinical studies and radiobiological models provide guidance for radiation oncology dose prescription.

Radiation therapy side effects are typically classified as acute or late. Acute side effects may include mucositis, dermatitis, nausea, and fatigue, dependent upon the target area, and are typically predictable with predictable recovery. Acute side effects are most often seen during radiation treatment. Late tissue toxicity may occur months to years after treatment, is limited to the tissue radiated, and may not be recognized, or alternatively can be quite severe. Examples would include secondary malignancies and normal tissue necrosis. Fortunately, with carefully prescribed radiation fields and dose delivery, late tissue effects are uncommon.

Assessing Patients Appropriate for Radiation Therapy

Radiation therapy may be indicated in the following clinical scenarios:

1. As adjuvant treatment following breast-conserving surgery (BCS);
2. As adjuvant treatment following mastectomy, when the patient has documented increased risk for local recurrence based on clinical/pathologic factors;
3. For palliative inoperable disease with pain/bleeding control;
4. Locally recurrent malignancy in a radiation-naïve patient or previously radiated patient.

A multidisciplinary discussion following the initial biopsy-confirmed breast cancer is our standard format prior to discussing treatment recommendations with the patient. For the radiation oncologist, pathologic confirmation of malignancy is required. Histological confirmation of invasive versus in situ disease is important as well as tumor receptor (Estrogen [ER]/Progesterone [PR]) findings and HER2 status. Cancer staging may also include CT or PET scan. Documentation of collagen vascular disease and autoimmune disease as well as any prior breast radiation may represent contraindications to radiation therapy. This latter information should be available prior to a decision regarding breast conservation as it may influence a preference for mastectomy.

In the early multidisciplinary evaluation discussion, an experienced breast surgeon should assess the likelihood of achieving negative margins following breast-conservation surgery. If multicentric disease is present or suspected by the radiologist, mastectomy may be the preferred surgical option. In addition cosmetic considerations following adequate surgical resection are important, and in some cases mastectomy with reconstruction provides a better cosmetic outcome than breast conservation with radiation.

A staging workup may include PET scan, brain MRIs, and so on when appropriate depending on the clinical stage. Oncotype DX and other predictive studies may be obtained and will determine whether adjuvant chemotherapy will be beneficial/indicated. Unless neoadjuvant chemotherapy (NACT) is indicated, adjuvant guidelines sequence chemotherapy following surgical recovery and prior to any radiation treatment. We currently recommend any adjuvant hormonal antiendocrine therapy (e.g., aromatase inhibitors, tamoxifen) to follow radiation treatment. In younger fertile patients pregnancy testing is virtually mandatory and, when positive, may represent a barrier for offering radiation therapy without some delay until the pregnancy has been completed.

Based on initial workup and pathology, the patient meets with the radiation oncologist to discuss the indication for adjuvant breast radiation therapy. In the situation of a postmenopausal/elderly patients with low-risk (ER-positive, node-negative, margin clear) disease, omitting radiation therapy may be considered if the patient is committed to the prescribed course of antiendocrine therapy. Technical decisions by the radiation oncologist include volume of tissue irradiated, i.e., partial breast versus whole breast, and treatment of axillary/supraclavicular/internal mammary nodes. We also advocate cardiac-sparing radiation techniques when treating the (typically left) breast, as discussed later in this chapter. The spectrum of treatment duration can range from 1 week to 6 weeks dependent on the volume of tissue encompassed and stage of disease

Consent is also important, with relevant treatment risks being discussed, including acute toxicity, late-term toxicity, cosmetic outcome, financial cost to the patient, and logistics.

Consultation by a radiation oncologist prior to definitive surgery is strongly encouraged to avoid confusion and confirm expectations of treatment duration. In our experience this early meeting with the patient enhances the patient's experience.

We will lay out our typical treatment process based on multidisciplinary decision-making later in this chapter.

General Clinical Radiation Therapy Concepts

Pathology is very important to the radiation oncologist, as a malignant diagnosis is required for radiation treatment. Upfront imaging including MRI and mammograms may be useful for radiation treatment planning. A radiation oncologist should be involved in the initial management discussion of newly diagnosed breast cancer patients and may influence decisions regarding breast conservation versus mastectomy, as well as extent of axillary lymph node staging. After initial surgery, pathology is again reviewed, and in some cases reoperation may be required to achieve negative margins. Again, the radiation oncologist should provide input at this decision point. Surgical clips placed at the time of initial/subsequent surgery may help define an area for radiation boosting and should be included in the surgical technique whenever possible. Patients who develop large treatment bed seromas may require tapping, which may delay radiation planning. We typically initiate radiation treatment within 8 weeks of surgery when chemotherapy is not indicated, or within 1 year of surgery if adjuvant multicycle chemotherapy is delivered.

Radiation Side Effects Following Treatment of Breast Cancer

Radiation side effects from breast radiation are limited to the radiated tissues, which includes the targeted breast/chest wall, lymph nodes, underlying lung, and skin. Contralateral breast tissue may be partially in field as well. For left-sided tumors cardiac tissue/coronary arteries/pericardium may be in field, requiring additional radiation planning for avoidance. For some right-sided breast cancer patients, the right coronary artery may be at risk for radiation exposure, requiring assessment at the time of planning.

Acute side effects of breast radiation include dermatitis in the radiation field. Tanning may also be a sequelae of radiation treatment as well as telangiectasia. Fibrosis may occur, especially, but not limited to, the surgical bed, and systemic fatigue is a transient side effect, although not typically as pronounced as with chemotherapy. Radiation pneumonitis is uncommon and can occur when larger volumes of underlying lung are included within the radiation field. Current techniques that limit lung volume minimize this risk. Patients who present with a dry cough post radiation may require a course of steroids (usually prednisone) with taper for management.

Late tissue toxicity from radiation could include lymphedema of the ipsilateral arm, but is only typically seen following extensive lymph node surgery.

Secondary malignancies from radiation are well documented in the literature. Radiation-induced cancer risk for all sites ranges between 0.2% and 1% per year in cancer survivors after radiotherapy. A bimodal distribution of secondary malignancies is noted, with the first peak within 3 years of treatment (typically leukemia in those receiving chemotherapy). A second peak typically involves solid tumors and occurs more than a decade out.[5]

An increased risk of secondary malignancy was reported in a meta-analysis involving more than 42,000 breast cancer patients (some treated with radiation and some not).[6]

Radiation-induced sarcomas typically originate 5–20 years after radiation and are typically more aggressive than spontaneously occurring sarcomas.[7]

Ironically young patients with Hodgkin's disease who received thoracic radiation, and unavoidably had exposed breast tissue, are reportedly 75 times more likely to develop invasive breast cancer than the general population. These patients were typically young at the time of successful treatment, and their long life expectancy produced a long latency period for cancer development.[8]

An excellent review article is referenced for a more comprehensive description of complications from chest radiation.[9]

Radiation Therapy Technical Definitions

Radiation therapy is given using highly calibrated LINACs that produce high-energy X-rays (called photons) that can be directed to an anatomically defined area. Various technical radiation deliveries are available, including three-dimensional delivery or IMRT, the latter of which effectively "shapes" the radiation field. IMRT or three-dimensional surface compensation technique represents appropriate considerations when treating the left breast, as it allows for avoidance of cardiac tissue and minimizes the volume of lung exposure, and is often delivered in conjunction with breath hold by the patient and automated positioning by the machine, further enhancing accuracy and cardiac tissue avoidance.

LINACs also produce electron beams, which are charged particles that interact with tissue at very limited depths. Electron beam treatment is typically used for boosting small volumes of the surgical tumor bed (a "boost"). Radiation therapy is typically given 5 days per week, each treatment called a "fraction" and delivered over a typically 10-minute time frame per fraction. Prior to the start of radiation, a treatment planning session is carried out, called a "simulation," which includes a noncontrast CT scan, and this is sometimes done using a motion-monitoring technique (Figs. 8.5 and 8.6). Permanent markers may be used on the patient's breast/chest wall called "tattoos" to allow for reproducible daily set up. In addition, a body cast or immobilization device is used at the time of simulation, which is used for daily treatment. Once the simulation is complete planning follows, allowing the radiation oncologist to define the overall target, tissue avoidance, boost volume, and technical treatment aspects. A dosimetry plan is subsequently generated and reviewed by the radiation oncologist and approved following a medical physicist's final technical review.

We typically schedule radiation planning simulation 1 week prior to the desired start of treatment. Imaging is obtained daily or weekly on the linear accelerator to confirm

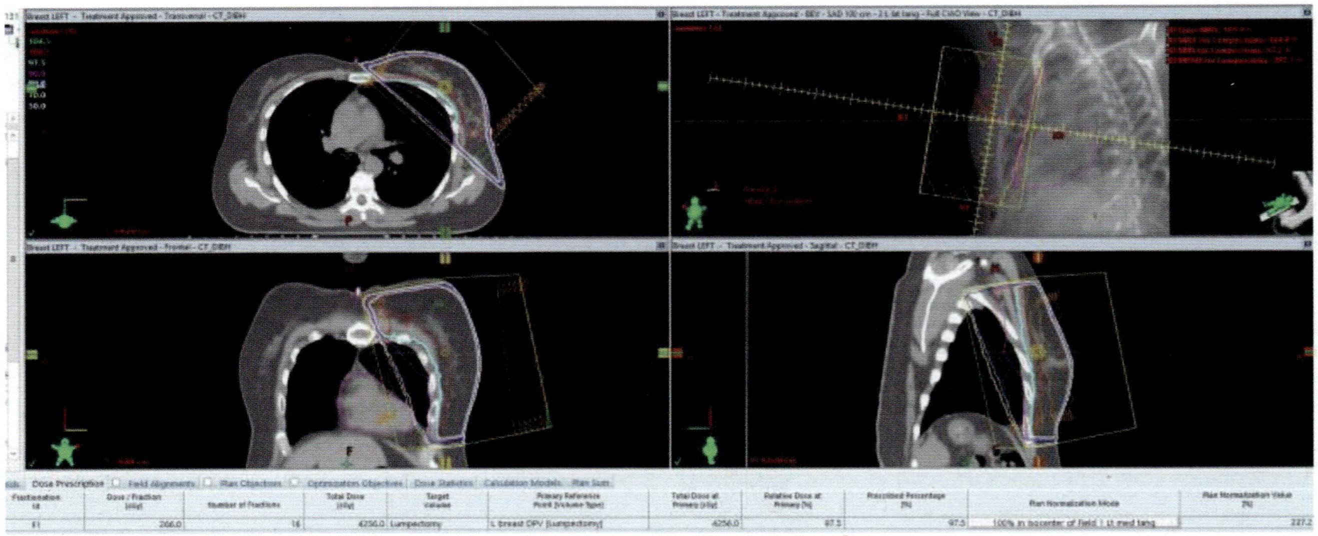

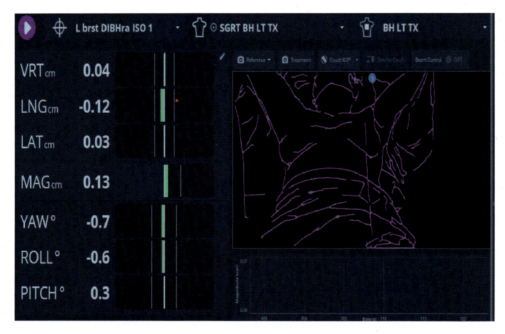

• **Fig. 8.5** Tangential radiation fields with isodose fields superimposed on computed tomography simulation. Axial, coronal, and sagittal fields demonstrate coverage of the whole breast.

• **Fig. 8.6** Chest wall/breast surface-guided treatment using monitoring with comfort breath hold and producing automatic adjustment of the radiation field (Align RT, Vision RT). Note dynamic, real-time, multiple sub-centimeter adjustments in the column.

set up accuracy. The overall goal of our radiation therapy technology is to provide a highly calibrated and accurate, tightly anatomically delivered radiation dose covering a limited volume of normal tissue. Finally, clinical assessment of the patient is done on a weekly basis, more frequently if needed, to monitor patient tolerance or toxicity.

Ductal Carcinoma In Situ

Ductal carcinoma in situ (DCIS) is a heterogeneous disease, found in 20–25% of newly diagnosed breast cancer patients.[10] Pathologists classify DCIS into low-, intermediate-, or high-grade categories, the latter demonstrating a higher likelihood of developing into invasive breast cancer.[11] We recommend a surgical margin of at least 2 mm when possible, and surgical clips to define the surgical bed. Given the lower mortality of DCIS versus invasive breast cancer, studies were performed to determine the relative value of offering postoperative breast radiation. In the landmark NSABP B-17 trial, a standard course of breast radiation reduced the risk of local recurrence in the ipsilateral breast by more than 50%.[12] A large meta-analysis published in 2010 showed a reduction of 15% at 10 years when using radiation for DCIS.[13] The data does not show a survival benefit with radiation therapy postoperatively in these patients, possibly attributed to salvage options at the time of documented recurrence. We typically recommend a course of hypofractionation (e.g., 4256 cGy in 16 fractions or 4000 cGy in 15 fractions) with or without a boost to the primary surgical bed. We do not include lymph node stations in the radiation field, given their very low risk of probable involvement. Left-sided DCIS is managed with cardiac-sparing technique, as previously shown. In elderly patients over 65–70 years of age with low-grade DCIS with ER-positive receptors, observation with tamoxifen or aromatase inhibitors is a viable option and is typically presented to the patient along with postoperative radiation options.[14] In some instances, microinvasive carcinoma is found at the time of pathology postoperatively, requiring reconsideration of treatment including sentinel lymph node assessment. A multidisciplinary discussion is thus required with this pathological upstaging and should be completed prior to any initiation of radiation planning.

Lobular carcinoma in situ has a very different biological behavior than DCIS and, absent any microinvasive findings, is not treated with radiation.

Invasive Breast Cancer, Breast-Conserving Adjuvant Radiation Treatment

The Early Breast Cancer Trialists' Collaborative Group (EBCTCG) published a meta-analysis of 17 randomized trials and determined that radiation therapy following BCS reduced the 10-year recurrence risk of ipsilateral breast cancer by 15.7% and reduced the risk of breast cancer death by 3.8% at 15 years. The meta-analysis, however, included node-positive and node-negative patients with different risk features and surgery. In this analysis, the benefit of adjuvant radiation therapy varied according to stratification, prompting additional trial-based studies.[15] These studies provide the framework for the recommendation of adjuvant radiation therapy for breast cancer and is referred to in the consent process following diagnosis or when breast conservation versus mastectomy is being considered.

The PRIME-II study, published in *The Lancet* in 2015, randomized women aged 65 years and older with T1 or T2 invasive breast cancer (maximum 3 cm) with hormone receptor–positive, axillary node–negative, surgical margin–negative breast cancer to receive endocrine therapy only versus adjuvant radiation with endocrine therapy. At 5 years the radiated breast tumor recurrence was 1.3% versus 4.1% in the endocrine-only arm, but there was no difference in the development of distant metastasis, contralateral breast cancer, or survival. The authors concluded that omission of radiotherapy may be considered for some patients.[16]

National Comprehensive Cancer Network (NCCN) Guidelines 4.2023 currently recommend the hypofractionated course of 4256 cGy in 16 fractions whole-breast treatment, with boost when there is an expected increased risk of recurrence in the tumor bed.

A more hypofractionated course of five fractions has been advocated for select cases. The FAST Forward study from the United Kingdom was published in 2020 and randomized these patients to various treatment arms including 26 Gy in five fractions, 27 Gy in five fractions, or 40 Gy in 15 fractions. Eligibility included patients at least 18 years of age with invasive carcinoma of the breast (pT1–3, pN0–1, M0). The study was not blinded because of the nature of the delivery, but the five-fraction course delivered in 1 week was noninferior to 40 Gy in 15 fractions for local control and normal tissue toxicity at 5 years.[17]

NCCN guidelines also note 28.5 Gy in five fractions as a hypofractionated option; however additional updates in hypofractionated clinical studies will be needed to clarify the optimal treatment prescription.[18]

In addition, select patients may be candidates for accelerated partial breast irradiation (APBI), which is also delivered in just five fractions. Instead of targeting the whole breast, the radiation dose is limited to the tumor bed plus a margin for microscopic disease, acknowledging that the index quadrant is the most common location for local recurrence after lumpectomy. The ABPI-IMRT-Florence Trial randomized patients to conventional whole-breast irradiation (WBI) versus APBI delivered in five fractions totaling 30 Gy versus 25 fractions totaling 50 Gy plus boost. At 10 years, the cumulative incidence of ipsilateral breast tumor recurrence (IBTR) was not statistically different between the arms; however the APBI arm had less acute and late toxicity, as well as better patient-reported cosmetic outcomes.[19]

Adjuvant radiation therapy follows a multidisciplinary process, delivered following surgical clearance; medical oncology assessment of adjuvant chemotherapy benefits; presentation to the patient involving radiation treatment side effects and benefits, i.e., treatment versus observation; and patient input regarding treatment location and duration. Ideally, the radiation oncologist would consult the patient prior to the initial breast-conservation surgery to discuss these issues.

Post-Mastectomy Radiation Therapy

Total breast mastectomy is potentially indicated for any number of circumstances including large tumor size, small breast size with expected unsatisfactory conservation cosmesis, multicentric disease, or patient preference. For large and higher-risk disease, NACT may be administered prior to mastectomy.

Radiation therapy may typically be omitted in post-mastectomy patients with negative nodes and clear margins from a T1 or T2 primary breast cancer.

Indications for post-mastectomy radiation include positive or very close (<1 mm) margins and/or tumor size typically greater than 5 cm. Treatment of regional lymph nodes is indicated for positive lymph node spread. The chest wall is normally treated to 45–50.4 Gy in 25–28 fractions and the relevant regional lymph nodes to the same dose. Internal mammary nodes are often considered based on risk features such as inner quadrant primary tumor location or when involved in a staging workup (CT scan or PET scan; Fig. 8.7). Skin bolus, which is essentially artificial tissue placed over the mastectomy incision or chest wall, will increase the radiation dose to that superficial tissue and is employed when there is concern for increased local recurrence. A mastectomy scar boost dose may be delivered with superficial electron therapy in typically five fractions, bringing the total dose to that site to approximate 60 Gy. In patients undergoing post-mastectomy reconstruction we rely upon the surgical team to give clearance before proceeding with radiation.

We employ a cardiac-sparing technique whenever cardiac tissue is determined to be at risk from radiation delivery (left- or right-sided primary breast cancer), or when internal mammary node coverage increases heart exposure to radiation. Optical surface management system technology can be used to monitor the patient's surface anatomy in real time to improve accuracy and facilitate breath-hold technique.

Other Radiation Therapy Indications

Male breast cancer (sex determined at birth) is treated similarly to female breast cancer in terms of treatment technique and dose. Given the infrequent diagnosis of male breast cancer, a multidisciplinary discussion and updated review of guidelines are indicated.

Occasionally neglected breast cancer will be diagnosed, and if significant pain or bleeding is present, a short course of palliative radiation may be beneficial. These patients typically have consultations with the breast surgeon, medical oncologist, and possibly palliative care team.

Recurrent breast cancer, with or without prior radiation, may be treated with radiation depending upon timing from the last treatment course and tentative treatment and surgical options. A metastatic workup is routinely performed, and multidisciplinary discussion follows.

Intraoperative Radiation Therapy as Adjunctive Treatment of Breast Cancer

This section discusses the role of intraoperative radiation therapy (IORT) in the treatment of breast cancer patients who are eligible for breast-conserving therapy (BCT). BCT is a listed option by the NCCN in their guidelines. BCT typically requires daily (5 days/week) radiation treatments for 3–6 weeks. Patients who travel far to radiation treatment centers may face transportation challenges, and in one report BCT compliance was shown to be inversely proportional to the distance of the closest radiation center.[20] One option to shorten the postoperative radiation course, in the appropriate low-risk woman, is IORT.

IORT represents direct targeting of the tumor bed during surgery after surgical removal of the tumor with sufficient margins, typically 2 mm. For breast cancer, IORT can be used as a substitute for a boost to the tumor bed, or in low-risk patients, as the only radiation treatment the patient will receive (IORT APBI).

Two modalities can deliver IORT in the operating room (OR): mobile LINACs that treat with electron beams; and mobile 50-kV low-energy X-ray units. There are currently two 50-kV systems used for IORT breast cancer treatment: Intrabeam (Carl Zeiss, Saarbrucken, Germany) and Xoft (iCad, Burlington, MA, USA). The Intrabeam applicator consists of different-sized plastic spheres ranging in diameter from 1.5 cm up to 5 cm, in 5-mm increments in sizes that fit over a rigid X-ray tube. The Xoft applicator is a double-lumen balloon used with balloon brachytherapy systems. Four balloons are currently available, depending on the

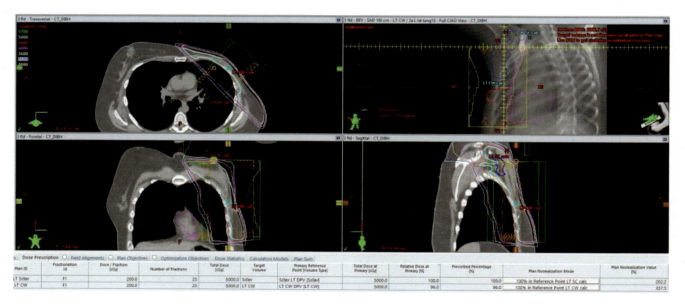

• **Fig. 8.7** Radiation isodose curves on a computed tomography simulation reconstruction showing axial, coronal, and sagittal coverage of radiation fields.

tumor size and shape: 3–4 cm, 4–5 cm, 5–6 cm, and a 5 × 7 cm elliptical balloon. The Xoft X-ray tube is on a flexible cable that can be inserted into the catheter of the double-lumen balloon. The Xoft system was designed to replace balloon brachytherapy devices but can also be used for IORT. Both devices require the use of mobile radiology shields to protect the personnel operating the equipment during the radiation procedure. There are also two commercial devices used for IORT with electrons: the Mobetron® (IntraOp Medical, Sunnyvale, CA, USA), which has a built-in beam shield so it can be used in most ORs without additional shielding; and the Liac (Sordina, Padova, Italy), which usually requires multiple mobile shields to be positioned around and under the surgical bed so it can be safely used in the OR. IORT when delivered with electrons is referred to as electron IORT or IOERT. These IORT modalities require specialized equipment and can be used in community cancer centers.

IORT as a Boost

External-beam radiation therapy (EBRT) boost is generally delivered in five fractions, following 3–5 weeks of WBI. The EBRT boost is intended to irradiate the excision cavity postoperatively, whereas an IORT or IOERT boost uses the direct visualization of the tumor bed during surgery and minimizes the risk of missing the tumor cavity.

IORT boost and IOERT boost have several similarities, despite having very different radiation distributions. Both treat subcutaneously, reducing skin toxicity with potentially better cosmesis, and both substitute for 1 week of EBRT boost treatment.

IORT boost for breast cancer was impractical prior to the development of mobile IORT technology, as patients had to be physically transported from the OR to the radiation oncology department, adding an hour or more to the surgical time.

Clinical Results for IOERT as a Boost

Montpellier[21] reported on long-term results for 50 patients treated with IOERT boost. Margins were assessed during the operation by frozen section, and all patients underwent a complete axillary lymph node dissection. The median dose delivered was 10 Gy to the 90% line. After IOERT, the temporary retaining sutures were removed and the tumor cavity was remodeled. The EBRT dose was 50 Gy in 25 fractions, delivered with cobalt radiation. Nodal irradiation was given as required. With a median follow-up of 9.1 years (range 5–15 years), they observed two local recurrences, one at 8 years and one at 14 years. Six additional patients had distant metastases, and 45 patients are alive, one with disease, giving a 10-year OS of 94%. All patients in their series had good to excellent cosmesis.

The University of Salzburg[22] treated two consecutive series of patients with stage I and II breast cancer. Group I consisted of 188 patients treated with BCS and postoperative

WBI, followed by a postoperative EBRT boost to the tumor bed. Group 2 comprised 190 patients treated with BCS, IOERT boost directly to the tumor bed, and postoperative WBI. The groups were comparable in regard to age, menopausal status, tumor size, histological type, grading, and axillary lymph node status. Applicators with diameters of 50–60 mm were used and a dose of 9 Gy was delivered to the 90% reference isodose using the appropriate energy for the tumor thickness. After median follow-ups of 81.0 and 51.1 months in Groups 1 and 2, respectively, no local recurrence was observed in the IOERT boost patients, while 12 IBTRs (6.4%) occurred in Group 1. The 5-year actuarial rates of IBTR were 4.3% and 0.0%, respectively (p = 0.0018). Distant metastases occurred in 24 patients (12.8%) and 8 patients (4.2%) in Groups 1 and 2, respectively, for 5-year actuarial rates of distant recurrence of 8.6% and 4.2% (p = 0.08). The 5-year disease-free survival (DFS) in Group 1 was 90.9% and in Group 2 was 95.8% (p = 0.064). With a more mature median follow-up period of 12.6 years for the patients treated with conventional BCT (Group 1), and 10.7 years for those receiving the IOERT boost (Group 2),[23] the IOERT group had an IBTR of 1.6% versus 7.2% (p = 0.0023) for the EBRT group. IOERT also had more favorable results for distant metastases and DFS, although with the small numbers in the study it did not achieve statistical significance.

A pooled analysis from seven European centers[24] combined and analyzed patients who were treated using IOERT boost plus 5 weeks of postoperative EBRT. There were 1109 patients treated between October 1998 and October 2005, 52% of whom had one or more risk factors for recurrence: young age (<40 years), positive nodes, high grade of tumor (G3), or larger tumors (T3). The patients in the study were all treated similarly to those in the Salzburg approach. With a median follow-up of 72.4 months, there were just 16 IBTRs (1.44%). DFS, disease-specific survival (DSS), and OS were 88.6%, 94.0%, and 91.3%, respectively. Young age is a risk factor, but the 5-year recurrence rate of 3.8% for the 53 women under the age of 40 years still compares very favorably with historical rates of 10% for this age group. In fact, IOERT boost results in lower recurrence rates in every age group compared to historic controls (Table 8.1).

San Felipi Neri Hospital[25] conducted a randomized trial comparing IOERT boost with EBRT boost. Women with T1–T2 breast cancer underwent conservative surgery and were randomly assigned to receive either IOERT boost (10 Gy) and postoperative EBRT (50 Gy), or postoperative EBRT (50 Gy) plus a 10-Gy EBRT boost. Patients with DCIS, invasive lobular carcinoma, or extensive intraductal component were excluded. IOERT was delivered using a single dose of 10 Gy with a radial margin of 2 cm and to a target depth of between 1.4 and 1.9 cm, using applicators with a 4–8-cm diameter. Surgical clips were positioned at the edge of irradiated areas in all patients. Following wound healing, patients received an additional 50 Gy EBRT to the whole breast, with 6–10 MeV photons. In the non-IOERT arm, a boost of 10 Gy in five fractions with a 6–12-MeV

TABLE 8.1	IOERT Boost Results by Patient Age Compared With Best EBRT Boost Results				
Age (Years)	Number of Patients	Follow-Up (Months and Range)	LR: Number of Patients	Annual Rate	Best EBRT Annual Rate
<40	53 (4.8%)	74.5 (15.5–126.0)	2 (3.7%)	0.64%	1.8%
40–49	234 (21.1%)	75.9 (4.8–187.9)	5 (2.1%)	0.34%	1.5%
50–59	326 (29.4%)	72.9 (3.8–208.5)	4 (1.2%)	0.21%	1.0%
<60	496 (44.7%)	73.0 (3.5–215.0)	5 (1.0%)	0.16%	0.6%

From the International Society of Intraoperative Radiation Therapy boost pooled analysis, modified from Fastner G et al.[6] Best EBRT rate is taken from data cited in Fastner G et al.[6] Note that IOERT boost provides lower local recurrence rates for every age group compared to EBRT boost.
EBRT, External-beam radiation therapy; *IOERT*, intraoperative electron radiotherapy.

electron beam was administered. From April 1999 to December 2004, 234 patients were randomized, 126 in the IOERT arm (with 131 treatments due to five bilateral neoplasms) and 118 in the non-IOERT arm. The mean age was 56.3 years (range, 29–75 years) in the IOERT arm, and 56.2 years (range, 34–75 years) in the non-IORT arm; 88 patients in the IOERT arm and 79 in the non-IOERT arm were premenopausal. Margins were negative in all patients. One local recurrence was observed in the IOERT arm (0.8%) and four in the non-IOERT arm (3.4%). Patients were salvaged with mastectomy. The Felipi Neri IOERT boost experience was updated at the Groupe Européen de Curiethérapie (GEC)-European Society for Radiotherapy and Oncology (ESTRO) Meeting in 2009.[26] With a median follow-up now of 68.8 months (range, 4–124 months), 223 patients had received an IOERT boost. There was one local failure (0.4%). DFS, DSS, and OS were 87.8%, 96.4%, and 94.6%, respectively. Distant metastases occurred in 16 patients (7.2%). Cosmetic evaluation was excellent or good in 88.3% of patients. Both acute and late toxicity were low (6.5% and 4.5%, respectively).

Fastner et al.[27] compared patients with locally advanced breast cancer treated with NACT followed by BCS and either an IOERT boost followed by WBI—Group I, or WBI followed by an EBRT boost—Group II. After a median follow-up of 59 months in Group I and 67.5 months in Group II, Group I had higher local control rates, locoregional control rates, and metastasis-free survival, and comparable rates for DSS and OS. Only two IBTRs occurred in Group I (2.5%), which compares favorably with an expected IBTR rate of 8% in studies[27] using NACT that did not include IOERT.

Clinical Results for IORT as a Boost

Vaidya et al.[28] reports on long-term results of IORT boost with 50 kV using the Intrabeam system. Three hundred cancers (299 patients) underwent BCS and 20 Gy as a boost to the tumor bed. A dose of 20 Gy to the surface of the applicator was administered, delivering 5–7 Gy of radiation 1 cm from the applicator surface. No tumors exceeded 4 cm in diameter and there was no restriction on tumor type, tumor grade, receptor status, or axillary node involvement. Of the 242 patients in whom systemic therapy was analyzed, 94 patients (31%) required adjuvant chemotherapy, and 195 patients (81%) received adjuvant hormonal therapy. All patients received 45–50 Gy of EBRT in 25 fractions over 5 weeks. If adjuvant chemotherapy was required, EBRT was delivered at its completion. With a median follow-up of 60.5 months (range, 10–122 months), eight patients have had an ipsilateral recurrence. The 5-year Kaplan-Meier estimate for recurrence was 1.73%, with five of eight recurrences identified within the tumor bed.

Many studies to date show that IORT boost with Intrabeam appears to provide an acceptable local control rate when compared with standard BCT. Long-term data requiring further follow-up is still needed in order to adequately assess cosmetic results.

There have also been several positive reports of IORT boost used after NACT.[29–31] Results are comparable with patients receiving conventional radiotherapy. There is currently no long-term data or follow-up from the iCad Xoft system when used as an IORT boost. Table 8.2 compares IORT/IOERT boost with conventional EBRT boost.

IORT as the Sole Radiation Treatment (IORT APBI)

Professional societies have provided guidelines to select which BCS patients may be suitable for APBI. APBI is a shortened radiation treatment for breast cancer, typically completed in 1 week or less. Both IORT and IOERT APBI are delivered before the final margin and nodal status is known. IORT APBI addresses this by treating the tumor as a boost if the final margin or nodal status is unfavorable. With IOERT APBI, there is no consensus on how to treat patients who are found to have unfavorable pathology, with each institution having its own approach. While both IORT and IOERT have been used in IORT APBI, there are significant differences in the two approaches (Table 8.3). In IOERT, the surgical remodeling of the breast parenchyma morphologically transforms the at-risk breast tissue so that it is compactly placed under the electron applicator.

TABLE 8.2 Comparison of IORT/IOERT Boost vs. EBRT Boost

Feature	IOERT/IORT Boost	EBRT Boost	Advantages of IOERT/IORT Boost
Skin dose	None with IOERT/IORT	Substantial	Subcutaneous delivery of IOERT/IORT eliminates skin boost dose
Size of boost volume	Typically, 25 mm^3 for a 1.5-cm tumor with IOERT[a]	Typically, 50 mm^3 for a 1.5-cm tumor	Smaller CTV should result in less toxicity
Number of fractions	1 treatment; IOERT adds 15–30 min to the surgical time; IORT 40–60 min	5 treatments; does not impact surgical time	IOERT/IORT eliminates ~1 week of treatment
Accuracy of radiation delivery	No chance for geometric miss of CTV[b]	Depends on imaging and varies center to center	Direct visualization of target makes IOERT/IORT superior method
Time of radiation boost	During surgery	9–40 weeks postsurgery	IOERT/IORT boost provides 1–2 log cell kill, reducing tumor burden for postoperative radiation
Breast size	Irrelevant with IOERT, as delivered directly to tumor bed. IORT may not be suitable for small-breasted women	Large-breasted women more challenging to boost	If volume to boost is deep-seated, more normal tissue must be irradiated with EBRT boost, compromising cosmesis
Dose uniformity	Excellent with IOERT. IORT is more nonhomogeneous but is compensated by postoperative EBRT	Excellent	Excellent
Ipsilateral recurrence	IOERT: <0.5% at 6 years; <1% at 10 years. IORT: 1.73% at 5 years	Typically, 3–4% at 5 years; Typically, 7–8% at 10 years	IOERT and IORT has a lower recurrence rate than EBRT boost
Cosmesis	90% good to excellent at 5 years+	70–85% long-term good to excellent cosmesis	30%+ of EBRT women unhappy with breast appearance after BCT

[a]With IORT, CTV is smaller than with EBRT boost. With IOERT, 2–3 cm of tissue adjacent to the tumor is included.
[b]Postoperative pathology administration of IORT requires reoperation and insertion of an applicator into the residual seroma from the excision cavity.
BCT, Breast-conserving therapy; *CTV*, clinical treatment volume; *EBRT*, external-beam radiation therapy; *IOERT*, intraoperative electron radiotherapy; *IORT*, intraoperative radiotherapy.

TABLE 8.3 Intraoperative Radiotherapy Versus Intraoperative Electron Radiotherapy

Method	Meets TV Concept of Holland	Homogeneity of Radiation Distribution	Can Treat Asymmetric PTV	Treatment Time	Added OR Time	Shielded OR
IORT	No	Poor[a]	No[b]	25–50 min[c]	~1 h	No
IOERT	Yes	Excellent	Yes	1–3 min[d]	15–30 min	No[e]

[a]20-Gy dose at the surface of the applicator falls to 5 Gy at 1 cm from the applicator surface.
[b]iCad Xoft has an elliptical balloon available that can account for some asymmetry.
[c]Treatment time is a function of applicator size.
[d]Treatment time is about 1 minute for boost and about 2 minutes for APBI. Conventional units take about twice as long.
[e]Depending on the OR, Liac and Novac often require about 1 ton of mobile shields to be positioned around and under the surgical bed prior to treatment. Conventional units always require a heavily shielded OR.
IOERT, Intraoperative electron radiotherapy; *IORT*, intraoperative radiotherapy; *OR*, operating room; *PTV*, planning treatment volume; *TV*, treatment volume.

Together with the temporary reapproximation of the tumor bed, which also places all of the tumor margins toward the center of the radiation field, irradiation of the microscopic disease that may extend 2–3 cm beyond the original tumor is delivered, consistent with the work of Holland et al.[32] and Faverly et al.,[33] ensuring that all margins receive a minimum dose of 18 Gy. This should be sufficient to sterilize any microscopic disease that remains.[34,35] IOERT adequately covers the tumor and tissue at risk, irrespective of the tumor shape.

Electron beam radiation generates more uniform dose distributions than those produced with 50-kV X-rays or brachytherapy. Treatment times are very short, only 1–2 min, compared with 30 or more minutes with 50-kV X-rays or brachytherapy. IOERT is the only APBI method that lends itself to immediate oncoplastic reconstruction, as the target volume receives all the radiation in the treatment.

Clinical Results for IORT/IOERT APBI

There have been two randomized studies comparing IORT (TARGIT-A)[28,36] and IOERT (ELIOT)[37] with conventional treatment.

The results for ELIOT[37,38] showed local recurrence for the IOERT group at 5 years and 10 years of 4.4% and 8.1%, respectively, and local recurrence for the EBRT group of 0.4% and 1.1%. (p < 0.0001). There was no difference in OS or DSS. While there were no differences for fibrosis, retraction, pain, or burning, there was a higher incidence of radiologically determined fat necrosis in the ELIOT group at 5% versus 2% for the EBRT group (p = 0.04).

Investigators did find a group of low-risk women who received IOERT APBI that had equivalent IBTRs to the EBRT group,[37] providing encouragement that in properly selected women and with proper IOERT technique, there may be a group of women suitable for IOERT APBI. In fact, a number of single-institution, nonrandomized publications have shown relatively low IBTR rates, comparable to those achieved with EBRT.

The University of Verona[39] treated 226 low-risk women with IOERT APBI. Only very low-risk patients were included, mostly women ≥50 years with biopsy-proven invasive ductal carcinoma who had low-grade G1 and G2 tumors ≤2 cm, and were N0, estrogen receptor-positive, and progesterone receptor-positive. The prescribed dose was 21 Gy to the 80% isodose line, ensuring that the entire target received at least 16.8 Gy, a dose they calculated had an equivalent biologically effective dose of 6 weeks of EBRT. The authors conclude that their data suggests that single-dose IOERT in highly selected patients with early-stage breast cancer can be safely delivered with good results. Long-term recurrence rates were low and 5-year median OS and local recurrence free survival rates were comparable with data in the literature on EBRT, thus encouraging the use of IOERT in low-risk patients with early-stage breast cancer.

Bergamo[40] treated 758 patients with BCS and IOERT. With a median follow-up of 5.2 years, the 360 patients who they considered low risk or suitable for this approach (age >50 years, tumor size ≤2 cm, pN0 or Nmic, Ki67 ≤20%, G1–G2, nontriple-negative and nonlobular cancer) had a 5-year local failure of 1.8% versus 11.6% for those who were unsuitable. The 116 patients who were American Society for Radiation Oncology (ASTRO) suitable had an even lower level of IBTR of 1.2%.

At ESTRO 2020, Bordet[41] reported on 681 women treated with IOERT. With a 5-year median follow-up, there were 24 relapses (3.2%) but only 8 (1.2%) true recurrences.

APBI Clinical Results: Orthovoltage (50-kV X-rays) Prospective Randomized Results

The TARGIT-A Trial[36] was an intent-to-treat, noninferiority trial in which 2232 patients from 33 centers in 11 countries were randomized to either TARGIT or 5 weeks of EBRT with or without an EBRT boost, depending on the treatment policy of the individual treatment center. The TARGIT arm allowed conversion from IORT APBI to IORT boost if the patient presented with adverse factors after randomization. They call this approach "risk-adapted IORT."

The 2014 Lancet publication[42] demonstrated a local failure rate in the TARGIT group 2% higher than in the EBRT group, and this difference was statistically significant (p = 0.042). The TARGIT group also did worse than the EBRT group for locoregional recurrence (p = 0.02) and showed a worsening trend for overall recurrences (ipsilateral, contralateral, axilla, and distant). There were 69 breast events in the TARGIT arm versus 48 in the standard arm. Postpathology TARGIT patients had worse local recurrence than prepathology TARGIT patients, compared to their respective EBRT group (5.4% vs. 1.7%). For prepathology TARGIT patients, the local recurrence was 2.1% versus 1.0% in the EBRT group.

The TARGIT study had 33 centers in 11 countries and lasted more than 12 years. When the TARGIT-A study was updated with a longer follow-up,[43] the 5-year recurrence rate was 2.11% for TARGIT-IORT versus 0.95% for EBRT. Sasieni and Sawyer[44] argue that the evidence remains insufficient for the use of IORT in women with early-stage breast cancer outside of a clinical trial. They see no reason to change the ASTRO consensus statement "low-energy X-ray IORT should continue to be used [only] within the context of a prospective registry or clinical trial to ensure long-term local control and toxicity outcomes are prospectively monitored."[18] They further argue that promoting the superiority of IORT because the 5-year local recurrence is <3.5% is meaningless, since no radiotherapy for women over the age of 65 years[16] has the same difference between those receiving surgery alone and those receiving radiotherapy.

Consistent with GEC-ESTRO guidelines, it is recommended that IORT photon therapy be used only in a clinical trial or in a prospective registry setting.[45]

A new Phase II trial for a low-risk group of women 70 years and older, TARGIT-E, is now recruiting patients. It is based on the TARGIT-A trial and allows both pre- and postpathology patients and conversion of prepathology patients from IORT APBI to IORT boost. Since each participating institution has the option to modify the entry criteria and the criteria to convert patients to IORT boost, this study contains the same design flaws already pointed out in the TARGIT-A analysis. The study intended to accrue patients through 2015 and expects 10 years of follow-up. The primary end point is local recurrence, and the stopping point at 5 years is 4% (which, interestingly, is the same recurrence that has been obtained in the trial of BCS + tamoxifen, with or without radiotherapy).[46]

There have been no randomized studies using the iCad Xoft system. Xoft does have the advantage over the

Intrabeam device in that, similar to balloon brachytherapy devices, it can be used postoperatively in APBI treatments.

Most reported Xoft IORT studies have few patients and very immature follow-up (12–30 months). One long-term study with 5-years median follow-up,[47] reported at an ASTRO meeting, had only 68 patients, reporting a recurrence rate of 5.8%. Silverstein et al.[48] does report on a more mature and robust study of Xoft IORT. Patients over the age of 40 years with invasive ductal carcinoma, invasive lobular carcinoma, or DCIS and tumors with a maximum tumor extent of 3 cm as determined by mammography, ultrasonography, or MRI were allowed. To be eligible for IORT as the sole radiation treatment, final histopathology had to confirm tumor extent ≤3 cm, tumor margins ≥2 mm, no extensive lymphovascular invasion, negative axillary lymph nodes, and skin-to-balloon spacing of at least 8 mm. Patients who exhibited one or more of these exclusionary parameters were referred to additional surgery (excision or mastectomy) and/or whole breast radiation therapy, with the IORT becoming the boost. If a positive lymph node was discovered intraoperatively, IORT was not performed and these patients were not included in the analysis. For the entire cohort of patients, the probability of local recurrence at 4 years was 3.9%. There were only two (1.3%) recurrences in the 164 patients that did not receive IORT as their sole treatment. The analysis was updated in 2022.[49] With 1400 tumors (33 bilateral) and a median follow-up of 62 months, the local recurrence rate for the 1175 patients treated with IORT alone had a 5-year recurrence rate of 5.98%, while those treated by adding whole breast radiation therapy had a 5-year recurrence rate of <1%. The 5-year probability of local recurrence for ASTRO-suitable patients was 4.31%, for Grade 1 tumors it was 2.91%, and for patients aged ≥70 years it was 2.41%. These authors state that their data support stricter selection criteria for IORT.

Conclusion

Both IORT and IOERT, delivered as a boost, provide good cosmetic results and potential cost savings for patients. ASTRO guidelines say that patients choosing IOERT APBI should be used only in patients meeting ASTRO APBI guidelines and cautioned that the recurrence rate may be slightly higher than with conventional approaches, although the survival will be comparable. ASTRO guidelines also recommend that IORT APBI be given only as part of a study or registry. This is consistent with the National Institute for Health and Care Excellence recommendations that limit IORT APBI participants to trials and registries.

References

1. Becquerel H. Emission of the new radiations by metallic uranium. *CR Acad Sci*. 1896;122:1086–1088.
2. Roentgen WC. Uber eine neue art von strahlen. Sitzgsber Physik-Med Ges. Wuerzburg. 1895;137:132–141.
3. Curie P, Curie MS. Sur une substance nouvelle radioactive, contenue dans la pechblende. *CR Acad Sci*. 1898;127:175–178.

4. Hutchinson F. Molecular basis for action of ionizing radiations. *Science*. 1961;134:533–538.
5. Hoskin P. The price of anticancer intervention. Secondary malignancies after radiotherapy. *Lancet Oncol*. 2002 Sep;3(9):577–578. [PubMed: 12233734].
6. Clarke M, Collins R, Darby S, et al. Effects of radiotherapy and of differences in the extent of surgery for early breast cancer on local recurrence and 15-year survival: an overview of the randomised trials. *Lancet*. 2005;366(9503):2087–2106.
7. Jerkehagen B, Smeland S, Walberg L, et al. Radiation induced sarcoma: 25-year experience from the Norwegian Radium Hospital. *Acta Oncol*. 2008;47(8):1475–1482.
8. Swerdlow AJ, Barber JA, Hudson GV, et al. Risk of second malignancy after Hodgkin's disease in a collaborative British cohort: the relation to age at treatment. *J Clin Oncol*. 2000;18(3):498–509.
9. Benveniste MF, Gomez D, Carter BW, et al. Recognizing radiation therapy-related complications in the chest. *Radiographics*. 2019;39(2):344–366.
10. Kerlikowske K. Epidemiology of ductal carcinoma in situ. *J Natl Cancer Inst Monogr*. 2010;2010(41):139–141.
11. Cutuli B, Lemanski C, De Lafontan B, et al. Ductal carcinoma in situ: a French national survey. Analysis of 2125 patients. *Clin Breast Cancer*. 2020 Apr;20(2):e164–e172.
12. Fisher B, Dignam J, Wolmark N, et al. Lumpectomy and radiation therapy for the treatment of intraductal breast cancer: findings from National Surgical Adjuvant Breast and Bowel Project B-17. *J Clin Oncol*. 1998 Feb;16(2):441–452.
13. Early Breast Cancer Trialists' Collaborative Group (EBCTCG) Overview of the randomized trials of radiotherapy in ductal carcinoma in situ of the breast. *JCNI Monographs*. 2010;2010(41):162–177.
14. McCormick B, Winter KA, Woodward W, et al. Randomized phase iii trial evaluating radiation following surgical excision for good-risk ductal carcinoma in situ: long-term report from NRG Oncology/RTOG 9804. *J Clin Oncol*. 2021 Nov 10;39(32):3574–3582. https://doi.org/10.1200/JCO.21.01083.Epub 2021 Aug 18. PMID: 34406870; PMCID: PMC8577682.
15. Early Breast Cancer Trialists' Collaborative Group (EBCTCG) Darby S, McGale P, Correa C, et al. Effect of radiotherapy after breast conserving surgery on 10-year recurrence and 15-year breast cancer death: meta-analysis of individual patient data for 10,801 women in 17 randomized trials. *Lancet*. 2011 Nov 12;378(9804):1707–1716.
16. Kunkler IH, Williams LJ, Jack WJL, Cameron DA, Dixon JM. PRIME II investigators. Breast-conserving surgery with or without irradiation in women aged 65 years or older with early breast cancer (PRIME II): a randomised controlled trial. *Lancet Oncol*. 2015 Mar;16(3):266–273. https://doi.org/10.1016/S1470-2045(14)71221-5.Epub 2015 Jan 28.
17. Murray Brunt A, Haviland JS, Wheatley DA. Hypofractionated breast radiotherapy for 1 week versus 3 weeks (FAST-Forward): 5-year efficacy and late normal tissue effects results from a multicentre, non-inferiority, randomised, phase 3 trial. *Lancet*. 2020;395(10237):1613–1626.
18. Correa C, Harris EE, Leonardi MC, et al. Accelerated partial breast irradiation: executive summary for the update of an ASTRO Evidence-Based Consensus Statement. *Pract Radiat Oncol*. 2017 Mar-Apr;7(2):73–79. https://doi.org/10.1016/j.pro.2016.09.007.Epub 2016 Sep 17. PMID: 27866865.
19. Meattini I, Marrazzo L, Saieva C, et al. Accelerated partial-breast irradiation compared with whole-breast irradiation for early breast cancer: long-term results of the randomized phase III APBI-IMRT-Florence trial. *J Clin Oncol*.

20. Athas WF, Adams-Cameron M, Hunt WC, Amir-Fazli A, Key CR. Travel distance to radiation therapy and receipt of radiotherapy following breast-conserving surgery. *J Natl Cancer Inst.* 2000;92:269–271.

21. Lemanski C, Azria D, Thezenas S, et al. Intraoperative radiotherapy given as a boost for early breast cancer: long-term clinical and cosmetic results. *Int J Radiat Oncol Biol Phys.* 2006;64(5):1410–1415.

22. Reitsamer R, Peintinger F, Kopp M, Menzel C, Kogelnik HD, Sedlmayer F. Local recurrence rates in breast cancer patients treated with Intraoperative electron-boost radiotherapy versus postoperative external beam electron-boost irradiation. A sequential intervention study. *Strahlenther Onkol.* 2004;180(1):38–44.

23. Fastner G, Reitsamer R, Kopp M, et al. *IOERT versus conventional boost during breast conserving therapy: 10-year results of a matched pair analysis.* Scottsdale: Presented at the ISIORT meeting; 2010.(now in publication).

24. Fastner G, Sedlmayer F, Merz F, et al. IORT with electrons as boost strategy during breast conserving therapy in limited stage breast cancer: long term results of an ISIORT pooled analysis. *Radiother Oncol.* 2013;108(2):279–286.

25. Ciabattoni A, Petrucci A, Palloni T, et al. IORT in breast cancer as boost: preliminary results of a pilot randomized study. *Suppl Tumori.* 2005;4(6):S53–S58.

26. Ciabattoni A, Ciccone V, Palloni T, et al. *IORT as anticipated boost in stage I and II breast cancer: long term follow-up results.* Barcelona: Presented at the GEC ESTRO meeting; 2009.(in publication).

27. Fastner G, Reitsamer R, Ziegler I, et al. IOERT as anticipated tumor bed boost during breast-conserving surgery after neoadjuvant chemotherapy in locally advanced breast cancer-results of a case series after 5-year follow-up. *Int. J. Cancer.* 2015;136(5):1193–1201.

28. Vaidya JS, Baum M, Tobias JS, et al. Long-term results of targeted intraoperative radiotherapy (Targit) boost during breast conserving surgery. *Int J Radiat Oncol Biol Phys.* 2011;81(4): 1091–1097.

29. Kolberg HC, Lövey G, Akpolat-Basci L, et al. Targeted intraoperative radiotherapy tumour bed boost during breast-conserving surgery after neoadjuvant chemotherapy: a subgroup analysis of hormone receptor-positive HER2-negative breast cancer. *Breast Care (Basel).* 2017 Oct;12(5):318–323.

30. Kolberg HC, Loevey G, Akpolat-Basci L, et al. Targeted intraoperative radiotherapy tumour bed boost during breast-conserving surgery after neoadjuvant chemotherapy. *Strahlenther Onkol.* 2017 Jan;193(1):62–69.

31. Kolberg HC, Loevey G, Akpolat-Basci L, et al. Targeted intraoperative radiotherapy tumour bed boost during breast conserving surgery after neoadjuvant chemotherapy in HER2 positive and triple negative breast cancer. *Rev Recent Clin Trials.* 2017;12(2):93–100.

32. Holland R, Veling SHJ, Mravunac M, Hendriks JHCL. Histologic multifocality of tis, T1–2 breast carcinomas implications for clinical trials of breast-conserving surgery. *Cancer.* 1985;56(5):979–990.

33. Faverly DR, Hendricks JH, Holland R. Breast carcinomas of limited extent: frequency, radiologic-pathologic characteristics, and surgical margin requirements. *Cancer.* 2001;91(4):647–659.

34. Nairz O, Deutschmann H, Kopp M, et al. A dosimetric comparison of IORT techniques in limited-stage breast cancer. *Strahlenther Onkol.* 2006 Jun;182(6):342–348.

35. Guenzi M, Fozza A, Blandino G, et al. Focus on the actual clinical target volume irradiated with intraoperative radiotherapy for breast cancer. *Anticancer Res.* 2012 Nov;32(11):4945–4950.

36. Vaidya JS, Joseph DJ, Tobias JS, et al. Targeted intraoperative radiotherapy versus whole breast radiotherapy for breast cancer (TARGIT-A trial): and international, prospective, randomised, non-inferiority phase 3 trial. *Lancet.* 2010;376(9735): 91–102.

37. Veronesi U, Orecchia R, Maisonneuve P, et al. Intraoperative radiotherapy versus external radiotherapy for early breast cancer (ELIOT): a randomized controlled equivalence trial. *Lancet Oncol.* 2013;14(13):1269–1277.

38. Orecchia R, Veronesi U, Maisonneuve P, et al. Intraoperative irradiation for early breast cancer (ELIOT): long-term recurrence and survival outcomes from a single-centre, randomised, phase 3 equivalence trial. *Lancet Oncol.* 2021 May;22(5):597–608.

39. Maluta S, Dall'oglio S, Marciai N, et al. Accelerated partial breast irradiation using only intraoperative electron radiation therapy in early stage breast cancer. *Int. J. Rad. Onc. Biol. Phys.* 2012;84(2):145–152.

40. Takanen S, Gambirasio A, Gritti G, et al. Breast cancer electron intraoperative radiotherapy: assessment of preoperative selection factors from a retrospective analysis of 758 patients and review of literature. *Breast Cancer Res Treat.* 2017 Sep;165(2): 261–271.

41. Philippson C, Simon S, Vandekerkhove C, et al. Early invasive ductal breast cancer: review after 5-year median follow-up of the first 681 patients treated by partial breast irradiation with intraoperative electron radiation therapy. *Eur J. Cancer.* 2020;138(Suppl 1):Poster 334.

42. Vaidya JS, Wenz F, Bulsara M, et al. Risk-adapted targeted intraoperative radiotherapy versus whole-breast radiotherapy for breast cancer: 5-year results for local control and overall survival from the TARGIT-A randomized trial. *Lancet.* 2014;383:603–613.

43. Vaidya JS, Bulsara M, Baum M, et al. Long term survival and local control outcomes from single dose targeted intraoperative radiotherapy during lumpectomy (TARGIT-IORT. for early breast cancer: TARGIT-A randomised clinical trial. *BMJ.* 2020;370:m2836.

44. Sasieni PD, Sawyer EJ. Intraoperative radiotherapy for early stage breast cancer-insufficient evidence to change practice. *Nat Rev Clin Oncol.* 2020(12):723–724.

45. Kirby AM. Updated ASTRO guidelines on accelerated partial breast irradiation (APBI): to whom can we offer APBI outside a clinical trial? *Br J Radiol.* 2018 May;91(1085):20170565.

46. Hughes KS, Schnaper LA, Berry D, et al. Eastern Cooperative Oncology Group. Lumpectomy plus tamoxifen with or without irradiation in women 70 years of age or older with early breast cancer Radiation Therapy Oncology Group. *N Engl J Med.* 2004;351(10):971–977.

47. Dickler A, Ivanov O, Syed AM, et al. Five year results of a multicenter trial utilizing electronic brachytherapy to deliver intraoperative radiation therapy in the treatment of early-stage breast cancer. *Int J Radiat Oncol Biol Phys.* 2015;93:E24–E25.

48. Silverstein M, Epstein M, Kim B, et al. Intraoperative radiation therapy (IORT): a series of 1000 tumors. *Ann Surg Oncol.* 2018;25:2987–2993.

49. Silverstein M, Epstein M, Chen P, et al. Recurrence and survival rates for 1400 early breast tumors treated with intraoperative radiation therapy (IORT). *Ann Surg Oncol.* 2022;29(6): 3726–3736.

9
Systemic Therapy for Breast Cancer

SIGRUN HALLMEYER, RUBINA QAMAR, AND COREY J. SHAMAH

Introduction

As the reader will see in this chapter, systemic treatment for all stages of breast cancer is complex and rapidly changing. There are many "approved" therapies that can be submitted to insurance companies for approval in determining treatment for a given patient. One of the reasons why our group has made the decision to follow pathways in the selection of treatments for cancer patients is to prioritize clinical trials (to gain new knowledge) and to offer patients the best evidence-based care. As a group, we have been following the Elsevier ClinicalPath system, formerly known as Via Oncology Pathways. After reviewing different pathways programs, this system was selected for several reasons:

- The evidence-based pathways were prioritized and selected by practicing community and academic oncologists.
- Each disease-specific committee has both academic and community oncologist chairs and members.
- Committee meetings are held virtually every quarter for review of the pathways. Changes can be made at these meetings if new evidence is available. Urgent meetings can be held if new field-changing information is released.
- All of our oncologists who regularly treat patients with any given disease are encouraged to attend and actively participate in the disease-specific committees.
- The pathways allow clinical trials to be prioritized as the first recommendation.
- Pathways are ranked by efficacy (most), toxicity (lesser), and cost (least), prioritized in this order.
- In addition to a clinical trial option, for each stage of disease there are several "recommended" pathways from which the physician can select. They can also choose to treat "off-pathway" if they believe this is in the best interest of the patient.

Unlike guidelines, such as National Comprehensive Cancer Network where multiple recommendations are listed, we felt it was most important to have recommendations prioritized so that we could collect and evaluate the data of a large number of similarly staged patients treated the same way. This has also allowed us to offer and accrue a large number of patients to clinical trials to help move the field forward.

Oncologists in our group are encouraged to follow the recommended pathways, always offering their patients the ability to participate in clinical trials and to be involved in the decision-making process. The physicians have the opportunity to deviate from the recommended pathway if they believe there are reasons why the recommended treatment is not the best for a given patient. For most diseases, between 85% and 92% of patients are treated on pathway. This chapter is broken down into three main parts:

1. Neoadjuvant therapy
2. Adjuvant therapy
3. Treatment of metastatic disease

Neoadjuvant Therapy for Breast Cancer

Introduction

Historical Perspective

The term *neoadjuvant therapy for breast cancer* is used in a setting where systemic therapy is utilized prior to definitive surgery. Historically, this treatment approach has been reserved for patients who had clinically unresectable disease, or for locally advanced patients who require a mastectomy to appropriately resect the entire tumor. For patients desiring breast conservation, neoadjuvant chemotherapy has been used to convert from mastectomy to lumpectomy for patients who achieve sufficient response. For this purpose, the treatment had been largely limited to the administration of neoadjuvant multiagent *chemo*therapy and has been largely limited to serve surgical outcomes.

Current Goals of Neoadjuvant Therapy

With the advent of more targeted agents, additional goals of neoadjuvant therapy have been identified. Beyond the surgical goal of transforming a patient for mastectomy to lumpectomy or from unresectable to resectable, the goal of neoadjuvant therapy is now also to quantify the tumor's response to neoadjuvant therapy to prognosticate short and long-term outcomes, and to delineate adjuvant therapy strategies after surgery. Based on the response achieved, the best adjuvant

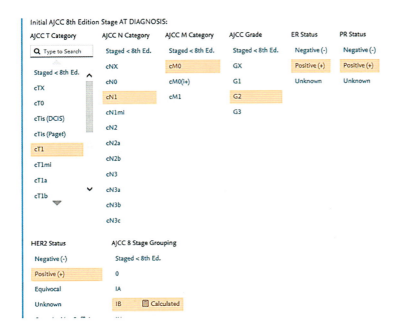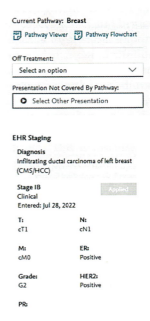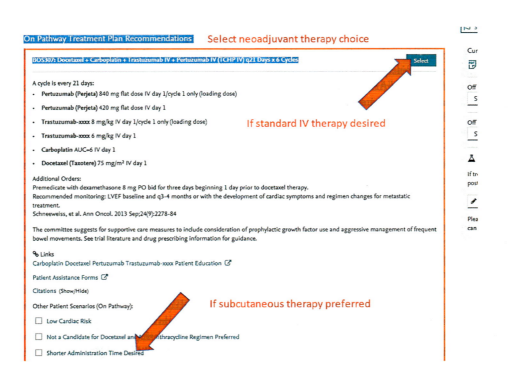

CHAPTER 9 Systemic Therapy for Breast Cancer

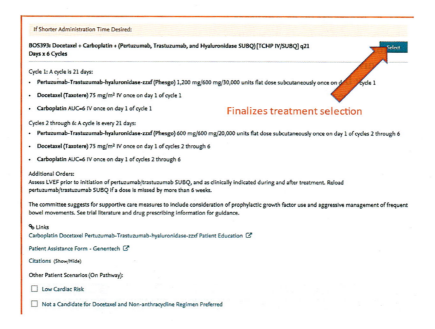

New formulations of the monoclonal antibodies targeting the HER2 domain have recently been developed and FDA approved, and are readily available in our pharmacies. These products are available for subcutaneous injection as single-agent preparations for trastuzumab, or as combination preparations for trastuzumab and pertuzumab. These formulations are considered interchangeable to the IV formulations and have quickly become part of our repertoire for patients in the neoadjuvant and adjuvant setting.

An example of the pathway that can be used in this setting is shown below:

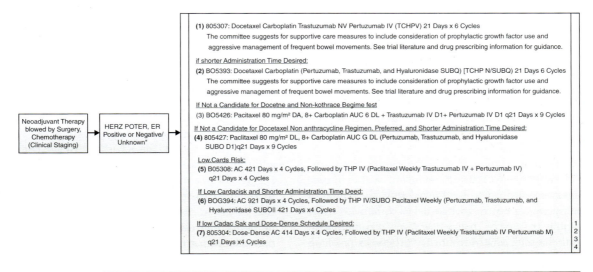

Endocrine Therapy

The approach to neoadjuvant therapy with endocrine agents has been studied in both the premenopausal and postmenopausal setting, with significant and notable differences. Much of the comparison of the neoadjuvant approach in treatment (principally chemotherapy vs. endocrine therapy) is based on the toxicity profile and response rates achieved, and many clinical trials are designed around these two endpoints and do not give a lot of information in regard to long-term outcomes such as event-free or OS.

Several clinical trials have shown that neoadjuvant endocrine therapy is inferior in producing high rates of clinical and pathologic response in premenopausal patients. However, this is in contrast to other data that show quite comparable response rates and breast-conservation rates in postmenopausal patients receiving either neoadjuvant endocrine therapy or neoadjuvant chemotherapy, as demonstrated in a meta-analysis including almost 3500 patients.[8] Based on this available data, one can anticipate a response rate to neoadjuvant endocrine therapy in the 60–70% range; however the complete pathologic response rate is only 1–3% after 3 months of exposure. This does not differ significantly from neoadjuvant chemotherapy outcomes for these ER-positive postmenopausal patients. Long-term follow-up in this clinical dataset shows no significant difference in local recurrences, and toxicity rates are significantly improved with endocrine therapy compared to chemotherapy, which is of course not surprising.

Based on this data, neoadjuvant endocrine therapy is typically reserved for patients who are treated in the postmenopausal setting. In the rare setting of a premenopausal patient presenting to our institutions with indication for neoadjuvant endocrine therapy, we typically strive to utilize ovarian suppression (OFS) with aromatase inhibitor (Ai)-based endocrine therapy as our treatment approach.

It is well understood that the full benefit of neoadjuvant endocrine therapy may not be achieved until at least 3–4 months of therapy, and in many instances not until even later. At our institutions, we typically administer neoadjuvant endocrine therapy in the appropriate setting for at least 4 months, and in many settings much longer. Much of the data that was accumulated more recently during the COVID-19 pandemic was driven by the fact that definitive surgical interventions had to be delayed to spare ventilator use in the operating room, and to delay patient exposure to the hospital setting. In that, we have used neoadjuvant endocrine therapy in patients that may otherwise not have qualified for neoadjuvant therapy (e.g., smaller tumors, node-negative disease) and have seen quite significant responses even in small tumors. With that, the indication for neoadjuvant endocrine therapy has broadened and is typically utilized in patients who meet criteria for endocrine therapy and do not have clinical, pathologic, or molecular evidence of benefiting from chemotherapy (Oncotype, MammaPrint), but would benefit from a neoadjuvant treatment approach based on disease extent or based on a desire to delay definitive surgical intervention. The treatment we utilize are AIs, which we use essentially interchangeably in this setting (anastrozole, letrozole, exemestane). Although there is some preliminary data on the efficacy of fulvestrant, this is not routinely used at our institutions in the neoadjuvant setting.

Immunotherapy

The addition of immunotherapy to neoadjuvant treatment has been explored in multiple settings and achieved FDA approval based on the KEYNOTE-522 trial in June 2021.[9]

This trial showed that the addition of pembrolizumab to neoadjuvant multiagent chemotherapy containing Taxol, carboplatin, Adriamycin, and Cytoxan improves the pathologic complete response rates from 51% to 65%, regardless of the PD-L1 status. This translated to a 37% improvement in event-free survival at the subsequent updated analysis, and a measurable benefit was seen across patients with either node-positive or node-negative presentation. With this data emerging, the KEYNOTE-522 regimen has become the standard of care at our institutions, and at this time is considered for all patients fit for this treatment and considered to be good candidates for neoadjuvant therapy in the triple-negative setting.

The IMpassion031 clinical trial utilized atezolizumab in addition to nab-paclitaxel, Adriamycin, and Cytoxan in the neoadjuvant setting, and showed very promising results with respect to improvement in complete pathological response rates that increased from 41% to 58%. This clinical trial was not powered to assess long-term differences in event-free survival rates. This stands in contrast to the NeoTRIPaPDL1 trial,[10] which showed no improvement with the addition of atezolizumab to carboplatin and nab-paclitaxel-based neoadjuvant chemotherapy. With that, atezolizumab is not currently the standard of care in the neoadjuvant triple-negative breast cancer setting at our institutions.

As much as immunotherapy has very recently changed the paradigm in the treatment of neoadjuvant therapy for triple-negative breast cancer, it has also created some additional complexities, including questions in the adjuvant setting after surgery. The KEYNOTE-522 regimen utilizes additional therapy with pembrolizumab in the adjuvant setting, and that competes with other current standards of care that include the recommendation for adjuvant therapy with Xeloda in patients having significant residual disease after neoadjuvant treatment (CREATE-X trial),[11] and adjuvant poly(adenosine diphosphate–ribose) polymerase (PARP) inhibitor therapy for patients carrying the BRCA mutation (Olympia trial).[12] This means that adjuvant therapy in triple-negative disease is highly individualized after neoadjuvant therapy followed by surgery. The treatment selection is based on multiple disease and patient-specific characteristics, and is typically managed in consultation with the multidisciplinary team that includes a surgeon, radiologist, radiation oncologist, medical oncologist, geneticist, pathologist, and often a plastic surgeon.

Post-Treatment Assessment and Management

Since one major goal of neoadjuvant therapy is to aid in surgical resection, we typically aim to proceed with definitive surgical resection within 4–6 weeks after completion of neoadjuvant treatment. The same clinical and radiographic evaluation utilized pretreatment should be repeated at that time, and typically includes a contrast-enhanced breast MRI, unless the radiologist feels that the pretreatment ultrasound was more effective in assessing the true extent of the disease. The role of repeat radiographic assessment is less clear in patients who had pretreatment evidence of multicentric disease or other medical or surgical contraindications for breast conservation, in which setting pursuit of mastectomy without post-neoadjuvant treatment imaging is reasonable.

Principles of Surgery in the Neoadjuvant Setting: Management of the Primary Tumor and the Axilla

Whether the patient is ultimately a candidate for breast conservation following neoadjuvant therapy depends on the response to this treatment and the size of the residual disease in relation to the patient's breast size. In the event of multicentric disease at presentation, breast conservation is not recommended even if a complete clinical/radiographic response is noted. Of course, a multitude of personal and other medical/surgical factors will influence the choice for mastectomy versus breast conservation. The surgical management of the primary breast tumor is discussed in the surgery chapter, and generally also applies here in the post-neoadjuvant setting.

Patients with initially clinically and radiographically node-negative disease typically are subjected to sentinel lymph node biopsy at the time of definitive breast surgery following neoadjuvant treatment.

Patients who initially present with radiographically suspicious lymph nodes undergo pathologic evaluation of those lymph nodes via core biopsy prior to neoadjuvant treatment in our institutions. The biopsied lymph nodes are marked with a radiopaque device and the marked and pathologically involved lymph node is required to be surgically removed at the time of axillary staging. Pre-neoadjuvant sentinel lymph node biopsy is generally discouraged, but in rare circumstances is indicated to clarify the pretreatment staging.

For patients who have extensive nodal involvement prior to neoadjuvant therapy (cN2 or cN3 disease), we generally still perform more generous axillary dissections at the time of definitive surgical intervention even if clinically and radiographically significant or even complete responses are encountered. However in the setting of N1 disease, the management of the axilla depends on the response to treatment. Patients who still have clinically and/or radiographically evident lymph node involvement are typically subjected to an axillary dissection, whereas patients who have clinically and radiographically excellent responses to neoadjuvant therapy are assessed with sentinel lymph node biopsy. In that setting, we require that the previously biopsied and involved

lymph node (identified by radiopaque marker) needs to be part of the axillary/sentinel lymph node sampling. In order to aid in that requirement, it has become our standard practice to mark involved lymph nodes with a Savi scout that can be intraoperatively detected by the surgeon.

Principles of Radiation in the Neoadjuvant Setting

Adjuvant radiation therapy is offered to all patients undergoing breast conservation following neoadjuvant therapy, as would be considered the standard of care in any other breast-conserving setting. For patients with persistent lymph node involvement after neoadjuvant treatment, comprehensive nodal radiation is offered to all patients as well. We offer sentinel lymph node biopsy only in patients who had limited (N1) clinical/pathologic evidence of lymph node involvement prior to neoadjuvant therapy but were successfully downstaged at the time of surgery (ypN0). The role of nodal radiation therapy in this setting remains unclear at this time and multiple clinical trials are currently ongoing that are investigating the role of radiation versus observation in this particular setting. Many of our radiation oncology groups are participating in those trials.

Pathology Assessment Post-Neoadjuvant Therapy

The pathologist plays a key role in the assessment of the patient's specimen following neoadjuvant therapy. With the advent and rapid adoption of neoadjuvant therapy in breast cancer, the American Joint Committee on Cancer updated its staging system to include a category of staging criteria specifically designed to assess disease extent following neoadjuvant therapy (ypT and ypN staging).

In addition to the anatomic staging assessment, residual cancer burden (RCB) calculators have been developed. These provide a standardized approach to the assessment of residual disease in the tumor bed and lymph nodes following neoadjuvant therapy. Scores calculated utilizing this tool are known to correlate tightly with recurrence-free survival at 10 years and are divided into RCB-0, which is synonymous with a complete pathologic response, and then range from RCB-I through RCB-III. We recently updated the requirements for our system-wide pathology reporting to include the RCB score in all patients receiving neoadjuvant therapy. Using the RCB to estimate a patient's risk of disease recurrence helps the medical oncologist tailor additional adjuvant therapy.

Adjuvant Therapy After Neoadjuvant Treatment

For most patients undergoing neoadjuvant therapy, systemic treatment does not stop at the time of surgery.

Patients with ER-positive disease typically receive at least 5 years of adjuvant endocrine therapy regardless of their response to the neoadjuvant treatment. For premenopausal patients, especially those under the age of 35 years and who resume menstrual periods following neoadjuvant therapy, we also recommend ovarian function suppression as part of the endocrine therapy. In patients with significant lymph nodal involvement, the addition of abemaciclib has been shown to benefit patients in the adjuvant setting and is typically included for 2 years following their definitive surgery, in addition to the routine standard endocrine therapy.

Patients with triple-negative disease who still have residual disease following neoadjuvant treatment are commonly subjected to additional adjuvant therapy with either Xeloda, pembrolizumab, or a PARP inhibitor. The systemic adjuvant therapy chosen depends on several factors: if they received neoadjuvant chemoimmunotherapy following the KEYNOTE-522 regimen (pembrolizumab), if they have significant residual disease (Xeloda based on the CREATE-X trial), or if they are BRCA mutation carriers (PARP inhibitor).

In patients with HER2/neu-positive disease, the adjuvant therapy routinely includes continued HER2/neu-targeted monoclonal antibody therapy with either trastuzumab and pertuzumab or TDM1 for the total duration of 1 year. Based on the KATHERINE clinical trial, TDM1 is the preferred agent in patients who have residual disease following neoadjuvant therapy.

Adjuvant Treatment of Breast Cancer

Adjuvant therapy is an additional cancer treatment given after the primary treatment to lower the risk of cancer recurrence. The adjuvant therapy decision is based on tumor characteristics and its impact on the risk of cancer recurrence with local therapy, any prior neoadjuvant therapy, as well as the benefit and toxicity of the adjuvant therapy and the patient comorbidities.

The adjuvant systemic therapy decision in breast cancer is based on hormone receptor (HR) and HER2 status, as well as the risk of cancer recurrence based on anatomic and pathologic characteristics. In this section, we will discuss systemic adjuvant therapy including chemotherapy and endocrine therapy, as well as HER2-targeted therapy. Recently approved PARP inhibitors and cyclin-dependent kinase (CDK)4/6 inhibitors will also be discussed. Briefly, the supportive role of bisphosphonates in the adjuvant setting and the role of immunotherapy will also be discussed.

The HR-positive and HER2-negative breast cancer subtype is the most common subtype, with an age-adjusted rate of 87.4 new breast cases per 100,000 women based on 2015–2019 cases. This is followed by the HR-negative/HER2-negative subtype with an age-adjusted rate of 13.2 new cases per 100,000, HR-positive/HER2-positive with an age-adjusted rate of 12.9, and HR-negative/HER2-positive with an age-adjusted rate of 5.2.[13]

Hormone Receptor–Positive and HER2-Negative Subtype

Most patients with HR-positive/HER2-negative breast cancer will not derive benefit from the addition of adjuvant chemotherapy to endocrine therapy. Several gene expression assays are commercially available to help select women who will benefit from the addition of chemotherapy to adjuvant endocrine therapy.

Multigene Assays

Multigene assays are approved in HR-positive and HER2-negative, node-negative as well as in one to three node-positive groups and include 21-gene (Oncotype Dx), 70-gene (MammaPrint), 50-gene (Prosigna), and EndoPredict 21-gene recurrence assays. OncotypeDx is the only assay that provides predictive information regarding chemotherapy benefit as well as prognostic information, with all other assays providing prognostic information only and their ability to predict chemotherapy benefit is unknown. The Breast Cancer Index predicts the benefit of extended adjuvant endocrine therapy.

The 21-gene recurrence score (RS) assay is based on a 21-gene (16 cancer-related genes and five reference genes) panel performed on paraffin-embedded tumor tissue and remains the most validated assay. The RSs range from 0 to 100, with higher scores indicating a greater risk of recurrence.

The OncotypeDx assay was studied in TAILORx, a prospectively conducted clinical trial that enrolled 10,273 patients between April 7, 2006 and October 6, 2010 with tumors of 1.1–5.0 cm in the greatest dimension and also included tumors measuring 0.6–1.0 cm in the greatest dimension with intermediate or high tumor grade.[14] Patients with a RS of 0–10 were assigned to receive endocrine therapy alone, and those with a RS of 26 or higher were assigned to receive chemotherapy plus endocrine therapy. The patients with a RS of 11–25 were randomized to endocrine therapy or chemoendocrine therapy. In total, 15.9% of women had a RS of 0–10 and were treated with endocrine therapy alone. The trial confirmed that a low RS (0–10) has a low rate of distant recurrence when patients were treated with endocrine therapy alone, with a rate of 5-year invasive disease–free survival (IDFS) of 93.8% (95% confidence interval [CI], 92.4–94.9), a rate of freedom from recurrence of breast cancer at a distant site of 99.3% (95% CI, 98.7–99.6), and a rate of OS of 98.0% (95% CI, 97.1–98.6).[14] An update in 2018 showed a low percentage of women with distant recurrence (3%) at 9 years with endocrine therapy alone if the RS was 0–15, irrespective of age.[15]

In 2018, results in patients with a mid-range RS of 11–25 showed that endocrine therapy was noninferior to chemoendocrine therapy in the analysis of IDFS.[15] At 9 years, the two treatment groups had similar rates of IDFS (83.3% in the endocrine therapy group and 84.3% in the chemoendocrine therapy group), freedom from disease recurrence at a distant site (94.5% and 95.0%) or at a distant or locoregional site (92.2% and 92.9%), and OS (93.9% and 93.8%). The chemotherapy benefit for invasive disease–free survival varied with the combination of RS and age ($P = .004$), with some benefit of chemotherapy found in women 50 years of age or younger with a RS of 16–25 (chemotherapy benefit of 1.6% with a RS of 16–20 and 6.5% with a RS of 21–25). A secondary analysis of the TAILORx trial was performed to determine whether the patient's age, tumor size, and histologic grade add prognostic information to the 21-gene RS and predictive information regarding the benefit of chemotherapy.[16] This analysis showed that clinical risk stratification provided prognostic information that, when added to the 21-gene RS, could be used to identify premenopausal women who could benefit from more effective therapy.[16]

The OncotypeDx assay was studied in HR-positive and HER2-negative breast cancer patients with one to three metastatic nodes in the RxPONDER trial.[17] This was a large, prospective trial that randomized 5083 women (33.2% premenopausal) with a RS of 25 or less to endocrine therapy alone or to chemoendocrine therapy. The premenopausal women who received chemoendocrine therapy had longer IDFS and distant relapse-free survival (DRFS) than those who received endocrine-only therapy, whereas postmenopausal women with similar characteristics did not benefit from adjuvant chemotherapy. However, it is somewhat controversial regarding how much benefit there was for premenopausal women in the chemoendocrine arm because of OFS caused by chemotherapy rather than the direct cytotoxic effect of the chemotherapy alone. Also, in clinical practice, this data is to be used with caution in patients with the high-grade disease with three positive nodes, as only 10.3% of patients had high-grade disease and 9.2% had three involved nodes.[17]

The 70-gene assay (MammaPrint) has also been studied in a prospective phase III randomized trial, MINDACT. This trial, which enrolled 6693 early breast cancer (N0 or one to three nodes positive) patients demonstrated that the 70-gene assay (MammaPrint) can identify a subset of patients who have a low likelihood of distant recurrence despite high-risk features based on size, grade, and nodal status (1.5% chemotherapy benefit in 5-year survival when added to endocrine therapy).[18] In this trial, women at low clinical and genomic risk did not receive chemotherapy, whereas those at high clinical and genomic risk did receive such therapy. In patients with discordant risk results, either the genomic risk or the clinical risk was used to determine the use of chemotherapy.[18] With a more mature follow-up approaching 9 years, the 70-gene signature shows an intact ability to identify among women with high clinical risk a subgroup with low genomic risk, with an excellent distant metastasis–free survival when treated with endocrine therapy alone.[19] For these women, the magnitude of the benefit from adding chemotherapy to endocrine therapy remains small (2.6%) and is not enhanced by nodal positivity. However, in an underpowered exploratory analysis, this benefit appears to be age dependent, as it is only seen in women younger than 50 years, where it reaches a clinically relevant threshold of 5%.[19] However like the 21-gene RS assay, the concern is that the noted benefit could be due to chemotherapy-induced ovarian function suppression rather than the direct effect of chemotherapy. This needs to be part of informed, shared decision-making with the patient.

Adjuvant Endocrine Therapy

Patients with invasive breast cancer that is ER- or PR-positive should be considered for adjuvant endocrine therapy regardless of the patient's age, lymph node status, or whether adjuvant chemotherapy was given. The endocrine options for women depend on whether they are in menopause or not. Menopausal status cannot be determined in patients receiving ovarian function suppression. There are no evidence-based criteria for the diagnosis of menopause. The National Comprehensive Cancer Network defines menopause as:

- Women 60 years and older
- Women less than 60 years are postmenopausal if one of the following conditions is met:
  - They previously underwent a bilateral oophorectomy.
  - Amenorrhea for 12 months or more in absence of tamoxifen, toremifene, prior chemotherapy, or OFS, and serum estradiol and follicle-stimulating hormone (FSH) is in the postmenopausal range.
  - They are amenorrheic on tamoxifen and serum estradiol and FSH are in the postmenopausal range.
  - Chemotherapy-induced amenorrhea for 12 months or more with estradiol and FSH levels in the postmenopausal range on serial assessments.

Only tamoxifen and AIs are approved medications for adjuvant treatment of breast cancer.

Tamoxifen is a selective estrogen receptor modulator (SERM) and can be used in ER-positive premenopausal and postmenopausal women. SERMs are competitive inhibitors of estrogen binding to the ER and have mixed agonist and antagonist activity. Tamoxifen has a prominent antagonist effect in breast cancer and is the only SERM approved to be used in the adjuvant setting.

Tamoxifen is converted to its active metabolites by CYP2D6 and UGT2B7. Some selective serotonin reuptake inhibitors such as fluoxetine and paroxetine inhibit CYP2D6 and decrease the formation of endoxifen, 4OH-tamoxifen, and active metabolites of tamoxifen, which may impact the efficacy of tamoxifen. Serotonin and norepinephrine reuptake inhibitors appear to have minimal impact on tamoxifen. These drug interactions should be considered when prescribing these medications but are not a contraindication. Studies have failed to demonstrate a survival difference with the use of selective serotonin reuptake inhibitors among patients taking tamoxifen.[20]

Side effects of tamoxifen include hot flashes, sexual dysfunction, venous thromboembolism (two- to threefold increase in relative risk), abnormal uterine bleeding, as well as increased risk of endometrial cancer and uterine sarcoma and a slight increase in the risk of stroke. Tamoxifen is also associated with fatty liver disease in over one-third of patients despite a favorable effect on cholesterol levels. There has been an increased risk of cataracts and less commonly reversible corneal pigmentation and irreversible retinal deposits that can be associated with macular edema and vision loss. Premenopausal women can remain fertile during tamoxifen treatment and should be strongly advised to use effective contraception while on tamoxifen treatment. Tamoxifen is related to birth defects and women planning to get pregnant should stop tamoxifen 2 months prior to attempting pregnancy.[21]

Duration of Treatment

A total of 5 years of tamoxifen decreases the annual odds of recurrence by 39% and annual odds of death by 31% irrespective of use of chemotherapy, age, lymph node status, and menopausal status, and was significantly more effective than 1–2 years' use.[22]

A meta-analysis of the results of 88 trials involving 62,923 women with ER-positive breast cancer who were disease free after 5 years of scheduled endocrine therapy showed that the breast cancer recurrences continued to occur steadily throughout the study period from 5 to 20 years.[23] The risk of distant recurrence was strongly correlated with the original tumor and nodal status, with risks ranging from 10% to 41%, depending on tumor and nodal status and tumor grade.[23]

In trials of 5 years of tamoxifen therapy versus no endocrine therapy, the recurrence rate in the tamoxifen group was approximately 50% lower than that in the control group during the first 5 years (the treatment period) and approximately 30% lower during the next 5 years.[24] The rate of death from breast cancer in the tamoxifen group was approximately 30% lower than that in the control group during the first 15 years (i.e., including 10 years after the cessation of therapy).[24]

Clinical trials comparing 5 or 10 years of tamoxifen include ATLAS and the aTTom trials. The ATLAS trial randomized women to 5 or 10 years of adjuvant tamoxifen, and the risk of recurrence during years 5–14 improved from 25.1% to 21.4% with 10 years of tamoxifen, with an absolute mortality reduction of 2.8%. There was an increased risk of endometrial cancer and pulmonary embolism.[25] The aTTom trial confirmed the significant reduction in recurrence with continuing tamoxifen to year 10. Breast cancer mortality was reduced by about one-third in the first 10 years following diagnosis and by half subsequently.[26]

Tamoxifen, when used with chemotherapy, should always be used sequentially with chemotherapy given first followed by tamoxifen, based on SWOG 8814 data.[27]

Role of Ovarian Suppression in Premenopausal Women

Before the availability of tamoxifen, OFS as a single treatment modality was utilized with some benefit. In contemporary medicine OFS alone is not considered standard-of-care adjuvant systemic therapy for breast cancer. For women with early-stage HR-positive breast cancer, adjuvant treatment with tamoxifen reduces their 15-year risk of death from breast cancer by about one-third. AIs are even more effective than tamoxifen in postmenopausal women but, used alone, are ineffective in premenopausal women due to compensatory ovarian estrogen production. Several trials have assessed whether, if administered with OFS, AIs may also be more effective than tamoxifen at preventing breast cancer recurrence in premenopausal women, but trial results have been inconsistent.

OFS has been used for multiple years in premenopausal women with controversial data. The 8-year update of the SOFT and TEXT trials compared 5 years of tamoxifen alone, tamoxifen with OFS, or exemestane with OFS. SOFT showed that the addition of OFS resulted in significantly higher (83.2% with OFS plus tamoxifen and 85.9% with OFS plus exemestane) 8-year disease-free survival (DFS) compared with tamoxifen alone (78.9%).[28] Among the women with cancers that were negative for HER2 who received chemotherapy, the 8-year rate of distant recurrence with exemestane plus OFS was lower than the rate with tamoxifen plus OFS (by 7% in SOFT and by 5% in TEXT). There were higher grade 3 toxicities with OFS.[28]

13 year median follow up update of the combinaed analysis of SOFT-TEXT trials in intention-to-treat population showed 12 year absolute improvement of 4.6% in disease free survival with 1.8% absolute improvement in distant recurrence free interval but no overall survival improvement in patients assigned to exemestane+OS over tamoxifen+OS. Among patients with HER2 negative tumors (86% of the intention-to-treat population) the absolute improvement in 12 year overall survival with examestane +OS was 2% and it was 3.3% in those who recieved chemotherapy (45.9% of the intention-to-treat population). Overall survival benefit was clinically significant in high-risk patients, eg, women age < 35 years (4.0%) and those with > 2 cm (4.5%) or grade 3 tumors (5.5%).[29]

A meta-analysis of 7030 women enrolled in four randomized trials evaluated AIs versus tamoxifen with OFS in premenopausal women. The 5-year absolute risk of breast cancer recurrence was 3.2% lower in the AI group than the tamoxifen group (6.9% vs. 10.1%) with no difference in breast cancer mortality.[30]

Aromatase Inhibitors

AIs suppress plasma estrogen levels by inhibiting or inactivating the enzyme aromatase, which is responsible for peripheral conversion of androgens to estrogens. AIs are only active in women with nonfunctioning ovaries.

There are three AIs available: anastrozole, letrozole, and exemestane. All three have shown similar antitumor efficacy and toxicity profiles in randomized trials. AIs are associated with hot flashes, night sweats, loss of bone density, musculoskeletal pains and stiffness, and sexual dysfunction. AI-associated musculoskeletal syndrome includes joint stiffness, arthralgias, bone pain, and carpal tunnel syndrome. These symptoms may be severe in up to one-third of the patients and lead to discontinuation of treatment in 10–20% of patients. There is data that exercise, nonsteroidal anti-inflammatory drugs, duloxetine, acupuncture, and brief interruption of the AI treatment may help.

If AIs are not tolerated, then a change to tamoxifen to complete the required adjuvant endocrine therapy is recommended.

Aromatase Inhibitors and Tamoxifen

The ATAC trial demonstrated anastrozole to be superior to tamoxifen with improved DFS (2.7% at 5 years and 4.3% at 10 years) with no difference in OS.[31]

Several studies have evaluated AIs as initial adjuvant therapy or sequential with tamoxifen. The BIG 1-98 study compared 5 years of tamoxifen alone, letrozole alone, or sequential use of the drugs and showed a 9% relative reduction in the hazard of a DFS event with letrozole compared with tamoxifen.[32] Outcomes achieved with the sequence of letrozole taken for 2 years followed by tamoxifen for 3 years were close to those with 5 years of letrozole monotherapy. This data is similar to the TEAM trial, where 5 years of the sequential regimen was similar to the AI-alone arm.[33]

Several trials have studied the use of tamoxifen for 2–3 years followed by AIs versus continued tamoxifen. A meta-analysis of the ABCSG-8, ARNO 95, and ITA studies showed significant improvement in DFS and OS with a switch to AIs.[34]

Duration of Endocrine Therapy

Similar to tamoxifen, there is evidence for benefit of extended adjuvant endocrine therapy in patients initially treated with tamoxifen. MA17 compared 5 years of tamoxifen compared with 5 years of tamoxifen followed by letrozole. The letrozole group showed improvement in DFS, but OS improvement was noted only in the lymph node-positive patients.[35] MA17-R evaluated extending AIs beyond 5 years. There was an improvement in 5-year DFS in patients on letrozole compared with placebo (95% vs. 91%), with no benefit in OS. However, there was an increase in bone fracture (14% vs. 9%), new-onset osteoporosis (11% vs. 6%), and bone-related events (18% vs 14%) with a longer duration of AIs.[36] A 10-year analysis of NSABP B-42 was presented at San Antonio Breast Cancer Symposium 2019 and also showed statistically significant improvement in DFS with an absolute improvement of 4% but no improvement in OS with the use of extended letrozole after 5 years of hormonal therapy.[37]

ABCSG-16/SALSA is a prospective, phase III trial that compared 2 versus 5 additional years of AIs in postmenopausal HR-positive women after 5 years of endocrine therapy.[38] After 10 years of follow-up, no benefit was noted for 5 additional years compared with 2 additional years of treatment with respect to DFS or OFS, or the risk of contralateral breast cancers. However, the majority of patients on this trial had low-risk T1 and N0 breast cancers that had been treated without adjuvant chemotherapy. Most patients had received tamoxifen alone (51%) or tamoxifen sequenced with an AI (42%) before trial entry.[38]

Role of Cyclin-Dependent Kinase 4 and 6 Inhibitors

Patients with breast cancer who have multinodal involvement, especially with four or more ALNs, have at least a 38% risk of relapse from 5 to 20 years. Patients with one to three ALNs and another poor prognostic factor are linked with a greater than 23% risk of relapse.[23] Despite successes observed with endocrine therapy for this patient population, there is an unmet need for identifying those who have primary endocrine resistance and preventing or delaying their recurrence with additional treatment.

CDK4/6 are important regulators of cell cycle progression in many cell types, including ER-positive breast cancer. In randomized trials, adding a CDK4/6 inhibitor to an AI or fulvestrant improves PFS and OS in both premenopausal and postmenopausal women.[39,40] Multiple clinical trials have evaluated the role of CDK4/6 inhibitors in high-risk early breast cancer.

Palbociclib was studied in a prospective, randomized, phase III PALLAS trial. A total of 5796 patients with HR-positive and HER2-negative early breast cancer were randomly assigned to receive 2 years of palbociclib (125 mg orally once daily, days 1–21 of a 28-day cycle) with adjuvant endocrine therapy or adjuvant endocrine therapy alone (for at least 5 years).[41] There was no improvement in IDFS or any other efficacy end point (4-year IDFS 84.2% vs. 84.5%; hazard ratio 0.96).[41]

PENELOPE-B is another double-blind, placebo-controlled, phase III study in which women with HR-positive HER2 – without a pathological complete response after taxane-containing NACT and at high risk of relapse were randomly assigned (1:1) to receive 13 cycles of palbociclib 125 mg once daily or placebo on days 1–21 in a 28-day cycle in addition to endocrine therapy. Palbociclib for 1 year in addition to endocrine therapy did not improve IDFS in women with residual invasive disease after NACT.[42]

MonarchE is the only positive trial showing the benefit of adding CDK4/6 inhibitors to high-risk breast cancer with adjuvant endocrine therapy.[43] This is a phase III trial that randomized 5637 adult women and men with HR-positive, HER2-negative, node-positive, resected, early high-risk breast cancer. Patients were randomized to receive either 2 years of abemaciclib plus their physician's choice of standard endocrine therapy for 5 years or greater (maximum 10 years) or standard endocrine therapy alone. The trial enrolled patients with four or more positive ALNs, or one to three positive nodes and either grade 3 disease or tumor 5 cm or larger in size, or one to three positive nodes and a centrally tested Ki-67 of 20% or greater.[43]

At the primary outcome analysis, with 19 months median follow-up time, abemaciclib plus endocrine therapy resulted in a 29% reduction in the risk of developing an IDFS event (hazard ratio, 0.71, 95% CI, 0.58–0.87; nominal $P = 0.0009$]. At the additional follow-up analysis, with 27 months median follow-up and 90% of patients off treatment, IDFS (hazard ratio, 0.70; 95% CI, 0.59–0.82; nominal $P < .0001$) and DRFS (hazard ratio, 0.69; 95% CI, 0.57–0.83; nominal $P < .0001$) benefit was maintained. The absolute improvements in 3-year IDFS and DRFS rates were 5.4% and 4.2%, respectively.[43] Whereas the Ki-67 index was prognostic, abemaciclib benefit was consistent regardless of Ki-67 index. Safety data were consistent with the known abemaciclib risk profile. OS data were not mature at the time of the IDFS analysis. The most common adverse reactions ($\geq 20\%$) were diarrhea, infections, neutropenia, fatigue, leukopenia, nausea, anemia, and headache. The risk of VTE was higher when used in combination with tamoxifen, with about 4% of patients in monarchE that received tamoxifen and abemaciclib experiencing a VTE.[43]

On October 12, 2021, the FDA approved abemaciclib with endocrine therapy (tamoxifen or an AI) for adjuvant treatment of adult patients with HR-positive, HER2-negative, node-positive early breast cancer at high risk of recurrence and a Ki-67 score $\geq 20\%$, as determined by an FDA-approved test.

Although exploratory analyses suggested similar hazard ratios in favor of abemaciclib regardless of Ki-67 status, there were relatively few Ki-67–low tumors in monarchE.[43]

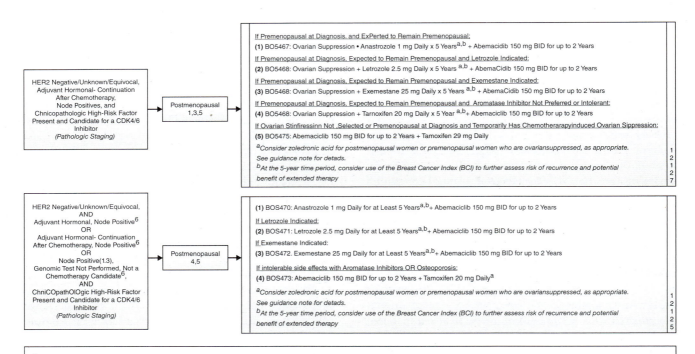

When discussing treatment options with patients, the potential benefits (improved IDFS) should be weighed against the potential harms (treatment toxicity, financial cost).

Adjuvant Chemotherapy

The decision to give adjuvant chemotherapy is made based on tumor characteristics including ER and or PR receptor and HER2 status, genomic analysis, as well as lymph node status, any prior neoadjuvant therapy, patient age, and comorbidities.

Once it is decided that the patient will benefit from chemotherapy, then the choice of the regimen depends on the characteristics of the tumor as well as the patient. Doxorubicin and taxanes remain a very important part of the chemotherapy regimens.

Regimen Selection

EBCTCG compared cyclophosphamide, methotrexate and 5-fluorouracil with the anthracycline-containing regimens, and anthracycline-based regimens produced somewhat greater reduction in recurrence and mortality (69% vs. 72% 5-year survival).[44] NSABP B-36 compared six cycles of fluorouracil, epirubicin, and cyclophosphamide (FEC) to four cycles of doxorubicin and cyclophosphamide (AC), and showed no difference in DFS with increased toxicity with FEC in node-negative patients.[45] This data has led to four cycles of AC as the standard anthracycline-based regimen. There has been no benefit of dose escalation of doxorubicin but there was a 5-year DFS (70% vs. 65%) and OS (OS) (80% vs. 77%) benefit by adding paclitaxel after AC.[46]

Sequential Use of Anthracyclines and Taxanes

A meta-analysis of phase III randomized trials to compare treatment outcomes for early-stage breast cancer patients receiving adjuvant chemotherapy with sequential or concurrent anthracyclines and taxanes included three eligible trials. Significant differences in favor of sequential regimens were seen in DFS (RR, 0.90; 95% CI, 0.84–0.98; $P = .01$) and in OS (RR, 0.88; 95% CI, 0.79–0.98; $P = .02$).[47] NSABP B-28 also showed improvement in DFS with AC followed by paclitaxel compared with AC alone (76% vs. 72%), with no difference in OS.[48]

Choice of Taxanes and Dose-Dense Data

The phase III EA1199 trial evaluated 4954 stage II and III breast cancer patients treated with four cycles of doxorubicin plus cyclophosphamide followed by randomization to paclitaxel or docetaxel every 3 weeks for four doses or weekly for 12 doses. When compared with the standard every-3-week paclitaxel arm, after a median follow-up of 12.1 years, DFS significantly improved, and OS marginally improved only for the weekly paclitaxel and every-3-week docetaxel arms. Weekly paclitaxel improved DFS and OS in triple-negative breast cancer.[49]

CALGB 9741 showed that dose-dense AC followed by taxol (paclitaxel) improved 4-year DFS (82% vs. 75%) when compared with the non-dose-dense arm.[50]

Non-Anthracycline Regimens

Anthracyclines are very effective in the treatment of breast cancer, but carry long-term side effects of cardiotoxicity and increased risk of acute leukemias and myelodysplastic syndrome. Myeloid neoplasms linked to doxorubicin-related therapy tend to have a latency period of 1–3 years after treatment and usually present with treatment related acute myeloid leukemia and rarely with treatment related myelodysplastic syndrome or treatment related myelodysplastic syndrome/myeloproliferative neoplasm. Cytogenetic alterations usually include abnormalities of 11q23 or 21q22 abnormalities.

Trials have been performed in search of an effective nonanthracycline regimen. Trials comparing four cycles of AC with six cycles of cyclophosphamide, methotrexate and 5-fluorouracil in premenopausal node-positive patients was equivalent in DFS and OS.[51]

A 7-year follow-up of the US Oncology Research Trial showed four cycles of docetaxel and cyclophosphamide (TC) has a better DFS at 7 years when compared with four cycles of AC (81% with TC and 75% with AC).[52] However, activity of TC relative to AC regimens with a taxane (TaxAC) is unknown.

In a series of three adjuvant trials (the ABC trials), women were randomly assigned to TC for six cycles (TC6) or to a standard TaxAC regimen.[53] The 4-year IDFS was 88.2% for TC6 and 90.7% for TaxAC ($P = .04$). The 4-year OS was high in both groups (~95%). Exploratory subgroup analyses suggested that TaxAC provides minimal if any benefit in ER-positive node-negative cohorts. There was a small benefit in ER-positive breast cancer with one to three positive nodes and in ER-negative and node-negative cohorts (2.0%–2.5%). Large benefit was seen in ER-positive breast cancer with four or more positive lymph nodes and ER-negative and node-positive cohorts (5.8–11%). Acute leukemia occurred as the first event in 0.24% of patients assigned to TaxAC and none assigned to TC.[53]

HER2-Positive Subtypes

The *HER2* gene encodes a tyrosine kinase receptor that mediates critical signaling functions in normal and malignant breast epithelial cells. An acquired alteration consisting of amplification and overexpression of the gene product occurs in approximately 20–25% of human breast cancers. HER2 overexpression is associated with an aggressive clinical phenotype that includes high-grade tumors, increased growth rates, early systemic metastasis, and decreased rates of DFS and OS. Preclinical data indicate that this adverse clinical picture results from fundamental changes in the biologic features of breast cancer cells containing the alteration, including increased proliferation, suppression of apoptosis, increased motility, greater invasive and metastatic potential, accelerated angiogenesis, and steroid hormone independence.[54]

triple-negative breast cancer. *N Engl J Med*. 2018 Nov 29;379(22):2108–2121.

128. Cortes J, Cescon DW, Rugo HS, et al. KEYNOTE-355 Investigators. Pembrolizumab plus chemotherapy versus placebo plus chemotherapy for previously untreated locally recurrent inoperable or metastatic triple-negative breast cancer (KEYNOTE-355): a randomised, placebo-controlled, double-blind, phase 3 clinical trial. *Lancet*. 2020 Dec 5;396(10265):1817–1828.

129. Bardia A, Hurvitz SA, Tolaney SM, et al. ASCENT Clinical Trial Investigators. Sacituzumab govitecan in metastatic triple-negative breast cancer. *N Engl J Med*. 2021 Apr 22;384(16):1529–1541.

130. Sledge GW, Neuberg D, Bernardo P, et al. Phase III trial of doxorubicin, paclitaxel, and the combination of doxorubicin and paclitaxel as front-line chemotherapy for metastatic breast cancer: an intergroup trial (E1193). *J Clin Oncol*. 2003 Feb 15;21(4):588–592.

131. Lipton A, Theriault RL, Hortobagyi GN, et al. Pamidronate prevents skeletal complications and is effective palliative treatment in women with breast carcinoma and osteolytic bone metastases—long term followup of two randomized placebo-controlled trials. *Cancer*. 2000;88:1082–1090.

132. Berenson JR, Rosen LS, Howell A, et al. Zoledronic acid reduces skeletal-related events in patients with osteolytic metastases. *Cancer*. 2001 Apr 1;91(7):1191–1200.

133. Himelstein AL, Foster JC, Khatcheressian JL, et al. Effect of longer-interval vs standard dosing of zoledronic acid on skeletal events in patients with bone metastases: a randomized clinical trial. *JAMA*. 2017 Jan 3;317(1):48–58.

134. Stopeck AT, Lipton A, Body JJ, et al. Denosumab compared with zoledronic acid for the treatment of bone metastases in patients with advanced breast cancer: a randomized, double-blind study. *J Clin Oncol*. 2010 Dec 10;28(35):5132–5139.

10

Breast Cancer Pathology for Precision Oncology

ANNA BERRY AND AMANDA MEINDL

Background

Breast carcinoma is the most common type of malignancy affecting women, aside from skin malignancy. It is the second most common cause of cancer deaths among women. Invasive breast carcinomas are a complex and heterogenous group of tumors, largely adenocarcinomas, with the majority falling into the category of invasive ductal carcinoma, not otherwise specified (NOS) [1,2] These tumors account for approximately 75% of all breast carcinomas.[1] The second most common type of breast carcinoma is invasive lobular carcinoma, accounting for up to 15% of breast cancers.[1,2] The terms "ductal" and "lobular" are not references to the cell of origin but rather how their associated in situ lesions affect lobular units. Ductal in situ lesions tend to expand and unfold lobular units, thus resembling ducts more than lobules. Lobular in situ lesions tend to expand but not distort the existing terminal duct lobular units (TDLUs). All breast carcinomas are thought to arise from the TDLU.[2]

The remaining tumor types are of "special type" and are named according to their specific cytologic features and growth patterns. These tumors include tubular carcinoma, mucinous carcinoma, cribriform carcinoma, papillary carcinoma, metaplastic carcinoma, adenoid cystic carcinoma, apocrine carcinoma, neuroendocrine carcinoma, and secretory carcinoma, among others. Histopathologic features remain the standard for classification of breast carcinomas; however, the emergence of molecular diagnostics has allowed us to further classify tumors based on their molecular features.

Hormone Receptors and HER2

The three main receptors that are evaluated in breast carcinoma are estrogen receptor (ER), progesterone receptor (PR), and human epidermal receptor-2 (HER2). Immunohistochemistry (IHC) analysis of these three biomarkers, combined with Ki-67 IHC analysis for proliferative rate, can be used to approximate molecular subtyping. The different molecular subtypes of breast carcinoma have variable immunophenotypes and will be discussed later in this chapter. Hormone receptors and HER2 should be evaluated on all invasive carcinomas to determine the immunophenotype of the tumor.

Hormone receptor status is also a useful tool in patient management. ER and PR expression by breast cancer cells is a weak prognostic factor for outcomes but a strong predictive factor for response to endocrine therapy.[1] Endocrine therapies include selective ER modulators (SERMs), aromatase inhibitors, and gonadotropin-releasing factor antagonists or refractory agonists. The most widely used endocrine therapy is tamoxifen, a type of SERM.[2]

The best way to score ER and PR is still not standardized among pathology institutions. However, studies have shown that patients with as little as 1% ER positivity may benefit from endocrine therapy.[2] Many institutions use a semiquantitative method for scoring ER and PR results, taking into account the percentage of tumor cells showing nuclear staining and the intensity (weak, moderate/intermediate, and strong intensity). The combination can be used to generate a score that can be used by clinicians in their treatment plans. The most widely used scoring system is the Allred scoring system. The most widely used cutoff percentages for ER and PR are 1% and 10% where less than 1% is a negative result, 1% to less than 10% is a low positive result, and ≥10% is a positive result.[1] It should be noted that in the Allred system, a result of less than 1% with moderate or strong staining intensity is still considered a positive result, and patients may benefit from endocrine therapy.[2] Hormone receptor markers are evaluated by staining the formalin-fixed paraffin embedded tumor samples using IHC and estimating the percentage of tumor cells staining and the intensity, under the microscope. This method of scoring remains relatively subjective, and many institutions have adopted the use of automated image analysis for the evaluation of ER and PR IHC results (Fig. 10.1).

HER2 is another prognostic marker that should be evaluated in all breast cancers.[1] It is a proto-oncogene present on chromosome 17q12. In HER2-positive breast carcinomas,

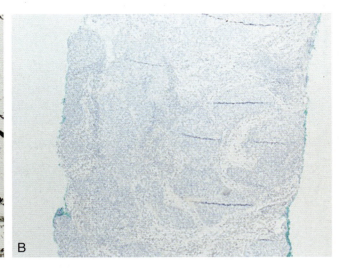

- **Fig. 10.1** Estrogen receptor (ER) by immunohistochemistry (images from left to right: (A) ER-positive, strong >95%; (B) ER-negative, <1%).

HER2 is overexpressed, usually due to gene amplification.[2,3] The HER2 protein is located on the surface of the tumor cells and makes a great target for therapy. HER2-targeted therapies include HER2-specific antibodies, such as trastuzumab, and small molecule inhibitors, such as the dual tyrosine kinase inhibitor lapatinib. Tumors that show HER2 overexpression or gene amplification have been shown to benefit greatly from treatment with trastuzumab and chemotherapy.[3]

The most commonly used methods for evaluating HER2 status are with IHC to assess for overexpression and/or in situ hybridization (ISH) to assess for gene amplification. The scoring system for HER2 IHC analysis is well established through recommendations from the College of American Pathologists (CAP) and the American Society of Clinical Oncology (ASCO).[4] Formalin-fixed paraffin-embedded tumor samples are stained using IHC for HER2 and evaluated under the microscope. Based on the staining pattern, the tumor is given an HER2 score of either 0 (negative), 1+ (negative), 2+ (equivocal), or 3+ (positive). A score of 0 is rendered when no staining is observed or membrane staining that is incomplete and is faint/barely perceptible and in ≤10% of tumor cells is present. A score of 1+ is rendered when there is incomplete membrane staining that is faint/barely perceptible and in greater than 10% of tumor cells. A score of 2+ is given when there is weak to moderate complete membrane staining observed in greater than 10% of tumor cells. Finally, a score of 3+ is given when there is circumferential membrane staining that is complete, intense, and in greater than 10% of tumor cells.[2,4] Again, this method of scoring can be subjective, and many institutions use automated imaging software to analyze samples (Fig. 10.2).

ISH analysis can be used in lieu of IHC; however, it is expensive and time-consuming. For cases that showed equivocal results by IHC, ISH should be performed on the sample to assess for the presence of gene amplification. The most widely used method for ISH analysis of HER2 gene amplification is using the dual probe method with a probe against the HER2 gene and the chromosome 17 centromere enumeration probe (CEP17). The number of HER2 signals and CEP17 signals per cell are evaluated and an HER2:CEP17 ratio is generated. The HER2:CEP17 ratio and HER2 copy number correspond to a "negative for gene amplification" or "positive for gene amplification" result with rare cases leading to an "equivocal" result. If an equivocal result is generated by ISH analysis, further testing is required.[2,4]

The protein Ki-67 is used as a biomarker correlated with cellular proliferation, as it is present during all phases of the cell cycle but is absent from resting cells. IHC assays are used to determine a proliferative index using the Ki-67 antibody stain. Positive tumor cells are counted and divided by the total number of tumor cells evaluated. This process is tedious and can be subjective. However, there are now several image analysis systems to assist with this task. Ki-67 expression is correlated with grade, but among lower-grade tumors, Ki-67 can serve as an independent prognostic variable. Ki-67 is also used as a companion diagnostic for the CDK 4/6 inhibitor abemaciclib, as described below.[5]

Molecular Classification of Breast Cancer

Gene expression profiling (GEP) studies have been able to identify several molecular subtypes for breast cancer through evaluation of DNA, mRNA, and proteins.[6] The most well-understood subtypes are based on mRNA expression studies, and include luminal (A and B), HER2, and basal-like. A fifth molecular subtype of breast carcinoma, the normal-like breast cancer subtype, has been identified and closely resembles luminal A breast tumors. This only accounts for a very small percentage of all breast carcinomas.[1,2]

These molecular subtypes show differences in clinical presentation, histopathologic features, response to therapy, prognosis, and molecular gene expression.[1,2] Molecular classification of breast carcinoma does show reproducible

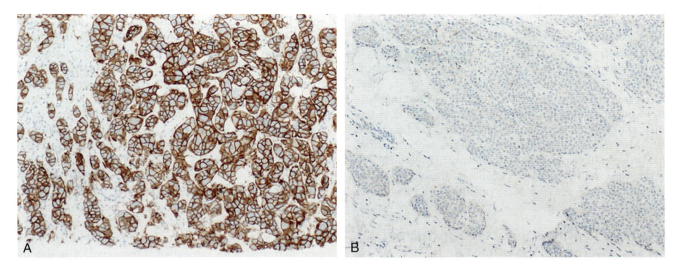

• **Fig. 10.2** Invasive breast carcinoma (images from left to right: HER2 positive, Score 3+; HER2 negative, Score 1+).

correlation with prognosis, compared to traditional prognostic factors alone. The molecular subtypes can be correlated with ER status. The ER-positive subgroups include luminal A and luminal B subtypes and ER-negative subgroups include the HER2 and basal-like subtypes.[2] While IHC staining as noted above can approximate these molecular subtypes, the agreement is not exact. Actual molecular subtyping is used in commercially available assays for prognosis, but a clinically reportable molecular subtype determination assay is not yet widely available.

Luminal Subtypes

The luminal A subtype of breast carcinomas accounts for ~55% of breast cancer and another ~15% of breast carcinomas fall into the luminal B subtype.[1,2] The luminal subtype of breast cancer typically shows a high level of hormone receptor expression. Luminal A types of breast cancer tend to show higher levels of ER expression, and expression of genes regulated and activated by ER, when compared to luminal B types, but lower levels of proliferation-related gene expression.[1,2] For this reason, Ki-67 IHC staining can be useful in approximating a luminal B phenotype. Luminal A subtypes are often PR positive by IHC, whereas luminal B subtypes are often PR negative or show low-level expression. HER2 is not typically expressed in luminal A cancers but can be expressed in up to 50% of luminal B cancers. The immunophenotype of luminal A tumors is often ER/PR positive and HER2 negative, whereas the immunophenotype of luminal B tumors is often ER/PR and HER2 positive (Fig. 10.3).[1-3]

Luminal A subtypes tend to be of lower histologic grade than luminal B subtypes, with a relatively indolent clinical course and better prognosis. These subtypes of tumors do tend to respond to endocrine therapy, with a more variable response to chemotherapy.[1-3] Luminal B tumors respond slightly better to chemotherapy, in general, than luminal A tumors. Even though luminal B tumors portend a somewhat worse prognosis than luminal A tumors, they are still considered to have a favorable prognosis, overall.[1,2]

HER2-Positive/HER2-Enriched Subtype

The HER2-positive subtype of breast carcinoma accounts for approximately 15% to 20% of breast carcinomas. These tumors show a high level of HER2 expression as well as overexpression of adjacent genes on the HER2 amplicon. These tumors do not generally show significant expression of ER or PR but do show a higher expression of genes related to proliferation. These tumors often have an ER/PR-negative and HER2-positive immunophenotype.[1-3]

HER2-positive carcinomas tend to be higher grade than luminal A or B tumors and are more often lymph node positive. They often have a more aggressive clinical course with a worse prognosis.[1,2] However, with the introduction of monoclonal antibody anti-HER2 therapy (Trastuzumab/Herceptin), the poor prognosis of these cancers can be altered, with many patients seeing complete pathologic response after therapy. In addition to anti-HER2 therapy, these tumors may respond to anthracycline-based chemotherapy.[2]

Basal-like Subtype

The basal-like subtype of breast carcinomas accounts for another 10% to 15% of breast tumors. These cancers are usually negative for expression of ER, PR, and HER2. These tumors often have a triple negative immunophenotype (ER/PR/HER2 negative by IHC). However, a small percentage of basal-like cancers show an ER-positive immunophenotype by IHC and another small percentage express HER2 by IHC. Basal-like tumors can be further characterized by their expression of basal cytokeratins (CK5/6, CK14, CK17) and basal epithelial genes like EGFR (Fig. 10.4).[1-3]

These are generally aggressive tumors and often present in much younger patients as well as African American women, to treating tumor biology alongside tumor morphology. For this reason, large-panel NGS testing of tumors in metastatic breast cancer (or in ctDNA if tumor tissue is unavailable) should be considered.

Breast cancer pathology is a complex and rapidly changing discipline, requiring specialized training and extensive continuing education. Interdisciplinary collaboration and cooperation are necessary to provide patients with the best diagnostic information and therapeutic options to improve survival and decrease the burden of disease.

References

1. Schnitt SJ, Collins LC. *Biopsy Interpretation of the Breast*. Wolters Kluwer Lippincott Williams and Wilkins: 249–322.
2. Hicks DG, Lester SC. Diagnostic Pathology. Breast. Salt Lake City, UT: Amirsys, 2012. Print.
3. Liu D. Plastic and Reconstructive Surgeon, CTCA Chicago. February 10, 2022. cancercenter.com/cancer-types/breast-cancer/types/breast-cancer-molecular-types.
4. Wolff AC, Hammond MEH, Allison KH, et al. Human Epidermal Growth Factor Receptor 2 Testing in Breast Cancer: American Society of Clinical Oncology/College of American Pathologists Clinical Practice Guideline Focused Update. *Arch Pathol Lab Med*. 2018;142(11):1364–1382. https://doi.org/10.5858/arpa.2018-0902-SA.
5. Liang Q, Ma D, Gao RF, et al. Effect of Ki-67 Expression Levels and Histological Grade on Breast Cancer Early Relapse in Patients with Different Immunohistochemical-based Subtypes. *Sci Rep*. 2020;10:7648. https://doi.org/10.1038/s41598-020-64523-1.
6. Yersal O, Barutca S. Biological subtypes of breast cancer: Prognostic and therapeutic implications. *World J Clin Oncol*. 2014;5(3):412–424. https://doi.org/10.5306/wjco.v5.i3.412.
7. Brett JO, Spring LM, Bardia A, et al. ESR1 mutation as an emerging clinical biomarker in metastatic hormone receptor-positive breast cancer. *Breast Cancer Res*. 2021;23:85. https://doi.org/10.1186/s13058-021-01462-3.
8. Johnston SRD, Harbeck N, Hegg R, et al. Abemaciclib combined with endocrine therapy for the adjuvant treatment of HR+, HER2-, node-positive, high-risk, early breast cancer (monarchE). J Clin Oncol. 2020;38(34):3987–3998. https://doi.org/10.1200/JCO.20.02514
9. André F, Ciruelos E, Rubovszky G, et al. Alpelisib for *PIK3CA*-Mutated, Hormone Receptor-Positive Advanced Breast Cancer. *N Engl J Med*. 2019;380(20):1929–1940. https://doi.org/10.1056/NEJMoa1813904.
10. Lord CJ, Ashworth A. PARP inhibitors: Synthetic lethality in the clinic. *Science*. 2017;355(6330):1152–1158. https://doi.org/10.1126/science.aam7344. Epub 2017 Mar 16.
11. Modi S, Jacot W, Yamashita T, et al. Trastuzumab Deruxtecan in Previously Treated HER2-Low Advanced Breast Cancer. *N Engl J Med*. 2022;387(1):9–20. https://doi.org/10.1056/NEJMoa2203690. Epub 2022 Jun 5.

11

Physical Therapy for Patients With Breast Cancer

LESLIE J. WALTKE

KEY POINTS

- Cancer physical therapy is the evidence-based, reimbursed medical care used to specifically examine, assess, and treat impairments related to cancer and cancer treatment.
- Though physical therapy is readily available to patients, it remains underutilized in most cancer programs.
- If a cancer physical therapy program is focusing solely on patients with lymphedema or postoperative breast surgery, it is missing the vast majority of its potential volume and value.
- Evidence suggests cancer physical therapy may impact quality of life, length of survival, recurrence risk, and overall survival in patients with cancer.
- Cancer physical therapy demonstrates outcome benefits for cancer patients and for cancer programs.
- Physical therapy for patients with cancer should begin during the peri-diagnosis period and continue through survivorship.
- Physical therapy for patients with breast cancer should start with first cancer treatment intervention whether it be neoadjuvant chemotherapy or surgery.
- Cancer physical therapy is a low-cost, low-risk, nonpharmacological intervention that may decrease length of hospital stays, decrease hospital readmissions, decrease emergency department visits, and decrease fall risk.
- This chapter is solely focused on physical therapy for patients with breast cancer. However, impairments in patients with cancer result from surgery, chemotherapy, and radiation. Therefore, a rehabilitation consult should be offered to all patients undergoing cancer treatment, regardless of cancer type.

An Introduction to Breast Cancer Physical Therapy

Medical management for malignant breast disease includes surgery, chemotherapy, radiation, hormonal therapy, immunotherapy, and biological therapy. Each of these antineoplastic interventions has potential negative impacts on the human physiological, cardiopulmonary, integumentary, and musculoskeletal systems. As a result, well-established short-term, long-term, and late morbidities are often present in patients exposed to these cancer treatments. These morbidities, in turn, may result in decreased functional performance, loss of activities of daily living (ADLs) capacity, decreased quality of life, impaired sexual health, impaired social function, and loss of vocational, recreational, and exercise capacity. Evidence exists also, that this overall decrease in functional, physical, and physiological performance may negatively impact life span.

Though common, these symptoms often go under addressed, and though some physical and functional loss with cancer surgery, radiation, and cytotoxic and cytostatic treatments for breast cancer is expected, much of this loss is unnecessary and preventable. Evidence suggests physical therapy can prevent, minimize, or eliminate many of these cancer treatment-related symptoms and impairments.[1]

Cancer rehabilitation is the medical modality used to specifically examine, assess, and treat the musculoskeletal, cardiopulmonary, physiological, integumentary, and functional impairments expected with cancer treatment, survivorship, advanced disease, and end of life. A vast body of quality studies show rehabilitation may increase quality of life, length of life, and that exercise may increase overall survival and decrease risk of recurrence in patients with breast cancer.[2] Breast cancer rehabilitation services are provided by physical therapists, occupational therapists, and physiatrists. In the case of metastatic breast cancer (MBC) impacting a patient's cognition, language, speech, breathing, or swallowing, a speech-language pathology consult may also be warranted.

Like other areas of specialization in physical therapy, such as orthopedics, neurology, geriatrics, etc., rehabilitation for patients with cancer is similarly evidence based and reimbursable. Physical therapists treat presenting impairments with the scientific application of therapeutic procedures with the goal of improving or preventing physical and physiological impairments and optimizing health and function. Skilled interventions used by rehabilitation therapists include, but are not limited to, therapeutic exercise, therapeutic activities, manual therapy, mechanical traction, ultrasound/phonophoresis, vasopneumatic devices, aquatic therapy, biofeedback, neuromuscular reeducation, orthotic/prosthetic use, cognitive performance testing, debridement, functional capacity evaluations, ADLs/self-care interventions, gait training, sensory integration, electrical stimulation, splinting/orthotics, prosthetic training, and wheelchair management. The most common of these interventions used in cancer rehabilitation include therapeutic exercise and manual therapy.

The National Accreditation Program for Breast Centers and the Commission on Cancer recognize the importance of cancer rehabilitation and have it as a required standard of a cancer care program. In its Optimal Resources for Cancer Care Guide, the Commission on Cancer states, "The availability of rehabilitation care services is an essential component of comprehensive cancer care, beginning at the time of diagnosis and being continuously available throughout treatment, surveillance, and, when applicable, through end of life." The National Comprehensive Cancer Network (NCCN) also recognizes the benefits of rehabilitation and in its Guidelines for Cancer-Related Fatigue, it recommends referral to rehabilitation from diagnosis to end of life.

An Overview of Breast Cancer Physical Therapy

Traditionally, patients with breast cancer are referred to rehabilitation for postoperative and lymphedema-related care. Postoperative breast surgery symptoms and impairments amenable to rehabilitation include regional pain and swelling, weakness, limited shoulder range of motion (ROM), soft tissue shortening and soft tissue restrictions, cording, decreased ADL, vocational and recreational capacities, and risk for the development of lymphedema. Rehabilitation is effective in minimizing or eliminating this symptomology. However, if rehabilitation therapists and cancer practitioners focus solely on the postoperative symptoms and discontinue physical therapy when these problems are resolved, patients continuing with adjuvant treatment will not benefit from best practice care. Patients additionally undergoing chemotherapy, radiation, hormonal, and/or biological antineoplastic therapies will be exposed to additional potential symptoms and impairments from each of these individual cancer treatments.

Surgery, chemotherapy, radiation, hormonal therapies, and biological therapies may each result in unique musculoskeletal, cardiopulmonary, physiological, and integumentary impairments (Table 11.1). Resultantly, symptoms and impairments amenable to rehabilitation will present at varying times throughout the cancer treatment continuum. To maximize best patient outcomes in breast cancer care, timely, seamless, evidence-based rehabilitation care across the cancer care continuum is recommended. The addition of rehabilitation therapists to the comprehensive oncology care team is pertinent for maximal patient health and outcomes during and after treatment for cancer.[3]

As a patient moves through medical treatments, cancer rehabilitation best practice involves the rehabilitation therapist providing active surveillance and rehabilitative treatment and education, based on the patient's symptom profile and functional needs (Fig. 11.1).

Impairments treated by oncology physical therapists include, but are not limited to, increased pain and symptoms, headaches, and impairments in posture, strength, ROM, scapulohumeral rhythm, muscle length and flexibility, tissue mobility, tissue and wound healing, joint mobility, gait, mobility, activity tolerance, balance, motor function/performance, coordination, sensory integration, body mechanics, bladder health, bowel health, and sexual health, as well as increased swelling and risk for falls.

Referring to Breast Cancer Physical Therapy

Oncology practitioners are encouraged to refer patients undergoing or pending cancer treatment to an oncology physical therapist in the peri-diagnosis period. Referrals from physicians, physician assistants, and nurse practitioners are generally third-party reimbursed. In some regional areas, payors and health systems may additionally offer direct access to physical therapists. If the patient is beginning breast cancer treatment with neoadjuvant chemotherapy, referral to oncology physical therapy should be made in the peri-diagnosis period, ideally prior to the onset of cycle one. If surgery is the patient's first anticancer intervention, physical therapy should begin as soon as possible postoperatively at the breast or reconstructive surgeon's discretion. If the patient is doing well postoperatively with pain control, is maintaining mobility and independence, and is on a walking program, physical therapy may begin as soon as possible after the drains are removed. If the patient does not have postoperative drains, is experiencing moderate to severe chest wall or axillary pain, has cording, or has less than 90 degrees of shoulder flexion/abduction with pending radiation, rehabilitation may begin at 1 to 2 weeks post breast surgery.

After a patient's injury or illness involving cardiology, neurology, or orthopedics, early mobilization with physical therapy is commonplace. Though not routine in oncology, this principle of early mobilization is also warranted. For example, even with the presence of postoperative restrictions, early referral to physical therapy post surgery remains beneficial. In this time, education and training in walking or aerobic exercise within postsurgical limitation can begin. Additionally, instruction in ADL modifications and safe strength exercises for the legs and nonsurgically affected muscles of the upper body can begin. If the patient is experiencing moderate to severe pain from cording or soft tissue restrictions or shortening, manual therapy and therapeutic exercise may be effective within

CHAPTER 11 Physical Therapy for Patients With Breast Cancer

TABLE 11.1 Indications for Rehabilitation Consult for Patients With Breast Cancer

Medical Intervention/ Disease Insult	Potential Resulting Physical/Physiological/ Functional Impairments Amenable to Rehab	Outcome(s) Expected With Rehabilitation
Neoadjuvant chemotherapy	Fatigue, cardiotoxicity, weight gain, barriers to exercise, functional loss, decreased performance status/ADL capacity	Minimized fatigue, weakness, functional loss
		Maximized performance status and cardiopulmonary function, minimized risk or amount of cardiotoxicity
SLNB (Sentinel lymph node biopsy)	Pain, limited arm/shoulder ROM, arm/shoulder weakness, cording, lymphedema risk, functional loss	Full preoperative pain-free mobility, strength, and function without limitation at involved upper quarter(s)
		Minimized risk of lymphedema
ALND (axillary lymph node dissection)	Pain, limited arm/shoulder ROM, arm/shoulder weakness, cording, lymphedema risk, functional loss	Full preoperative pain-free mobility, strength, and function without limitation at involved upper quarter(s)
		Minimized risk of lymphedema
Partial mastectomy	Pain, limited shoulder ROM, shoulder weakness, functional loss, expected pending radiation (see Acute Curative Radiation)	Full preoperative pain-free mobility, strength, and function without limitation at involved upper quarter(s)
Mastectomy	Pain, limited shoulder ROM, shoulder weakness, functional loss	Full preoperative pain-free mobility, strength, and function without limitation at involved upper quarter(s)
Breast reconstruction—tissue expander/implant	Pain, limited shoulder ROM, shoulder weakness, soft tissue tightness and restrictions, functional loss	Full preoperative pain-free mobility, strength, and function without limitation at involved upper quarter(s)
Breast reconstruction—tissue transfer	Pain, limited shoulder ROM, shoulder weakness, soft tissue tightness and restrictions, functional loss	Full preoperative pain-free mobility, strength, and function without limitation at involved upper quarter(s)
Cytotoxic chemotherapy	Fatigue, nausea, cardiotoxicity, weight gain, barriers to exercise	Minimized fatigue, weakness, functional loss
		Maximized performance status and cardiopulmonary function
Bone marrow support drugs (pegfilgrastim)	Pain, barrier to function and exercise	Educated in bone flair and alternative activity and exercise options
		Minimized functional loss
Acute curative radiation	Pain, fatigue, limited shoulder ROM and function, functional loss, barriers to full function and exercise	Minimized fatigue, weakness, functional loss
		Maximized performance status and cardiopulmonary function
Post curative radiation	Soft tissue tightness and restrictions, risk for lymphedema, soft tissue pain, fatigue, weakness	Minimized fatigue, weakness, functional loss
		Maximized performance status and cardiopulmonary function
Hormonal therapy (AI)	Arthralgias, myalgias, barriers to function and exercise	Good patient understanding of mechanism of arthralgia/myalgia
		Patient educated in adapted exercise as needed
		Patient compliant with 150 min/week exercise

(Continued)

Unlike other types of cancers, evidence does not support preoperative physical therapy for breast cancer operations as physical therapy interventions do not impact postoperative pain or function or decrease the length of the postoperative hospital stay. Breast surgeons and plastic surgeons should encourage patients to remain active, walk regularly after diagnosis, and after surgery as allowed within their restrictions. Referral of a patient to physical therapy in the postoperative phase and the associated postoperative patient restrictions is at the discretion of the referring surgeon. The most common factor impacting initiation of physical therapy is the presence of postoperative drains. Typically, physical therapy may start when the patient's drains are removed. If patients have postoperative drains yet are reporting moderate to severe chest wall pain, axillary pain, symptomatic cording or have active ROM less than 90 degrees at either shoulder with pending radiation, they should be referred to physical therapy after discussion with their surgeon. Studies suggest earlier intervention is ideal.[6]

Early rehabilitation in the presence of postoperative limitations and drains can still address modifications for ADLs, including a walking or aerobic program with a progressive resistive exercise prescription for noninvolved muscles. This intervention may minimize unnecessary distress, pain, and loss of function and help prepare them for any pending adjuvant systemic or local treatment.

Goals of Postoperative Breast Surgery Physical Therapy

The goals of physical therapy for patients after breast cancer surgery encompass three primary intents: (1) to return the entire upper quarter(s) to full or maximized pain-free preoperative tissue mobility and length, shoulder ROM, strength, and overall function; (2) to educate the patient in potential long-term and late effects of cancer surgery and how to minimize those risks, watch for them, and initiate an action plan if noticed; and (3) to promote patient compliance in a basic combined aerobic and resistive exercise program for pending chemotherapy, radiation, or survivorship and to ensure the patient understands the positive impact of this regular exercise on their treatment tolerability, overall health, cancer recovery, and decreased cancer recurrence.[7]

Post–Breast Cancer Surgery Physical Therapy Subjective History

After surgery for breast cancer, patients may or may not have postoperative pain or functional limitation but still may benefit from physical therapy. Scar tissue development over the next few months may create soft tissue shortening and restrictions, pain, and decreased shoulder ROM, which could be prevented with a chest wall and axillary stretch program. Patients receiving adjuvant chemotherapy and/or radiation may benefit from the development of a personalized exercise prescription to mitigate treatment-induced fatigue. Patients need to be educated about long-term effects, including lymphedema, and learn their role in preventing these sequelae. Exercise may improve quality of life post breast cancer and decrease the risk of breast cancer recurrence.[8]

Once the referral to oncology physical therapy is received, the physical therapist may consult with the referring clinician, the multidisciplinary cancer team, and the cancer nurse navigator, as well as complete a pertinent chart review. At the initial physical therapy evaluation, the therapist will take a subjective history and complaints, examine the patient, do tests and measures, and evaluate the results. Using these results, a determination can be made if the patient needs physical therapy treatment, and if so, what type of treatment, how much, and on what timeline.

In a standard subjective physical therapy evaluation, information is obtained on the patient's past medical history, living situation, home environment, work status, and social and recreational activities. They will be questioned about their evaluation-related complaints, concerns, pain level, physical and functional limitations, and other pertinent information that may be impactful to their rehabilitation and recovery. Attention should be directed at previous injuries or physical dysfunction in the involved upper quarter(s), primarily at the glenohumeral joint(s).

Information should also be gathered on the patient's past, current, and any pending cancer treatment. It is also of great importance to learn the patient's exercise literacy, history, experience, preferences, access to exercise equipment, modes of exercise, and safe places to exercise, as well as any co-morbidities potentially affecting exercise compliance and tolerance. Gathering clinical data with standardized outcome tools are also warranted. Though not specific to breast cancer, subjective outcome tools such as the Quick Disability of the Arm, Shoulder and Hand (DASH),[9] Lower Extremity Functional Scale (LEFS),[10] Timed Up and Go,[11] and the 6-Minute Walk Test[12] will provide functional information to help develop a comprehensive physical therapy plan of care.

Post–Breast Cancer Surgery Objective Examination

At the postoperative objective examination, the physical therapist will assess the involved upper quarter for wound/incision healing and for the presence of abnormal swelling or redness. Any abnormal finding or signs suggestive of potential abscess, infection, dehiscence, or blood clot warrant immediate notification of the referring surgeon.

Because breast cancer surgery involves removing soft tissues, ensuing postoperative tissue restrictions, tissue shortening, and scarring may present over the next few weeks to months. As such, physical therapists, in addition to assessing shoulder, neck, and elbow ROM, should also assess the soft tissues in the surgical area. This involves testing length and mobility of the skin, connective tissue, and muscle at the anterior chest wall, lateral chest wall, and axilla. If the patient had lymph node surgery, the objective examination should look for the presence of cording at the chest, axilla, arm, hand, and/or fingers. The postoperative physical therapy exam should also include strength and functional assessment of the ipsilateral chest wall, scapular, shoulder, and arm muscles.

Post–Breast Cancer Surgery Rehabilitation Assessment

After examination, the physical therapist can make an assessment. This should include the resulting clinical impression, differential impairment diagnosis, the patient's problem list, the patient's goals, and their goal potential or prognosis. If the patient is presenting with pain, the physical therapist should determine the pain source, if possible. Pain in the postoperative patient may be from postsurgical change, nerve, swelling, cording, soft tissue restrictions or shortening, chemotherapy, support drugs, orthopedic injury, or recurrence.

Post–Breast Cancer Surgery Physical Therapy Plan of Care, Interventions, and Treatment

Based on the initial evaluation of subjective and objective data and the assessment, a physical therapy treatment plan of care for the noted impairments and their resulting disabilities will be developed. For example, a postoperative patient may present with decreased ROM with the resulting disability of not being able to dress themselves independently or reach adequately for full ADLs function. With these findings, a stretching program can be developed to address the soft tissue tightness where the patient would be educated in compensatory ADL techniques to regain the ability to dress and reach.

After breast cancer surgery, treatment is directed to reverse and/or prevent any impairments and to optimize the patient's overall health and function. The most common of these interventions include therapeutic exercise (CPT code 97110) and manual therapy (CPT code 97140). Therapeutic exercise involves instructing a patient in specific exercises to address weakness or loss of joint mobility due to disease or injury. Manual therapy includes techniques such as manipulation, soft tissue mobilization, or joint mobilization.

A physical therapy plan of care should include treating any upper quarter integumentary or musculoskeletal dysfunctions like muscle weakness, cording, edema, soft tissue restrictions, limited ROM, and resulting loss of function. All breast surgery rehabilitation plans of care should include a walking program and strengthening for the core, arms, and legs if adjuvant chemotherapy, radiation, or hormonal therapies are pending.

The rehabilitative treatment frequency and duration can be determined in collaboration with the treating therapist, referring provider, and the patient and will be based on the type and severity of clinical findings (Fig. 11.2).

Resolving the Postoperative Breast Cancer Physical Therapy Phase

The postoperative rehabilitation phase can be resolved when the patient meets a variety of goals. These goals include a return to the patient's preoperative comfort and function, full or maximized tissue length and mobility, and full or maximized strength, and ROM. Pain should be controlled optimally. Additionally, patients should be independent in a home strength and stretching program for the upper quarter, knowledgeable in infection, and lymphedema risk reduction, be on an exercise prescription for cancer survivorship and should be ready and able to return to their precancer activities or vocation. They should also be ready for any pending adjuvant chemotherapy, radiation, and/or hormonal therapy.

A key component of a patient's successful return to their precancer activities and/or readiness for ensuing chemotherapy, radiation, or hormonal therapy is their demonstration of self-confidence and compliance with their home exercise prescription of stretching and strengthening to the upper quarter(s) and aerobic and resistive exercise. They should also understand the long-term and potential late effects of breast cancer surgery including the risk of pain, weakness, or soft tissue tightness, and restriction of motion. They should also be alert to signs of developing cellulitis or lymphedema.

Late scarring from breast cancer treatment can result in soft tissue pain, tightness, and decreased length and mobility at the involved upper quarter(s). This can occur even months or years after surgery or radiation. As a result, continued stretching and ROM monitoring for 1 to 2 years after surgery or radiation are recommended. Continued exercise including shoulder abduction with trunk rotation stretch helps ensure that the skin, connective tissue, and muscle maintain their length and mobility during posttreatment scar maturation. The maintenance of this mobility, length, and function may also contribute to decreasing the risk of lymphedema in the ipsilateral arm (Fig. 11.2).[13]

Lymphedema Risk Reduction and Risk Reduction Education

Axillary lymph node removal increases the risk for developing lymphedema in the ipsilateral breast, trunk, arm, hand, and/or fingers. Patients should be educated to avoid infections in the affected extremity, maintaining or achieving a normal body mass index (BMI) range, maximizing the soft tissue length, strength, and mobility at the involved upper quarter by continuing regular exercise.[14]

Healthy and normalized upper extremity lymphatic function can be enhanced by the movement of the ipsilateral arm, muscle contractions in the arm, increased heart rate, and increased respiratory rate.[15] With an increase in post breast cancer treatment BMI being a risk factor for lymphedema, a cancer physical therapy plan of care which includes and encourages long-term aerobic and resistive exercise and

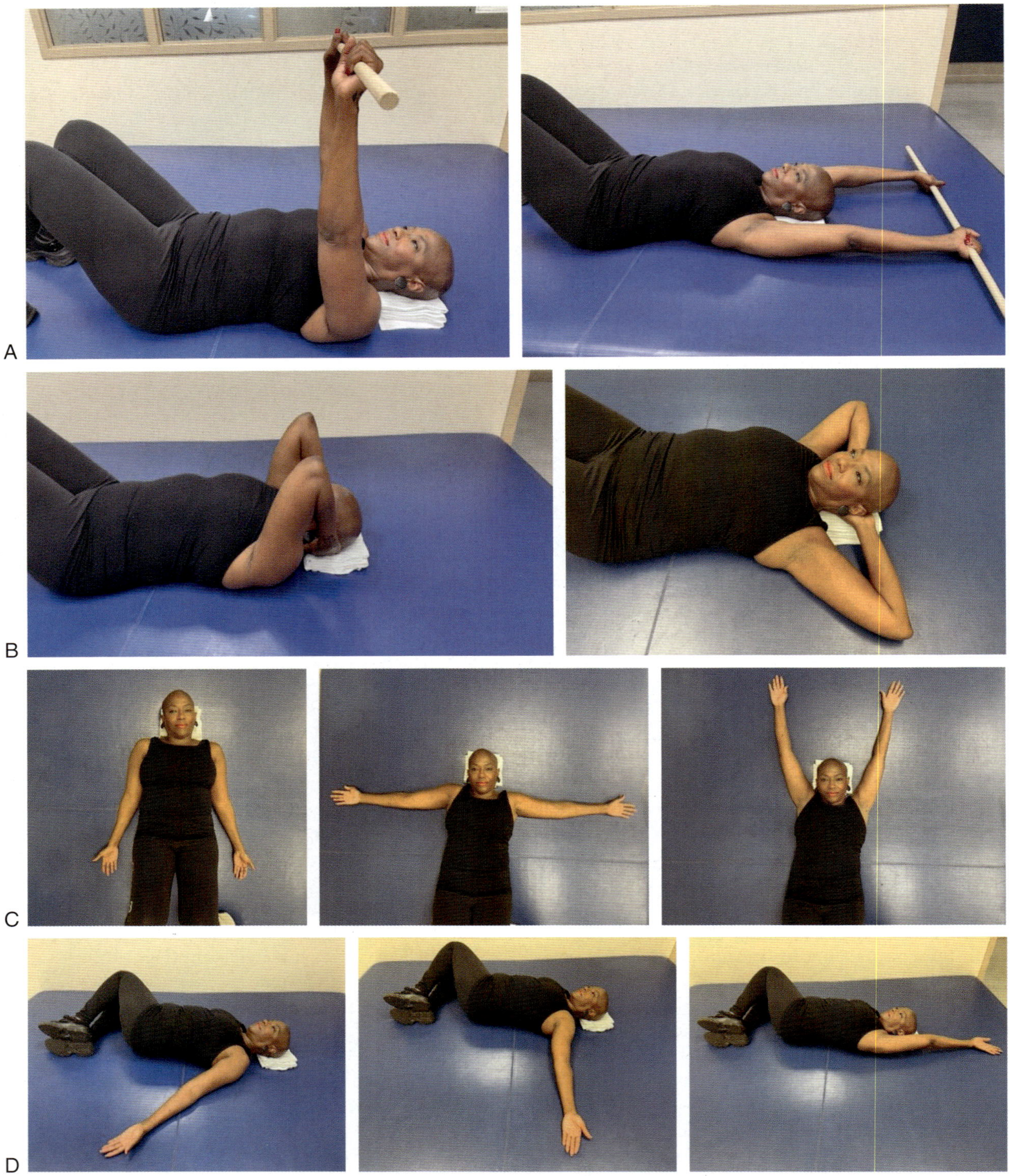

• **Fig. 11.2** Four Key Postoperative Stretches. (A) Shoulder flexion. (B) Shoulder abduction with external rotation. (C) Shoulder abduction in frontal plane. (D) Shoulder abduction with trunk rotation.

activity may benefit patients with BMI and weight management in the post cancer treatment phase where weight gain is common. Research also indicates patients post lymphadenectomy who engage in regular exercise have decreased lymphedema risk.[16,17]

Since infection is the most common precipitator of lymphedema after an axillary dissection or lymphatic channel interruptive surgery, a critical role of a physical therapist is to educate patients in infection risk reduction, in the signs of cellulitis, and an action plan to follow if they notice any of these signs. Decreased exposure to infection in an involved limb and rapid treatment of cellulitis if noted, may lead to decreased risk for lymphedema. Of importance to note, the decades long propagated, traditional lymphedema precautions, such as avoiding air travel, avoiding blood draws, avoiding blood pressure readings, and avoiding repetitive activity, are not evidence based.[18,19]

Chemotherapy: Implications for Rehabilitation Physical Therapy

Section Key Points

- Exercise is a well-established, effective, evidence-based treatment for cancer-related fatigue.
- Physical therapy is a critical intervention for chemotherapy-related cardiopulmonary, musculoskeletal, and functional loss.
- The NCCN in its fatigue guidelines recommends rehabilitation begin at diagnosis.
- Encouraging patients to exercise will benefit them during chemotherapy.
- Exercise during chemotherapy does not contribute to decreased immune cells or immunity.

Efficacy of Physical Therapy During Chemotherapy

Cytotoxic chemotherapy can cause significant and varied side effects including fatigue, muscle loss, nausea, weakness, neuropathy, cardiomyopathy, weight gain, weight loss, loss of overall ADL, decreased vocational and recreational function, and increased distress, anxiety, and depression. Ample evidence exists that physical therapy and exercise are effective treatments to prevent, minimize, or eliminate many of these side effects.[20] Early referral to rehabilitation and starting an exercise program prior to the onset or soon after the onset of neoadjuvant or adjuvant chemotherapy can improve patient outcomes.[21,22]

The NCCN in its guidelines for the treatment of cancer-related fatigue recommends rehabilitation begin at diagnosis. Referrals to rehabilitation during chemotherapy for breast and other cancers remain underutilized in most cancer centers.

Though the exact mechanism of action of the effects of exercise on cancer-related fatigue is not yet clearly defined, physical therapy during chemotherapy is feasible and not associated with adverse events, and multiple studies have shown it to be an effective treatment for cancer-related fatigue.[23] Chemotherapy with certain drugs has been shown to have a deleterious effect on ejection fraction and performance status, both of which can be reduced with exercise.[24]

In addition to their positive impact on cancer-related fatigue, rehabilitation and exercise may improve cognition, chemotherapy-induced peripheral neuropathy (CIPN), inflammation, immunity, cardiovascular function, VO_2max, physical strength, stamina, and maintain or improve BMI.[25] Exercise during treatment may help

maintain adherence to the chemotherapy treatment schedule and completion of the patient's full prescribed chemotherapy regimen.[26]

A physical therapy evaluation and assessment for patients beginning or undergoing chemotherapy will assess the patient's living environment, comorbidities, musculoskeletal or medical restrictions, access to exercise equipment, exercise experience and literacy, motivation and understanding, and access to supportive resources. This assessment may help the patient successfully complete systemic chemotherapy.

A key to maintaining, gaining, or minimizing physical and functional loss and mitigating symptom burden during chemotherapy is by partaking in regular exercise. There is a plethora of evidence supporting exercise as an effective tool in improving patient outcomes during chemotherapy. Effective types of exercise include aerobic exercise, resistive exercise, and combined aerobic and resistive exercise.[27] Research-based dose recommendations range from 30 minutes three times a week during treatment to 150 to 300 minutes per week, including twice-weekly resistive exercise in survivorship (Fig. 11.3).[28]

Patients undergoing cytotoxic chemotherapy tend to have varying symptoms and side effect profiles based on their cycle and dose timeline. Therefore, it is important to note that as symptom burden elevates and subsides, what constitutes "moderate" exercise may also change. During days nearing the end of a chemotherapy cycle, patients may feel stronger and less sick. In this scenario, "moderate" intensity may require longer, more intense activity. If earlier in the chemotherapy cycle, when patients are experiencing more significant symptoms such as extensive fatigue, dehydration, nausea, or neuropathy, to reach "moderate," the exercise dose required may be significantly less to achieve the same perceived exertion. For example, a patient in cycle 1, day 7 of a cytotoxic chemotherapy course may walk 2 miles and do 3 sets of 10 repetitions of quadricep, hamstring, gluteal, biceps, triceps, and upper back strengthening. This same patient in cycle 5, day 3 may achieve a "moderate" perceived exertion by sitting to standing from a chair five times and walking slowly for 2 to 3 minutes. Physical therapists can help support patients during this timeframe by teaching them to adjust their daily routine to what makes their aerobic and resistive exercise feel moderate based on their current symptomology. Evidence suggests that even in the presence of significant symptoms, patients should be encouraged to continue moderately perceived exercise.[29]

Completing the full dose of prescribed chemotherapy for breast cancer is more likely to provide better outcomes. Evidence suggests patients with good muscular strength and cardiovascular fitness are more likely to complete their full course of chemotherapy. A 2021 analysis of two multicenter trials found that using exercise during chemotherapy to increase or maintain cardiovascular and muscular strength in patients with early breast cancer, improved treatment tolerability, and higher rates of chemotherapy completion were achieved.[30]

Effects of Exercise on Health-Related Outcomes in Those with Cancer

What can exercise do?

- **Prevention of 7 common cancers***
  Dose: 2018 Physical Activity Guidelines for Americans: 150-300 min/week moderate or 75-150 min/week vigorous aerobic exercise
- **Survival of 3 common cancers****
  Dose: Exact dose of physical activity needed to reduce cancer-specific or all-cause mortality is not yet known; Overall more activity appears to lead to better risk reduction

*bladder, breast, colon, endometrial, esophageal, kidney and stomach cancers
**breast, colon and prostate cancers

Overall, avoid inactivity, and to improve general health, aim to achieve the current physical activity guidelines for health (150 min/week aerobic exercise and 2x/week strength training).

Outcome	Aerobic Only	Resistance Only	Combination (Aerobic + Resistance)
Strong Evidence	Dose	Dose	Dose
Cancer-related fatigue	**3x**/week for **30** min per session of moderate intensity	**2x**/week of **2** sets of **12-15** reps for major muscle groups at moderate intensity	**3x**/week for **30** min per session of moderate aerobic exercise, plus **2x**/week of resistance training **2** sets of **12-15** reps for major muscle groups at moderate intensity
Health-related quality of life	**2-3x**/week for **30-60** min per session of moderate to vigorous	**2x**/week of **2** sets of **8-15** reps for major muscle groups at a moderate to vigorous intensity	**2-3x**/week for **20-30** min per session of moderate aerobic exercise plus **2x**/week of resistance training **2** sets of **8-15** reps for major muscle groups at moderate to vigorous intensity
Physical Function	**3x**/week for **30-60** min per session of moderate to vigorous	**2-3x**/week of **2** sets of **8-12** reps for major muscle groups at moderate to vigorous intensity	**3x**/week for **20-40** min per session of moderate to vigorous aerobic exercise, plus **2-3x**/week of resistance training **2** sets of **8-12** reps for major muscle group at moderate to vigorous intensity
Anxiety	**3x**/week for **30-60** min per session of moderate to vigorous	Insufficient evidence	**2-3x**/week for **20-40** min of moderate to vigorous aerobic exercise plus **2x**/week of resistance training of **2** sets, **8-12** reps for major muscle groups at moderate to vigorous intensity
Depression	**3x**/week for **30-60** min per session of moderate to vigorous	Insufficient evidence	**2-3x**/week for **20-40** min of moderate to vigorous aerobic exercise plus **2x**/week of resistance training of **2** sets, **8-12** reps for major muscle groups at moderate to vigorous intensity
Lymphedema	Insufficient evidence	**2-3x**/week of progressive, supervised, program for major muscle groups does not exacerbate lymphedema	Insufficient evidence
Moderate Evidence			
Bone health	Insufficient evidence	**2-3x**/week of moderate to vigorous resistance training plus high impact training (sufficient to generate ground reaction force of **3-4** time body weight) for at least **12** months	Insufficient evidence
Sleep	**3-4x**/week for **30-40** min per session of moderate intensity	Insufficient evidence	Insufficient evidence

Citation: bit.ly/cancer_exercise_guidelines

Moderate intensity (40%-59% heart rate reserve or VO₂R) to vigorous intensity (60%-89% heart rate reserve or VO₂R) is recommended.

ExeRcise is Medicine
AMERICAN COLLEGE of SPORTS MEDICINE.

• **Fig. 11.3** Cancer Exercise Guidelines. (bit.ly/cancer_exercise_guidelines. From American College of Sports Medicine. Copyright © 2019 by ACSM. Reprinted by permission.)

A 2020 randomized controlled trial demonstrated some improvement in CIPN-related pain in the upper extremities and some sensory function preservation with exercise during chemotherapy.[31] While receiving neurotoxic chemotherapy agents, physical therapists can also support patients with symptom management. By assisting patients with physical functioning, activity modifications, adaptations, desensitization techniques, and exercise modifications, patients may experience less distress, fewer falls, less loss of ADL function, and maintain activity levels. This may also positively impact a patient's ability to continue chemotherapy.[32]

Like many other types of cancers, chemotherapeutic agents used to treat breast cancer come with potential cardiac toxicity. Exercise has been shown to be cardioprotective in the presence of chemotherapy.[33] A systematic review by the American Physiological Society reveals exercise to be protective to the heart during anthracycline use. Although the mechanisms of exercise-related protections are unclear, studies point to benefits of exercise in reducing oxidative stress and causing more rapid clearance of the cardiotoxic drug from the heart muscle.[34]

For physical therapists, a sustained clinical relationship with their patient during chemotherapy is warranted. Physical therapists can provide strategies and treatments to increase functionality, quality of life, confidence, and exercise compliance during a very difficult time for the patient.[35] A physical therapy evaluation for patients undergoing or pending neoadjuvant or adjuvant chemotherapy should acquire pertinent past medical history, pertinent comorbidities, and subjective and objective data. A standard subjective assessment should include information of living situation, vocational status, support, previous, current, and future cancer treatment, as well as exercise literacy, experience, and available equipment.

Objective data may include outcome tools such as the LEFS, the 6-Minute Walk Test, functional strength testing, stand tolerance, walk tolerance, and balance testing. Frequency and duration of outpatient rehabilitation visits may be based on the patient's starting physical, functional, and exercise capacities, as well as their exercise literacy, experience, and resource availability.

As they progress through their months-long systemic treatment, patients should be taught the important skill set of modifying their aerobic, resistive, and balance exercise based on their symptoms that day. Home exercise prescriptions should involve both basic and advanced aerobic and resistive exercise options for patients to choose from based on how they feel.

Breast Cancer Radiation Therapy: Implications for Physical Therapy

Section Key Points

- Moderate intensity aerobic exercise during radiation therapy minimizes fatigue in patients.
- Progressive resistance exercise during radiation may reduce pain and fatigue.
- Physical therapy is effective in recovering losses of shoulder ROM after radiation therapy.

Overview of Physical Therapy During Radiation Therapy for Breast Cancer

Adjuvant radiation therapy to the breast, chest wall, axilla, and/or supraclavicular nodes as treatment for breast cancer, may present both acute and delayed fatigue, musculoskeletal, integumentary, lymphatic, and cardiopulmonary sequelae. Common radiation treatment-related impairments and disabilities include fatigue, pain, loss of ipsilateral shoulder ROM, upper quarter weakness, soft tissue pain, soft tissue shortening and restrictions, lymphedema, loss of ADL, vocational, social, recreational, and exercise capacity. This gives the physical therapist the opportunity to prepare for, minimize the impact of, and/or prevent many of these side effects with a rehabilitation plan of care.

Rehabilitation During Radiation Therapy for Breast Cancer

The transition phase prior to the patient starting radiation therapy is a valuable timeframe for the physical therapist and patient. In this typically 4-week period between breast surgery or chemotherapy and radiation, the physical therapist has the opportunity to improve the course of both the patient's care and the patient's tolerance of the pending radiation dose.

If the patient has recently completed surgery, assessing postoperative ROM at the shoulders and identifying and addressing any deficits, will help ensure the patient can achieve and maintain the positioning for the radiation planning session and the ensuing radiation treatments. Because the typical patient positioning for radiation to the upper quarter requires both arms to be elevated overhead for a period of time, prior to the onset of radiation the physical therapist will assess the patient's available ROM at both shoulders. If current mobility is inadequate at either shoulder, the physical therapist can alert the radiation oncology team of a potential delay, and increase the frequency of the patient's physical therapy treatments and home exercise

prescription to minimize the risk of delay in the start date. Initiating an exercise program in the postoperative period will also help the patient maintain or regain their preoperative activity levels and not enter radiation with energy or functional deficits. For patients beginning radiation after completing chemotherapy, this time between cancer treatment modalities may be used to initiate and/or support compliance of a new or existing exercise prescription. Doing so, may help minimize the potential for treatment-related fatigue, weakness, and functional loss, and minimize the risk of treatment interruptions.

As the patient begins and continues radiation, whether recovering from surgery or chemotherapy, they should continue their exercise prescription of combined resistive and aerobic exercise. Research strongly supports the use of exercise during radiation to minimize treatment-related fatigue, weakness, and functional loss.[36]

For patients continuing to exhibit soft tissue shortening or restrictions within the radiation field, manual therapy and stretching should be put on hold during radiation therapy. Manual therapy can be resumed, if needed, post radiation when the skin demonstrates adequate healing after consultation with the radiation oncologist. During this period, other areas of physical therapy may continue. If the patient is exhibiting arm weakness, cording, or edema, or continues to have postchemotherapy dysfunctions such as fatigue, weakness, CIPN, or related balance or functional loss, continued physical therapy is warranted and feasible during radiation.

If the skin reaction on the chest wall, breast, or axilla creates symptoms altering their ability to function normally or exercise at their accustomed level, the physical therapist can work with the patient to alter modes and types of exercise to help maintain their strength and energy while still protecting the skin.[37]

Rehabilitation After Radiation Therapy for Breast Cancer

After the conclusion of radiation therapy, the physical therapist should ensure patients continue their upper quarter stretching and continue their aerobic and resistive exercise prescription into survivorship.

In the weeks and months following radiation, the skin, connective tissue, and muscle in the treatment field may shorten, tighten, thicken, and potentially adhere to adjacent tissues. Therefore, patients should be strongly encouraged to continue their stretching program for the soft tissues in and around the radiation treatment field for at least 12 to 18 months.[38] Patients should understand that even if they are pain free with full shoulder ROM and tissue mobility, loss of shoulder mobility and tissue tightness may gradually occur due to late-onset radiation fibrosis. A patient's continued stretching may mitigate these changes. This in turn may minimize any loss of ROM at the ipsilateral shoulder, weakness at the chest or arm, or late onset of soft tissue pain. Maximizing tissue length and mobility at the upper quarter may also improve movement and strength of the arm and can lead to improved lymphatic function and decreased lymphedema risk.[39]

After radiation completion, as patients enter the survivorship phase, they again should be educated, encouraged, and supported in continuing their exercise prescription of 150 to 300 minutes a week of moderate intensity combined aerobic and resistive exercise lifelong.

Metastatic Breast Cancer: Implications for Physical Therapy

Section Key Points

- Patients with metastatic disease live with a plethora of disease and treatment-related physical burdens.
- Patient health, performance status, and ejection fraction are important factors in oncology physician decision-making. Most of these can be modified with physical therapy.[40]
- Resistive exercise is helpful for patients with cancer-induced cachexia.[41]
- Rehabilitation and exercise do not increase risk of fracture or adverse events in patients with bone metastases.[42]
- Skeletal muscle mass, functional energy loss, poor balance, and loss of mobility can negatively impact patient independence. Physical therapy can improve each of these impairments and disabilities.[43]
- Fatigue is prevalent in patients with MBC. Exercise is a proven modality to minimize cancer-related fatigue. Exercise in patients with MBC positively impacts quality of life, physical capacity, safety, and can decrease the risk of further health problems.[44]

Physical Therapy Efficacy in Metastatic Breast Cancer

Oncologists now have a larger and more varied arsenal of treatment options for patients with MBC. As a result, more people with MBC are living longer with a better quality of life. An important consideration for treatment addition or continuation for a patient with MBC includes their overall health, safety, performance status, and ejection fraction. As these factors are all modifiable, physical therapy for patients with advanced cancer can be a valuable tool for impacting the patient's health, longevity, and treatment decisions. As such physical therapists should collaborate with the oncology, palliative, and hospice teams to best heighten a patient's safety, quality of life, and overall care while living with metastatic cancer.[45]

Physical Therapy Interventions in Metastatic Breast Cancer

Common symptoms in MBC, include fatigue, pain, generalized weakness, decreased cardiopulmonary function, impaired balance, frailty, difficulty walking, cancer-related cachexia, and impaired functional capacity. Physical therapists can create plans of care to minimize or eliminate these burdens, directly leading to a capacity to better tolerate treatment and disease-related physical and physiologic stressors.

Fatigue is prevalent in patients with MBC. This fatigue may impact quality of life, vocational capacity, ADL function, independence, living situation, and treatment options and decisions. Even in the setting of metastatic disease, exercise is a mainstay in treatment for cancer-related fatigue. Patients involved in regular prescribed exercise have less frailty, better quality of life, less physical stamina loss, and less risk of further health issues.[46] Physical therapists will create therapeutic exercise prescriptions for patients with MBC based on their presenting mobility, pain level, treatment impacts, cardiopulmonary function, safety awareness, cognitive function, and preferences. Patients with poor performance status, whether from deconditioning, metastatic disease, or treatment, can be seen in the outpatient rehabilitation clinic if needed. Plans of care may focus on therapeutic exercise and activities to enhance patient safety, functional strength, balance, mobility, ADLs, and functional tolerance. Patients not requiring inpatient or outpatient rehabilitation will still benefit from physical therapist oversight and surveillance. Patients can be instructed to be independent with their exercise prescription and its progression or regression based on their current physical tolerance and symptomology. As their overall health and function may change from week to week on treatment, this skill is critical to continued exercise compliance and assistance of a physical therapist is warranted.[47]

MBC and its treatment may present a myriad of function-altering challenges to the patient. For patients being impacted by CIPN, aromatase inhibitor (AI)-related pains, or issues related to brain metastasis, physical therapists can work with the patient, the patient's family, and physician team to create a rehabilitation and exercise plan to minimize pain and disability while maximizing safety, independence, and function.

Bone is the most common area for breast cancer to metastasize. MBC in the bone most often impacts the spine, pelvis, femur, and humerus. These bony areas are integral for good, safe function, independence, and mobility. In collaboration with the physician and based on current imaging and the patient's subjective reports and objective performance, patients will be educated in safety, compensatory activities, safe strengthening, and assessed for safe gait and overall functional performance. Even in the presence of bone metastases and pain, patients can demonstrate improvements in fatigue, decreased pain, increased muscle strength, better balance, improved ADL function, and functional energy with rehabilitation and exercise.[48] Physical therapists can also alert the patient to signs and symptoms related to pain, bowel and bladder function, change in cognitive status or neurological function requiring a call to their physician or necessitating an emergency department visit.

Exercise led by a physical therapist in the presence of metastatic disease, including metastatic bone disease, is safe and feasible and is likely to result in decreased pain, increased lean muscle mass, and increased functional capacity. Exercise does not increase the likelihood of fractures in patients with metastatic bone disease when compared to nonexercisers.[49]

Physical Therapy Interventions for Late and End-Stage Metastatic Breast Cancer

As metastatic cancer progresses, patient's symptoms typically rise. In this scenario of advancing metastatic cancer, fatigue and weakness may become more devastating, balance and ambulation may become unsafe, endurance becomes problematic, and cachexia may develop. Physical therapy in the inpatient, outpatient, and home settings can positively impact safety, quality of life, pain, strength, fatigue, and function in patients entering their last months or weeks of life.

Physical therapists can develop simple energy-conserving exercises and safety programming to benefit patients and help to keep them at home and out of the hospital. With even incremental improvements in cachexia, muscle mass, and strength, patients can better maintain independence and transfer from supine to sit, roll, and go from sitting to standing. Patients maintaining mild strength may tolerate 5 to 10 minutes of standing, which may allow meal prep in the kitchen, self-grooming, and safer toileting. Maintaining the strength to stand, walk even 30 feet, navigate curb steps, and transfer in and out of a car, opens the opportunity for patients to continue oncology office visits, critical community functions, socialization, and quality of life.

Patients with end-stage disease are more likely to require hospitalizations. During hospitalizations, even when not required by medical or safety restrictions, patients tend to be in bed and less active. When entering this scenario with marginal strength and independence, hospitalization can be a negative, irreversible turning point. When patients with late-stage MBC experience an inpatient hospital stay, physical therapists can help with gentle in bed or bedside strengthening, create self-care, bathroom and toileting strategies, and walk programs as appropriate. By maximizing their strength, energy, and ADL and safety skill sets, patients may improve their options for independence, living situation, and discharge destination.

During their last weeks of life, rehabilitation continues to provide value to patients and their caregivers. Physical therapists can assess and instruct patients in the use of appropriate assistive ambulatory devices, proper transfer techniques, provide adaptive equipment for self-care, bathing, and toileting, and provide in-home safety assessments. These simple interventions may increase safety for the patient, family, and caregivers; decrease fear; decrease fall risk; and maximize self-control. In patients experiencing moderate to severe pain, physical therapists can work with physicians and nurses to provide nonpharmacological suggestions for pain control, including heat, ice, transcutaneous electrical nerve stimulation (TENS) and positioning.

Breast Cancer Survivorship: Implications for Physical Therapy

Section Overview

As of January 2022, there are an estimated 4 million breast cancer survivors in the United States, more than any other type of cancer survivor.[50] This alone makes survivorship issues for patients with breast cancer of paramount importance. The American Society of Clinical Oncology (ASCO) reported that upward of 40% of patients with a history of cancer continue to live with pain, fatigue, and weakness for years after the conclusion of treatment.[51] Studies also suggest that inactivity and impaired musculoskeletal and cardiopulmonary health in survivors impacts quality of life and overall survival.[52] Though patients posttreatment may know they should be active, the prevalence of residual side effects, lack of understanding and pain are barriers to being active and partaking in regular exercise. These issues not only impact the breast cancer survivor community but can also place burdens and strains on economic, societal, and health systems.[53]

Physical therapy will continue to have increasing importance for patients completing treatment for breast cancer. There are an increasing number of patients being diagnosed with breast cancer and surviving longer after treatment. Pain and disability resulting from chemotherapy are the main reasons patients discontinue therapy before it is complete—rehab and exercise can reverse some of these effects.

Regular exercise in cancer survivorship is known to decrease recurrence risk and mitigate cardiomyopathy. Finally, supervision in survivorship increases exercise compliance. Many of the long-term and late side effects impacting people living post breast cancer are amenable to physical therapy.[54]

Cardiorespiratory, musculoskeletal, and functional long-term and late side effects of cancer treatment are common after completing treatment for breast cancer. "Long-term side effects" starting during treatment and continuing after the conclusion of treatment include fatigue, weakness, loss of functional energy, CIPN, cardiorespiratory loss, anxiety, depression, and upper quarter stiffness, weakness, and loss of function. "Late effects," side effects from cancer treatment that present after the conclusion of treatment, include cardiomyopathy, bone mineral density loss, lymphedema, radiation fibrosis, and postsurgical scar tissue affecting upper quarter comfort, mobility, and function. Despite the value of exercise, most breast cancer survivors are not meeting the ACS's exercise guidelines of 150 to 300 minutes per week of exercise and are living below their physical, psychological, and functional optimum. Although cancer survivorship care plans may recommend an active lifestyle, patients are often not given the guidance, programs, or skills to ensure or maximize their success. Physical therapists contribute to patient outcomes in survivorship by continuing to address and treat these long-term and late cancer treatment effects and by helping patients comply with exercise prescriptions, overcoming barriers, and increasing confidence.

Physical Therapy for Long-Term Side Effects

Musculoskeletal pain, weakness, stiffness, and impaired function often follow people into survivorship after surgery of the breast and axilla. For patients treated with chemotherapy and/or radiation, early survivorship may also include fatigue, limited functional energy, neuropathy, cognitive impairment, anxiety, and depression. Each of these long-term post-cancer side effects is amenable to physical therapy.

Scarring, soft tissue shortening, and restrictions at the chest wall may remain or may progress with time causing continuing or worsening symptoms. This can lead to pain, limited ROM, decreased use, and muscle weakness. These symptoms may impact ADLs, social activity, inactivity, deter exercise, and can contribute to fear of recurrence and negatively impact lymphedema risk. In the early survivorship phase, physical therapists will continue to treat soft tissue dysfunction as it arises or changes with manual therapy and will continue to progress and monitor the patient's upper quarter stretching and strength program. Education about the possibility of scar tissue shortening and tightening in the future is important for the patient's understanding and compliance to help them eventually achieve and maintain normal strength, shoulder ROM, and normal tissue length throughout the chest wall and axilla. Home rehabilitation prescriptions for this population are patient dysfunction specific, but generally should include strengthening of the upper quarter muscles two to three times weekly along with stretching most days of the week.

Persistent posttreatment-related fatigue, chemotherapy-related skeletal muscle mass loss, and cardiopulmonary loss can be effectively treated under the care of a physical therapist with therapeutic exercise. Physical therapists will continue to support patients in maintaining their individual exercise prescriptions of combined aerobic and resistive exercise developed during their treatment.

When cancer therapy is complete, patients often discontinue their exercise prescriptions due to thinking they are "done" or are just too tired. During survivorship, patients will tend to be more compliant with their exercise with continued encouragement from their cancer doctors and nurses, if they have support resources and are engaging in goal-oriented exercise.

Though evidence suggests exercise may minimize some CIPN, it continues to be a significant issue for many cancer survivors, even those engaging in regular exercise. Neuropathy in patient's hands and/or feet causes a wide range of symptoms and impairments ranging from inconsequential to life altering. With late onset of CIPN, exercise may have limited to no impact on the amount of dysesthesia present in the extremities. However, if the patient's sensory symptoms are impairing their ability to move, function, be active and exercise they may develop secondary weakness and loss of dexterity in the muscles of the fingers, hands, arms, feet, and lower legs. This may lead to a limited ability to perform regular self-care, ADLs, social, and recreational activities and dissuade people from exercise. Patients with chemotherapy-related neuropathy in the feet and lower legs may have balance and tripping issues resulting in an increased risk of falling. Whether or not the current amount of sensory dysesthesia is permanent, will reduce with time, or can be reduced with exercise, physical therapy can provide immediate exercise for balance, lower leg, and foot strength to improve function, tolerance, and safety and decrease fall risk. Simple home programs of strength and balance exercise are effective, inexpensive, and do not require special equipment. Patients should learn that inactivity does not decrease the neuropathy but may lead to more weakness and loss of function. Physical therapists may also be helpful to patients living with long-term CIPN by assisting them in finding strategies to cope with the dysesthesia and still maintain social, recreational, ADL, and exercise function. This may include desensitization, finding alternate footwear or modified utensils, compensatory techniques, and finding safe enjoyable modes of exercise that minimally impact the patient's neuropathy-related symptoms.[55]

Physical Therapy for Late Effects

Late effects potentially occurring after breast cancer treatment include cardiomyopathy, lymphedema of the breast, chest wall, and arm, arthralgias and myalgias from aromatase inhibitor (AI) use, scar tissue, radiation fibrosis, and bone mineral density loss. With patient education, physical therapy as needed, and continued exercise, there is an opportunity to mitigate the risk of developing some of these late effects.

AIs are known to cause arthralgias and myalgias in patients ranging in severity from mild to severe. This pain is a common reason for patients to discontinue this important medication in recurrence avoidance. A home-based prescription of aerobic and strength exercise may be effective in lessening or eliminating this AI-related pain potentially increasing medication compliance.[56]

Because scar tissue maturation and radiation fibrosis can happen over months or years, patients should be made aware of their tissue mobility status, their shoulder ROM capacity, and their arm strength. Patients with mild residual deficits in soft tissue and shoulder mobility should continue on their prescription to maximize improvements. Knowing that scar tissue and radiation can insidiously develop slowly over time, even patients with pain-free normal mobility should periodically check their shoulder ROM, tissue length, and tissue mobility over the first several years post surgery and radiation.

Exercise as a modality itself can impact the likelihood and severity of multiple late effects from cancer treatment. Therefore, exercise prescriptions are crucial in cancer survivorship. A patient's exercise prescription is a valuable tool that can help minimize the risk or impact of cardiomyopathy, bone mineral density loss, fatigue, strength, and lymphedema. There is good evidence that exercise may improve quality of life and overall survival. Still compliance with continued, regular exercise in cancer survivorship is low. Physical therapists are a crucial component in a patient's success in maintaining regular exercise. Patients will be helped with encouragement, goal setting, oversight, direction, and support with questions and active surveillance.

Prior to discontinuing the patient's plan of care, they should be educated in their specific late symptom potential, the strategies to minimize risk if possible, how to watch for them, and an action plan to follow if these symptoms were to arise. At the time of physical therapy plan of care discontinuation, physical therapists should also reinforce the importance of their established relationship and offer lifelong care. Physical therapists may also do follow-up visits along the timeline of the physician or survivorship visits. Patients should be educated to call their physical therapist if they have questions, if they feel their home program is no longer adequate, or if their symptoms are reemerging or worsening. If they have new or unexplained symptoms, swelling, or signs of infection, abscess, or cellulitis, they should immediately contact their physician or physician extender.

Team Phoenix—An Innovative Tool to Redefine Cancer Survivorship

Our institution has supported an intense fitness program for women cancer survivors after completion of cancer treatment. Team Phoenix, originally started in 2011, is a 14-week medically overseen, goal-oriented exercise training program where multidisciplinary clinicians, triathlon coaches, and volunteers train and teach cancer survivors to regain endurance, strength, flexibility, and overall health and wellness by training for and completing a sprint-distance triathlon. The program has three major goals:

1. It empowers cancer survivors to improve their physical and mental fitness.
2. It redefines "survivorship" by teaching the joys of lifelong fitness and by removing physical and psychological barriers to maintaining exercise routines; and
3. The information from Team Phoenix athletes helps future survivors with data correlating the impact of exercise on inflammation, cancer-related fatigue, and cardiac function, which may be adversely affected by cancer treatment.

Now, with over 340 "alumnae" more than 70% of the athletes who participated continue with regular fitness activities including running, biking, swimming, or other exercise activities. Over 50% of the "alumnae" have continued with triathlons of varying distances and many have moved on to complete half-Ironman distances. Several have even completed a full Ironman distance triathlon. This innovative program has shown that with proper investment and training, cancer survivors can learn to engage in lifelong exercise and move on to live a more productive and healthier life after cancer.

Chapter Summary

Oncology physical therapy is an evidence-based, third-party reimbursed area of medical care known to positively impact morbidity and mortality associated with cancer treatment, cancer survivorship, and end of life care. Because cancer operations, systemic treatments, and radiation therapy present side effect profiles, including symptomology known to be amenable to physical therapy, the NCCN and ASCO recommend patients exposed to these modalities be referred for a physical therapy consult around the time of their cancer diagnosis. At the initial consult, physical therapists will examine the patient for musculoskeletal, cardiopulmonary, integumentary, and functional impairments and disabilities and create a plan of care involving treatments for the current symptoms, the development of and instruction in a comprehensive exercise prescription, and a surveillance plan for potential impairments as the patient progresses through their cancer treatment. The physical therapist's role in the care of a patient with breast cancer extends from diagnosis into survivorship or end of life care.

As well as improving outcomes for cancer patients, oncology physical therapy may improve outcomes for cancer programs. Physical therapy for patients with cancer has been shown to increase patient satisfaction, be cost effective, decrease fall risk, decrease hospital length of stay and readmissions, and decrease emergency department utilization.

Cancer physical therapy is low-cost, low-risk, high-value, evidence-based treatment that patients with cancer deserve. Because improved oncology outcomes are associated with physical therapy, referral at the time of cancer diagnosis is warranted and encouraged.

References

1. Kannan P, Lam HY, Ma TK, et al. Efficacy of physical therapy interventions on quality of life and upper quadrant pain severity in women with post-mastectomy pain syndrome: a systematic review and meta-analysis. *Qual Life Res*. 2021:1–23.
2. Haykowsky MJ, Scott JM, Hudson K, et al. Lifestyle interventions to improve cardiorespiratory fitness and reduce breast cancer recurrence. *Am Soc Clin Oncol Educ Book*. 2017;37:57–64.
3. Wilson CM, Mueller K, Briggs R. Physical therapists' contribution to the hospice and palliative care interdisciplinary team: a clinical summary. *J Hosp Palliat Nurs*. 2017;19(6):588–596.
4. Klein I, Kalichman L, Chen N, et al. Effect of physical activity levels on oncological breast surgery recovery: a prospective cohort study. *Sci Rep*. 2021;11(1):1–10.
5. Kannan P, Lam HY, Ma TK, et al. Efficacy of physical therapy interventions on quality of life and upper quadrant pain severity in women with post-mastectomy pain syndrome: a systematic review and meta-analysis. *Qual Life Res*. 2021:1–23.
6. Akram S, Ashraf HS, Umar B, et al. Comparison of health related quality of life among female patients who had received early versus delayed physiotherapy after modified radical mastectomy. *RMJ*. 2021;46(2):292–292.
7. Loprinzi PD, Cardinal BJ, Winters-Stone K, et al. Physical activity and the risk of breast cancer recurrence: a literature review. *Oncol Nurs Forum*. 2012;39(3):269–274.

8. Cormie P, Zopf EM, Zhang X, et al. The impact of exercise on cancer mortality, recurrence, and treatment-related adverse effects. *Epidemiol Rev*. 2017;39(1):71–92.

9. LeBlanc M, Stineman M, DeMichele A, et al. Validation of QuickDASH outcome measure in breast cancer survivors for upper extremity disability. *Arch Phys Med Rehabil*. 2014;95(3):493–498.

10. Mehta SP, Fulton A, Quach C, et al. Measurement properties of the lower extremity functional scale: a systematic review. *J Orthop Sports Phys Ther*. 2016;46(3):200–216.

11. Christopher A, Kraft E, Olenick H, et al. The reliability and validity of the Timed Up and Go as a clinical tool in individuals with and without disabilities across a lifespan: a systematic review: Psychometric properties of the Timed Up and Go. *Disabil Rehabil*. 2021;43(13):1799–1813.

12. But-Hadzic J, Dervisevic M, Karpljuk D, et al. Six-minute walk distance in breast cancer survivors—A systematic review with meta-analysis. *Int J Environ Res Public Health*. 2021;18(5):2591.

13. Campbell KL, Winters-Stone K, Wiskemann J, et al. Exercise guidelines for cancer survivors: consensus statement from international multidisciplinary roundtable. *Med Sci Sports Exerc*. 2019;51(11):2375.

14. Baumann FT, Reike A, Hallek M, et al. Does exercise have a preventive effect on secondary lymphedema in breast cancer patients following local treatment—a systematic review. *Breast Care*. 2018;13(5):380–385.

15. Lane K, Worsley D, McKenzie D. Exercise and the lymphatic system. *Sports Med*. 2005;35(6):461–471.

16. Simonavice E, Kim JS, Panton L. Effects of resistance exercise in women with or at risk for breast cancer-related lymphedema. *Support Care Cancer*. 2017;25(1):9–15.

17. Schmitz KH, Ahmed RL, Troxel AB, et al. Weight lifting for women at risk for breast cancer–related lymphedema: a randomized trial. *JAMA*. 2010;304(24):2699–2705.

18. Ahn S, Port ER. Lymphedema precautions: time to abandon old practices. *J Clin Oncol*. 2016;34(7):655–658.

19. Konishi T, Tanabe M, Michihata N, et al. Risk factors for arm lymphedema following breast cancer surgery: a Japanese nationwide database study of 84,022 patients. *Breast Cancer*. 2022:1–10.

20. Hutchison NA, Deval N, Rabusch S, et al. Physical therapy–based exercise protocol for cancer patients: evaluating outcomes for cardiopulmonary performance and cancer-related fatigue. *PM&R*. 2019;11(11):1178–1183.

21. An KY, Arthuso FZ, Kang DW, et al. Exercise and health-related fitness predictors of chemotherapy completion in breast cancer patients: pooled analysis of two multicenter trials. *Breast Cancer Res Treat*. 2021;188(2):399–407.

22. Mustian KM, Alfano CM, Heckler C, et al. Comparison of pharmaceutical, psychological, and exercise treatments for cancer-related fatigue: a meta-analysis. *JAMA Oncol*. 2017;3(7):961–968.

23. Hendricks T, Williams P. Exercise Testing and Prescription With Cancer Patients to Help Relieve Cancer-Related Fatigue (CRF); 2022.

24. Pinkstaff SO. Breast cancer and cardiovascular disease: defining the role of physical therapists. *Rehabil Oncol*. 2018;36(4): E10–E13.

25. Cave J, Paschalis A, Huang CY, et al. A systematic review of the safety and efficacy of aerobic exercise during cytotoxic chemotherapy treatment. *Support Care Cancer*. 2018;26(10):3337–3351.

26. An KY, Arthuso FZ, Kang DW, et al. Exercise and health-related fitness predictors of chemotherapy completion in breast cancer

patients: pooled analysis of two multicenter trials. *Breast Cancer Res Treat*. 2021;188(2):399–407.

27. Schmitz KH. *Exercise oncology: prescribing physical activity before and after a cancer diagnosis*. Springer; 2020;No. 180348.

28. Campbell KL, Winters-Stone K, Wiskemann J, et al. Exercise guidelines for cancer survivors: consensus statement from international multidisciplinary roundtable. *Med Sci Sports Exerc*. 2019;51(11):2375.

29. Johnsson A, Demmelmaier I, Sjövall K, et al. A single exercise session improves side-effects of chemotherapy in women with breast cancer: an observational study. *BMC Cancer*. 2019;19(1):1–9.

30. An K-Y, Arthuso FZ, Kang DW, et al. Exercise and health-related fitness predictors of chemotherapy completion in breast cancer patients: pooled analysis of two multicenter trials. *Breast Cancer Res Treat*. 2021;188(2):399–407.

31. Hammond A, Elizabeth MP, Steinfeld K, et al. An exploratory randomized trial of physical therapy for the treatment of chemotherapy-induced peripheral neuropathy. *Neurorehabil Neural Repair*. 2020;34(3):235–246.

32. Brayall P, Donlon E, Doyle L, et al. Physical therapy–based interventions improve balance, function, symptoms, and quality of life in patients with chemotherapy-induced peripheral neuropathy: a systematic review. *Rehabil Oncol*. 2018;36(3):161–166.

33. van der Schoot G, Ormel H, Westerink N, et al. Optimal Timing of a Physical Exercise Intervention to Improve Cardiorespiratory Fitness. *J Am Coll Cardiol CardioOnc*. 2022;4(4):491–503.

34. Chen JJ, Wu PT, Middlekauff HR, et al. Aerobic exercise in anthracycline-induced cardiotoxicity: a systematic review of current evidence and future directions. *Am J Physiol Heart Circ Physiol*. 2017;312(2):H213–H222.

35. van der Leeden M, Huijsmans RJ, Geleijn E, et al. Tailoring exercise interventions to comorbidities and treatment-induced adverse effects in patients with early stage breast cancer undergoing chemotherapy: a framework to support clinical decisions. *Disabil Rehabil*. 2018;40(4):486–496.

36. Drouin JS, Young TJ, Beeler J, et al. Random control clinical trial on the effects of aerobic exercise training on erythrocyte levels during radiation treatment for breast cancer. *Cancer*. 2006;107(10):2490–2495.

37. Schmidt ME, Meynköhn A, Habermann N, et al. Resistance exercise and inflammation in breast cancer patients undergoing adjuvant radiation therapy: mediation analysis from a randomized, controlled intervention trial. *Int J Radiat Oncol Biol Phys*. 2016;94(2):329–337.

38. da Silva Leal NFB, de Oliveira HF, Carrara HHA. Supervised physical therapy in women treated with radiotherapy for breast cancer. *Rev Lat Am Enfermagem*. 2016;24:e2755.

39. Kung TA, Champaneria MC, Maki JH, et al. Current concepts in the surgical management of lymphedema. *Plast Reconstr Surg*. 2017;139(4):1003e–1013e.

40. Leggio M, Fusco A, Loreti C, et al. Effects of exercise training in heart failure with preserved ejection fraction: an updated systematic literature review. *Heart Fail Rev*. 2020;25(5):703–711.

41. Kamel FAH, Basha MA, Alsharidah AS, et al. Resistance training impact on mobility, muscle strength and lean mass in pancreatic cancer cachexia: a randomized controlled trial. *Clin Rehabil*. 2020;34(11):1391–1399.

42. Sheill G, Guinan EM, Peat N, et al. Considerations for exercise prescription in patients with bone metastases: a comprehensive narrative review. *PM&R*. 2018;10(8):843–864.

43. Groen WG, Ten Tusscher MR, Verbeek R, et al. Feasibility and outcomes of a goal-directed physical therapy program for

44. Navigante A, Morgado PC. Does physical exercise improve quality of life of advanced cancer patients? *Curr Opin Support Palliat Care*. 2016;10(4):306–309.

45. Wilson CM, Mueller K, Briggs R. Physical therapists' contribution to the hospice and palliative care interdisciplinary team: a clinical summary. *J Hosp Palliat Nurs*. 2017;19(6):588–596.

46. Dittus KL, Gramling RE, Ades PA. Exercise interventions for individuals with advanced cancer: a systematic review. *Prev Med*. 2017;104:124–132.

47. Yee J, Davis GM, Hackett D, et al. Physical activity for symptom management in women with metastatic breast cancer: a randomized feasibility trial on physical activity and breast metastases. *J Pain Symptom Manage*. 2019;58(6):929–939.

48. Guo Y, Ngo-Huang AT, Fu JB. Perspectives on spinal precautions in patients who have cancer and spinal metastasis. *Phys Ther*. 2020;100(3):554–563.

49. Sheill G, Guinan EM, Peat N, et al. Considerations for exercise prescription in patients with bone metastases: a comprehensive narrative review. *PM&R*. 2018;10(8):843–864.

50. Miller KD, Siegel RL, Lin CC, et al. Cancer treatment and survivorship statistics, 2022. *CA Cancer J Clin*. 2022;1–23.

51. Paice JA, Lacchetti C, Bruera E. Management of chronic pain in survivors of adult cancers: ASCO clinical practice guideline summary. *J Oncol Pract*. 2016;12(8):757–762.

52. Elme A, Utriainen M, Kellokumpu-Lehtinen P, et al. Obesity and physical inactivity are related to impaired physical health of breast cancer survivors. *Anticancer Res*. 2013;33(4):1595–1602.

53. Potiaumpai M, Doerksen SE, Chinchilli VM, et al. Cost evaluation of an exercise oncology intervention: the exercise in all chemotherapy trial. *Cancer Rep*. 2022;5(3):e1490.

54. Ormel HL, Schröder CP, van der Schoot GGF, et al. Effects of supervised exercise during adjuvant endocrine therapy in overweight or obese patients with breast cancer: The I-MOVE study. *Breast*. 2021;58:138–146.

55. Brayall P, Donlon E, Doyle L, et al. Physical therapy–based interventions improve balance, function, symptoms, and quality of life in patients with chemotherapy-induced peripheral neuropathy: a systematic review. *Rehabil Oncol*. 2018;36(3):161–166.

56. Baglia ML, Lin IH, Cartmel B, et al. Endocrine-related quality of life in a randomized trial of exercise on aromatase inhibitor–induced arthralgias in breast cancer survivors. *Cancer*. 2019;125(13):2262–2271.

PART 4

Follow-Up and After Care

12
Nutrition

ELIZABETH DUCHAC AND SHANNON MCCARTHY

Introduction

Nutrition care is essential not only in after care or survivorship but also as a supportive resource throughout diagnosis and treatment of breast cancer. Patients often request nutrition advice early on in their care. Breast cancer patients in particular show interest in learning more about diet and lifestyle. Many want to learn all they can to ensure a good outcome. In our system, we focus on plant-based eating, as able, and promote physical activity as tolerated. When patients begin treatment, our first goal is for them to survive and thrive throughout treatment. We assist with symptom management throughout treatment, in addition to providing healthy eating and lifestyle information.

Role of Oncology Dietitians

Oncology dietitians have a specific focus on oncology patients and are encouraged to obtain designated certification. The Oncology Nutrition Dietetic Practice Group of the Academy of Nutrition and Dietetics has worked together with the Commission on Dietetic Registration to create a Board Certification credential (Certified Specialist in Oncology Nutrition [CSO]) for Registered Dietitians in Oncology Nutrition. CSO stands for Board Certified Specialist in Oncology Nutrition. A recommended minimum of 2 years of clinical practice with documentation of 2000 hours of practice experience in the oncology care setting is required.[1]

Oncology dietitians participate in multidisciplinary clinics where appropriate, including breast, head and neck, gastrointestinal, thoracic cancers, and survivorship. Oncology dietitians provide education to patients, family, and staff. We also present to the community for various events and participate in community health fairs regarding cancer prevention.

Oncology dietitians assess for malnutrition, as this is a common issue in the oncology population. We perform a Nutrition Focused Physical Assessment on our patients. We document this assessment in the electronic medical record (EMR) and update it throughout treatment. Preventing malnutrition and early intervention is always preferable and far more achievable than reversing severe malnutrition.

Documenting malnutrition in the outpatient setting helps support the acute care staff with malnutrition diagnoses in the hospital setting. Outcomes are affected by malnutrition status, so documenting this throughout a patient's care supports accuracy and efficacy, in addition to achieving best outcomes (Fig. 12.1).

During treatment, oncology dietitians support patients with food and fluid recommendations. We may suggest oral nutrition supplement drinks. Often patients are interested in making healthy changes during treatment, but other times their focus is survival or getting through treatment. It is imperative that the oncology dietitian meets the patient where they are with their own treatment goals.

Oncology dietitians support our colleagues' recommendations to start a walking program as soon as possible. We promote physical activity as able, and often suggest cancer rehabilitation for patients when appropriate. If patients are reluctant to try cancer rehab or therapies, additional encouragement from the dietitian to try these may be beneficial.

Certain patients may need nutrition support, such as enteral or parenteral nutrition. The oncology dietitian assesses the patient's needs and collaborates with the provider to prescribe the appropriate enteral or parenteral formula. Some oncology dietitians instruct patients on how to use their feeding tubes when needed. We monitor their intake and tolerance for nutrition support and ensure proper fluid intake.

Medical Nutrition Therapy

Medical nutrition therapy (MNT) is defined as "nutritional diagnostic, therapy, and counseling services for the purpose of disease management which are furnished by a registered dietitian or nutrition professional" (Medicare MNT legislation, effective January 1, 2022). MNT is a specific application of the Nutrition Care Process in clinical settings that is focused on the management of diseases. MNT involves in-depth individualized nutrition assessment and a duration and frequency of care using the Nutrition Care Process to manage disease.

MNT for oncology patients includes setting goals of care. These include addressing any nutrition impact symptoms resulting from the disease and its treatment; supporting the

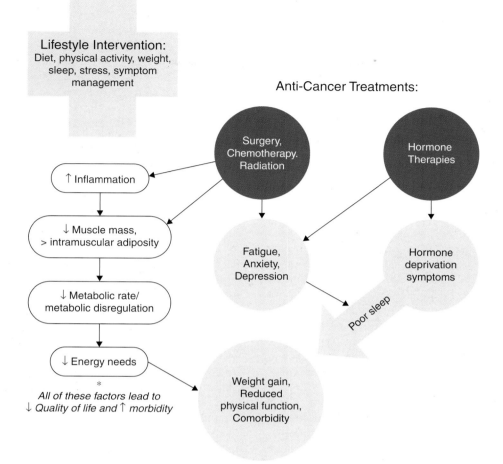

• **Fig. 12.1** Lifestyle Intervention for Symptoms Experienced by Cancer Survivors.

patient's goals while providing evidenced-based care; limiting unintentional weight loss during treatment to less than 1 to 2 pounds per week; and encouraging the patient to maintain and obtain a healthy body weight. Previous recommendations in oncology patients would have avoided any weight loss during treatment, even intentional, to improve other health outcomes and minimize additional cancer risk. More recent evidence in the overweight patient suggests slow, intentional weight loss while eating healthfully and increasing physical activity is considered safe. A study comparing women with breast cancer and women without breast cancer found no difference in resting energy expenditure between the two groups.[2]

Nutrition-related problems during breast cancer treatment include fatigue, vasomotor symptoms, lymphedema, bone loss, musculoskeletal symptoms from aromatase inhibitors, neuropathy, nausea and vomiting from chemotherapy, mucositis, taste changes, and weight gain.

A common issue for cancer patients, particularly breast cancer, is well-meaning family and friends providing their own suggestions for diet and supplementation. With information so easily accessible, this can oftentimes prove to be more of a hinderance than helpful. People are overloaded with information and may find it difficult to sift through facts or solutions that are effective. Food and supplement pills are two areas where patients get excessive information or suggestions. We can help them navigate this complicated part of their treatment with reliable, reputable resources.

Family members often would like to be able to do something to help their loved one who is suffering through a diagnosis and treatment. Food is an area they often feel they can help with. Part of our role as a dietitian is to help family members understand the complexity of symptoms, as well as gray areas. Things can change quickly in symptoms and side effects—something that worked last week, or last cycle, may not work today, or at this time. We can help patients and family members understand this changing flow, and realize it is to be expected and common. Family members work hard to prepare foods for their loved one that they request, usually like, and typically work well, but often the patient is unable to eat it as desired or finish a plate of food. As frustrating as this is to deal with, it is quite common. Sometimes reassuring patients and families that this experience is fairly common is a way to help them cope with this aspect of their disease. Sometimes a husband or a wife will feel this inability to eat or finish a plate of food is personal to the helper. It is important we remind them this is a normal challenge facing patients on cancer treatment.

Many nutrition supplement pills make claims they can speed up apoptosis, slow tumor growth, or prevent cancer altogether. As nutrition professionals we must help our patients and family members sift through this information as well. Some supplement pills may interact with certain chemotherapy or immunotherapy drugs, causing them to become less efficacious. Many of these pills are metabolized on the same pathway as the antineoplastic drugs, thus potentially interfering with the drugs' effectiveness. Oncology dietitians can recommend food sources of vitamins and minerals to help manage side effects, and potentially increase effectiveness of these therapies. These changes should be made in consultation with the patient's treating oncologist.

Evidence shows a diet made up mostly of minimally processed plants can lower the risk for cancer, in addition to other chronic diseases. Getting the health benefits of plant-based diet eating does *not* require one to completely remove all animal proteins (eggs, poultry, fish, and dairy) from one's diet. Instead, one should make plants the majority of each meal.[3] Decreasing consumption of red meat can decrease the risk of breast cancer. Including omega-3 fatty acids in the diet has been shown to decrease mortality in breast cancer patients.[2]

Phytonutrients are an important part of a plant-based diet. They provide color, flavor, fiber, and texture. Phytonutrients include carotenoids, lycopene, isoflavones, and anthocyanins. They may help prevent cancer through a variety of mechanisms, including preventing damage to cellular DNA. Different colors of plant-based foods provide different combinations of phytonutrients. The type and amounts of phytonutrients vary greatly between vegetables and fruits. We recommend including a wide variety of colorful plant foods to get the benefits from as many different phytonutrients as possible.[4]

Functional foods are foods that are eaten in the diet to provide beneficial properties that go beyond the basic nutritional function.[5] In relation to breast cancer, soy and flaxseed have been studied for the effects they can have on breast cancer risks and the effects their compounds have on tumors.

Soy

It is important to address the link between soy consumption and breast cancer risk. Many breast cancer patients feel that they need to avoid soy. Soy's role has been controversial because earlier animal studies suggested that the phytoestrogens contained in soy isoflavones may stimulate breast cancer growth. Newer studies have found that this is not the case and, in some cases, those phytoestrogens may lower the risk of breast cancer. These studies have found that it is safe to use soy in moderation in breast cancer patients. Some lab studies have shown that isoflavones could act like estrogen and promote tumor growth, and other studies found them to act against the effects of estrogen and have protective properties. Meta-analysis of the prospective cohort studies had previously shown that relationships between levels of dietary isoflavones and breast cancer risk was inconclusive, but newer meta-analysis explored all possible correlations between dietary isoflavone intake and the risk of breast cancer.[6] This analysis found that moderate intake of soy foods was not significantly related to breast cancer risk, but a high intake of soy foods correlated with reduced risk of breast cancer (RR = 0.87, P = .048). In this meta-analysis, it also found that isoflavones may inhibit aromatase synthesis by binding to the estrogen receptor (ER), possibly blocking the binding of more potent natural estrogens. The Zhao et al. meta-analysis found that high intakes of soy foods provide a beneficial role in reducing the risk of breast cancer but did not study the mechanisms of how soy compounds do this.[6]

While soy is not particularly common in the North American and European diets, it is a common protein in diets of Asian countries. Based on observational studies, soy food consumption may provide protection from breast cancer primarily in Asian countries but not Western countries.[7] It raises the question of the protective effects of soy foods based on genetic factors such as metabolic enzymes, timing of exposure, or intestinal metabolism by microbiota. In Asian countries, soy is introduced into the diet at a young age, and it is hypothesized that consumption during the prepubescent period can affect breast tissue morphology, decreasing overall risk of developing breast cancer.[8] Asian populations have the highest intake of isoflavones in the diet with 20 to 50 mg/day.[7] In Western countries, it is less common to eat whole soy foods, and it is usually introduced later in the life span, with North American populations consuming between 0.15 and 3 mg/day and European populations consuming even less at 0.49 to 1 mg.[5] The occurrence of breast cancer in the United States and Europe is two to four times higher than in Asia.[9] There have been many randomized controlled trials (RCTs) to study how introducing soy isoflavones into the diet can affect estrogen homeostasis and its effect on breast cancer risk.

With the promotion of plant-based diets, soy is an important protein because it has the complete amino acid profile that the body requires, making it an ideal substitute for animal proteins. It is also lower in calorie and fat content than some animal proteins, which can be helpful in weight management. Besides being a good source of protein, many soy foods are good sources of fiber and selenium. Soy isoflavones are also good source of antioxidants.[9]

Soy contains six different isoflavones with the three primaries being daidzein, genistein, and glycitein.[8,10] Isoflavones are phytoestrogens, and soy is the main source of phytoestrogens in the human diet. They are structurally like 17-β-estradiol and may bind to estrogen Erα and Erβ receptors. Genistein, the main isoflavone in soy, was shown to have a two-phase effect on the ER present on breast cancer cells in a study by researchers at Texas A&M University-Commerce.[8] At low concentrations, genistein stimulated the growth of positive-ER breast cancer cells, whereas at higher concentrations it inhibited the growth of ER positive breast cancer cells.[7,11]

Soy is considered a healthy food due to its many health-promoting compounds. Isoflavones exert antioxidant properties that protect breast cells from the damage of oxidative stress that can lead to cancer development through stimulation of inflammatory and proliferative pathways.[9] Other compounds such as phenolic acid, phytic acid, lignans, and saponins can provide more antioxidant and anti-inflammatory defense against cancer proliferation.[12] Soy is also a good source of folate helping maintain healthy deoxyribonucleic acid (DNA) and keep cancer-promoting genes inactivated. Half a cup of cooked soybeans contains 47 µg of folate while a quarter cup of soynuts contain almost half the daily recommended value of folate.[13]

Soy is considered safe to consume in moderation for breast cancer patients and survivors, including those with estrogen-sensitive breast cancers. Moderate consumption is one to two standard servings of whole soy foods. This is less than the average intake in Asian countries of up to three servings of soy foods that contribute up to 100 mg of isoflavones per day with no increased risk of breast cancer.[12] Whole soy foods are tofu, soy milk, edamame, or soy nuts. Each serving averages about 7 g of protein and 25 mg of isoflavones.[12]

Flaxseed

Flaxseed has also been extensively studied in relation to breast cancer. It is important to understand flaxseed and how to incorporate it into the diet before, during, and after treatment. It can be consumed as whole seed, ground seed, flaxseed oil, or as partially defatted flax meal. There are two species of flaxseed; golden flaxseed grown in colder climates; and brown flaxseed grown in warmer, humid climates.[14] There are four main bioactive compounds in flaxseed: alpha-linoleic acid (ALA), an omega-3 fatty acid, lignans, and fiber. Flaxseed is also a good source of magnesium, phosphorous, manganese, vitamin B1, selenium, and zinc.[14]

In both animal studies and human trials, dietary flaxseed has been proven protective against breast cancer.[15] Flax is the richest source of lignans, containing 100 times more than any other food.[14,16] These phytoestrogens can modify estrogen levels through estrogenic and anti-estrogenic effects due to rich compositions of ALA and secoisolariciresinol diglucoside (SDG), which makes up about 95% of flaxseed lignan content. Doses of 50 mg SDG have been shown to reduce tumors through the action of bacteria in the colon converting the SDG into enterolignans, enterolactone, and enterodiol, which bind to the estrogen receptors and affect tumor cell growth.[15] These metabolites are structurally like estrogen and have a weak estrogenic effect. SDG can reduce cancer mortality by 33% to 70%.[15]

Omega-3 fatty acids are important to the diet, as they are an essential fatty acid that the body cannot make on its own. Flaxseed is considered the best plant-based source of omega-3 fatty acids in the diet. The Western diet lacks in omega-3 fatty acids due to the extensive processing of foods and other agricultural practices. The recommendation for the ratio of polyunsaturated fatty acids (PUFAs) in the diet is 1:1 to 2:1 of omega-6 fatty acids to omega-3 fatty acids.[17] As mentioned earlier, the ALA is the omega-3 fatty acid present in flaxseed and is the precursor to eicosapentaenoic acid (EPA) and docosahexanoic acid (DHA). These compounds are anti-inflammatory and can be protective against cancer.[17] The recommendation for daily intake is one to four tablespoons (~13 to 51 g) of ground flaxseed per day, but more human studies are needed. Ground flaxseed is preferable, as it is easier for the body to access the nutrients in ground flaxseed over the whole seed.

There has been concern over interaction of flaxseed when patients are taking Tamoxifen. Per experimental studies, it is safe to consume flaxseed when taking Tamoxifen. Doing so can possibly have a protective effect.[14] Flax has also been studied with other breast cancer therapies and was found to downregulate the cardiotoxicity of Doxorubicin and Trastuzumab in mouse studies. This is likely attributed to the antioxidant effect decreasing reactive oxygen species (ROS) generation, but more studies are needed.[18]

Lymphedema

Lymphedema occurs in an estimated 20% to 64% of breast cancer patients.[19,20] The swelling from obstructed lymphatic vessels in the arm, shoulder, and trunk can be painful and affect a person's feeling of health and well-being on many levels. It is characterized by a progressive increase in inflammation, depositing of fat, and fibrosis in edematous tissues.[21] One of the major risk factors for breast cancer-related lymphedema (BCRL) after treatment is overweight status and obesity.[19] A meta-analysis found that there is an upward trend in BCRL with increasing body mass index (BMI). In this analysis, the odds ratio (OR) of obese (BMI >30 kg/m²) breast cancer patients to normal weight patients was 1.84, and 1.39 for obese versus overweight (BMI =25 to 29.9 kg/m²). This demonstrates a positive association between weight and the degree of lymphedema.[20]

A 5% to 10% weight loss can have a significant impact on health as well as lymphedema.[22] Studies have shown that weight loss is positively correlated to decreased volume of lymphedema and the impact of lymphedema on quality of life.[19,20,22] Currently there is no specific diet for lymphedema, and many diets have been studied including calorie restricted, ketogenic, intermittent fasting, and anti-inflammatory diets.[19-22] All have had some positive outcomes with weight loss and volume.

Anti-inflammatory Diet

An anti-inflammatory diet consists of foods that are rich in antioxidants, fiber, phytonutrients, plant-based and lean animal proteins, and anti-inflammatory spices. It can be helpful in managing weight and, in turn, reduce lymphedema.[20,23] The anti-inflammatory diet also focuses on mindful eating, which focuses on using senses during the eating experience. It also suggests slowing down when eating, taking time with the meal process. Mindful eating can help with weight loss as well as lowering cortisol levels.[23,24] Anti-inflammatory diets focus on a high variety of vegetables and fruits of a variety of colors. Protein is mostly plant-based but also includes fatty fish and lean animal protein, with little to no dairy. Healthy fats come from avocados, nuts, seeds, and olive oil. Herbs and spices are included for their anti-inflammatory properties, and there is focus on a healthy lifestyle.[24,25] Many diets have anti-inflammatory properties, and the Mediterranean diet is well known for its anti-inflammatory properties. The Nordic diet and the Okinawa diet also have been studied for their diversity of anti-inflammatory nutrients and health properties.[25] These types of diets fit in with the American Institute of Cancer Research and American Cancer Society dietary recommendations to reduce cancer risk and recurrence (Fig. 12.2).[26]

Cancer survivorship is an expanding area of clinical dietetics practice. Close to 70% of patients in whom cancer is diagnosed survive beyond the 5-year monitoring period, which is considered a benchmark for cancer treatment. The term "cancer survivor" encompasses individuals in active treatment and recovery as well as those with advanced disease commonly receiving palliative care.[6] Our focus in survivorship clinic visits is on those individuals who are living past their initial cancer therapy, are currently disease-free, or have stable disease. In the time soon after completing therapy, many people are highly motivated to make healthy lifestyle and diet changes.

Our oncology dietitians partner with providers to offer multidisciplinary support for survivorship. We educate patients on healthy diet and lifestyle as well as physical activity. The provider then can focus on the disease process, what the patient has been through and what they can expect in the future. We often bring in a support counselor if they haven't already met with the patient to further utilize that resource. We partner with our integrative medicine providers to assist patients in meeting their survivorship goals.

Our survivorship nutrition recommendations include the American Institute of Cancer Research's recommendations for cancer prevention, as well as the American Cancer Society's Stay Healthy guidelines. We offer plant-based diet information and focus on achieving and maintaining a healthy weight. We encourage physical activity, increasing as able toward the goal of 150 minutes of activity per week. Nutrition counseling in survivorship visits should address

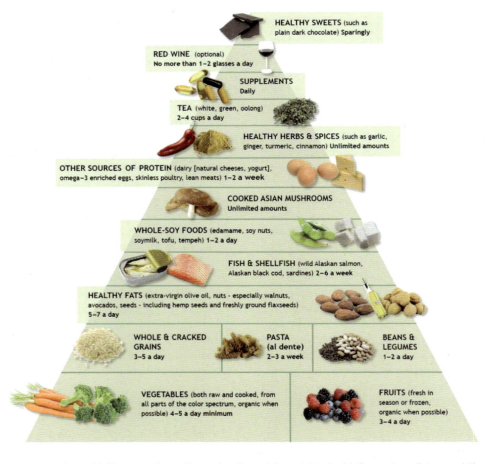

• **Fig. 12.2** Anti-inflammatory Diet Pyramid. (Courtesy: https://www.drweil.com/diet-nutrition/anti-inflammatory-diet-pyramid/dr-weils-anti-inflammatory-food-pyramid/)

the known modifiable risk factors for breast cancer. These include alcohol consumption, overweight and obesity status, and low levels of physical activity.[26]

Further survivorship recommendations include limiting dietary fat intake, especially for postmenopausal women with ER+, PR− breast cancer who followed a higher-fat diet before diagnosis. As part of a plant-based diet, we recommend adequate dietary fiber intake. According to a meta-analysis from 2012, women who eat more than 25 g of fiber per day have a lower risk of breast cancer.[19] Including foods rich in various natural colors also promotes a variety of nutrients to protect our bodies from harm.

Weight loss or maintaining a healthy weight is addressed especially in survivorship. Oncology dietitians include this in the survivorship visit, again meeting the patient where they are with their goals. We start with small, measurable goals. Some patients prefer to use a weight loss program that has worked for them in the past, such as Weight Watchers. We support any healthy eating program they feel works well for them or are willing to participate in. One key to helping with any program or lifestyle change is meal planning and preparation. We focus on this in detail during our visit for the best success. Focusing on behavior change in small increments, and having a plan helps build confidence and consistency.

References

1. Certification (CSO) General Information. *Oncology Nutrition, A Dietetic Practice Group of the Academy of Nutrition and Dietetics*. https://www.oncologynutrition.org/get-involved/certification-cso-general-information. Accessed April 29, 2022.
2. Coble Vos A, Williams V. *Oncology Nutrition for Clinical Practice*. 2nd ed. 2021:1–7, 279, 357–364.
3. AICR's Foods That Fight Cancer™ and Foods to Steer Clear of, Explained. American Institute of Cancer Research. https://www.aicr.org/cancer-prevention/food-facts/. Accessed April 29, 2022.
4. Plant-Based Diet. *Oncology Nutrition Handouts and Resources*. Academy of Nutrition and Dietetics; 2021.
5. Chauhan B, Kumar G, Kalam N, et al. Current concepts and prospects of herbal nutraceutical: a review. *J Adv Pharm Technol Res*. 2013;4(1):4–8. https://doi.org/10.4103/2231-4040.107494.
6. Zhao TT, Jin F, Li JG, et al. Dietary isoflavones or isoflavone-rich food intake and breast cancer risk: a meta-analysis of prospective cohort studies. *Clin Nutr*. 2019;38(1):136–145. https://doi.org/10.1016/j.clnu.2017.12.006.
7. Maskarinec G, Ju D, Morimoto Y, et al. Soy food intake and biomarkers of breast cancer risk: possible difference in Asian women. *Nutr Cancer*. 2016;69(1):146–153. https://doi.org/10.1080/01635581.2017.1250924.
8. Johnson KA, Vemuri S, Alsahafi S, et al. Glycone-rich soy isoflavone extracts promote estrogen receptor positive breast cancer cell growth. *Nutr Cancer*. 2016;68(4):622–633. https://doi.org/10.1080/01635581.2016.1154578.
9. Finkeldey L, Schmitz E, Ellinger S. Effect of the intake of isoflavones on risk factors of breast cancer: a systematic review of randomized controlled intervention studies. *Nutrients*. 2021;13(7):2309. https://doi.org/10.3390/nu13072309.

10. Kang X, Zhang Q, Wang S, et al. Effect of soy isoflavones on breast cancer recurrence and death for patients receiving adjuvant endocrine therapy. *Can Med Assoc J*. 2010;182(17):1857–1862. https://doi.org/10.1503/cmaj.091298.
11. Pabich M, Materska M. Biological effect of soy isoflavones in the prevention of civilization diseases. *Nutrients*. 2019;11(7):1660. https://doi.org/10.3390/nu11071660.
12. American Institute for Cancer Research. *Soy: Intake Does Not Increase Risk for Breast Cancer Survivors*; 2022. https://www.aicr.org/cancer-prevention/food-facts/soy/. Accessed April 29, 2022.
13. U.S. Soybean Export Council. *Soy Nutritional Content*; n.d. Nutrional-content-soy.pdf (ussec.org). https://ussec.org/wp-content/uploads/2015/10/Nutrional-content-soy.pdf. Accessed April 29, 2022.
14. Calado A, Neves PM, Santos T, et al. The effect of flaxseed in breast cancer: a literature review. *Front Nutr*. 2018;5:4. https://doi.org/10.3389/fnut.2018.00004.
15. Parikh M, Maddaford TG, Austria JA, et al. Dietary flaxseed as a strategy for improving human health. *Nutrients*. 2019;11(5):1171. https://doi.org/10.3390/nu11051171.
16. Ezzat SM, Shouman SA, Elkholy A, et al. Anticancer potentiality of lignan rich fraction of six Flaxseed cultivars. *Sci Rep*. 2018;8(1):544. https://doi.org/10.1038/s41598-017-18944-0.
17. Simopoulos AP. An increase in the omega-6/omega-3 fatty acid ratio increases the risk for obesity. *Nutrients*. 2016;8(3):128. https://doi.org/10.3390/nu8030128.
18. Bkaily G, Jacques D. Flaxseed as an anticardiotoxicity agent in breast cancer therapy. *J Nutr*. 2020;150(9):2231–2232. https://doi.org/10.1093/jn/nxaa213.
19. Vafa S, Zarrati M, Malakootinejad M, et al. Calorie restriction and synbiotics effect on quality of life and edema reduction in breast cancer-related lymphedema, a clinical trial. *Breast*. 2020;54:37–45. https://doi.org/10.1016/j.breast.2020.08.008.
20. Wu R, Huang X, Dong X, et al. Obese patients have higher risk of breast cancer-related lymphedema than overweight patients after breast cancer: a meta-analysis. *Ann Transl Med*. 2019;7(8):172. https://doi.org/10.21037/atm.2019.03.44.
21. Cavezzi A, Urso SU, Ambrosini L, et al. Lymphedema and nutrition: a review. *Veins Lymphatics*. 2019;8(1). https://doi.org/10.4081/vl.2019.8220.
22. Keith L, Rowsemitt C, Richards LG. Lifestyle modification group for lymphedema and obesity results in significant health outcomes. *Am J Lifestyle Med*. 2017;14(4):420–428. https://doi.org/10.1177/1559827617742108.
23. Ricker MA, Haas WC. Anti-inflammatory diet in clinical practice: a review. *Nutr Clin Pract*. 2017;32:318–3325. https://doi.org/10.1177/0884533617700353.
24. Nelson JB. Mindful eating: the art of presence while you eat. *Diabetes Spectr*. 2017;30(3):171–174. https://doi.org/10.2337/ds17-0015.
25. Stromsnes K, Correas AG, Lehmann J, et al. Anti-inflammatory properties of diet: role in healthy aging. *Biomedicines*. 2021;9(8):922. https://doi.org/10.3390/biomedicines9080922.
26. Springfield S, Odoms-Young A, Tussing-Humphreys L, et al. Adherence to American Cancer Society and American Institute of Cancer Research dietary guidelines in overweight African American breast cancer survivors. *J Cancer Surviv*. 2019;13(2):257–268. https://doi.org/10.1007/s11764-019-00748-y.

13

Breast Cancer Survivorship in Community Oncology Practice

JAMIE CAIRO

Breast cancer is the most commonly diagnosed cancer among women.[1] Recent improvements in healthcare, including earlier detection and effective treatment strategies, have significantly improved survival rates.[2,3] With more than 3.8 million breast cancer survivors in the United States, the 5-year survival rate is 90% and the 10-year survival rate is 80%. Therefore, most patients diagnosed with breast cancer will become long-term survivors. Breast cancer predominantly affects women, with less than 1% of all breast cancers occurring in men,[4] thus much of the information on breast cancer survivorship is geared toward women. Breast cancer survivors frequently experience a number of physical and psychosocial issues that can affect their health and wellbeing. Cancer programs and clinicians need to be prepared to address these long-term effects of cancer and its treatment. The term "cancer survivor" most commonly refers to any person who has been diagnosed with cancer, but the needs of patients with metastatic disease are different from those with curative intent disease. This chapter will review and discuss the essential elements of survivorship care in community oncology practice for breast cancer patients diagnosed with curative intent disease.

Surveillance

The primary goals of surveillance are to watch for recurrence of the original cancer or development of a second cancer. Patients with early-stage breast cancers (tumor <5 cm and fewer than four positive nodes) may follow up with their primary care provider 1 year after their diagnosis, according to the American Society of Clinical Oncology.[5] Crabtree et al. found that there are differing views regarding primary care's role in cancer survivorship care that includes a "lack of coherence" about the overall concept of survivorship.[6] The authors found that in spite of a growing number of cancer survivors in the United States as well as a shortage of oncologists, some primary care providers believe that care after cancer treatment has ended should continue to be done by the oncology team. Table 13.1 summarizes current surveillance recommendations for breast cancer survivors, as outlined in this section.

Regular assessment with history and physical examination, including a clinical breast examination, remains the mainstay of detecting breast cancer recurrence.[7] The physical examination should be performed by a clinician who is experienced in doing breast examinations and should include examination of the affected breast, if present, as well as the chest wall, the contralateral side, bilateral axillary regions, and the supraclavicular fossas. If lymphedema is present, circumferential measurement of both upper extremities should be done. It is also recommended that palpation of the spine, sternum, ribs, and pelvis for bone tenderness should be routinely performed. Cardiac evaluation, as well as assessment of the lungs and abdomen, and a neurologic assessment that evaluates balance, gait, and sensory and motor function are important as well. Routine gynecologic follow-up is recommended for women who have not undergone total hysterectomy, particularly patients who are prescribed tamoxifen, as they are at increased risk for developing endometrial cancer.[8] Follow-up recommendations for breast cancer survivors are summarized in Table 13.1.

Imaging

Mammography

Mammography continues to be the imaging standard for breast cancer screening. The use of digital breast tomosynthesis as opposed to full-field digital mammography reduces recall rate and improves sensitivity and specificity.[9] Variability exists in guideline recommendations for surveillance initiation, interval, and cessation. According to the National Comprehensive Cancer Network (NCCN),[10] American Cancer Society, and American Society of Clinical Oncology (ASCO),[11] annual mammograms are recommended for women who have had breast-conserving surgery (partial mastectomy or lumpectomy) and/or radiation. Women who have had a simple, modified radical or radical mastectomy should continue to have a yearly mammogram on the remaining breast.[11]

Magnetic Resonance Imaging

Breast magnetic resonance imaging (MRI) is not routinely recommended for surveillance due to insufficient evidence

TABLE 13.1 Surveillance Recommendations for Breast Cancer Survivors

Mode of Surveillance	Recommendation
History/physical examination	Every 3–6 months for the first 3 years after primary therapy, then every 6–12 months for the next 2 years, and then annually
Mammography	Mammography should be performed yearly
Pelvic examination	Regular gynecologic follow-up is recommended for all women. Patients who receive tamoxifen therapy are at increased risk for developing endometrial cancer and should be advised to report any vaginal bleeding to their physicians. Longer follow-up intervals may be appropriate for women who have had a total hysterectomy and oophorectomy
Bone density testing	Those at risk for developing bone loss due to medication should be screened with a bone density test every 2 years

that it is any better than mammography in detecting breast cancer recurrence. However, it can be a useful diagnostic tool, specifically for women with a known *BRCA1*, *BRCA2*, or other high-risk genetic mutation and/or those who have a strong family history.[8]

Genetics

If not already done by the time of survivorship, women who are at high risk of familial breast cancer syndromes and all men with breast cancer should be referred for genetic counseling. As an alternative to surveillance, women with a personal history of breast cancer and genetic mutation may want to consider bilateral mastectomy, which can be performed at the time of diagnosis or at a later point.[12] The criteria to recommend referral for genetic counseling includes:
- Ashkenazi Jewish heritage.
- History of ovarian cancer at any age in the patient or any first- or second-degree relatives.
- Any first-degree relative with a history of breast cancer diagnosed before the age of 50 years.
- Two or more first- or second-degree relatives diagnosed with breast cancer at any age.
- A patient or their relative with a diagnosis of bilateral breast cancer.
- History of breast cancer in a male relative.

Breast Cancer Tumor Marker Testing and Other Blood Tests

For routine surveillance, it is not recommended to test with CA 15-3, CA 27.29, and CEA tumor markers. In addition,

laboratory studies and other radiologic tests have not been shown to be helpful in breast cancer surveillance in asymptomatic patients.[8]

Bone Density Testing

Women with a history of breast cancer may be at increased risk of developing osteoporosis because of their prior cancer treatment, as well as the use of aromatase inhibitors (AIs) for prevention of recurrence in hormone receptor–positive breast cancer in postmenopausal women. NCCN guidelines recommend that women with breast cancer treated with an AI should have a baseline bone density test and then have periodic scans, although the frequency of long-term screening is not specified.[10] ASCO recommends that cancer survivors at risk for developing bone loss due to medication should be screened with a bone density test every 2 years, or more frequently if deemed medically necessary.[13]

Screening for Secondary Cancers

Screening for secondary malignancies related to diagnosis and treatment after breast cancer is an important part of survivorship. A second breast cancer in the opposite breast, or in the same breast for women who were treated with breast-conserving surgery, is the most common occurrence for these patients. Li et al. found that the cumulative incidence of developing second primary cancers after early-stage initial primary breast cancer was 7.43% at 10 years, 14.41% at 15 years, and 20.08% at 20 years.[14] Radiation therapy was also associated with increased risk of secondary cancers. Hormone status has been found to affect one's risk of secondary malignancy. Women with hormone-positive disease have a decreased risk of developing a secondary primary breast or ovarian cancer, but they have an increased risk of urinary tract cancers, possibly due to hormone use. Smoking history, obesity, and high blood pressure are also risk factors for the development of second primary cancers, underscoring the need for counseling about healthy lifestyle habits.[15] Aside from physical examination and yearly mammograms, there are no recommended screening tests for secondary cancers. Breast cancer survivors should be educated to watch for the following symptoms:
- New lumps in the breast
- Changes to the skin of the breast, including inflammation and redness
- Nipple discharge
- Thickening along or near the mastectomy scar
- Swollen lymph nodes
- New and unexplained pain, especially chest, back, or hip pain
- Persistent cough and/or difficulty breathing
- Loss of appetite and/or weight loss without trying
- New and/or progressive headaches
- New or increased seizure activity

Assessment and Management of Physical and Psychosocial Long-Term and Late Effects of Breast Cancer and Treatment

Body Image

Studies have found that over 50% of all breast cancer patients experience issues with body image.[16,17] The loss of one or both breasts, weight changes, and hair loss are just a few of the changes that can lead to body image distress and subsequent depression and anxiety. Poor body image perceptions can also negatively impact personal relationships and sexual functioning.[18] The negative impact on self-image and self-esteem can pose a significant challenge for patients and lead to diminished quality of life.[19] In 2021, Morales-Sanchez et al. conducted a systematic review of interventions to improve body image and self-esteem in breast cancer survivors.[20] They identified group therapy and support, physical activity programs, and cosmetic-focused interventions as helpful with alleviating body image distress, to varying degrees of effectiveness.

Lymphedema

Breast cancer lymphedema, defined as a progressive swelling of either the proximal portion or the distal digits of the arm, is a potentially irreversible complication of breast cancer and its treatment. It is caused by the disruption of lymphatic flow after axillary surgery and radiation. A 2013 meta-analysis found an estimated risk of 17% among patients with breast cancer, with risk increasing up to 2 years after surgery. The risk of developing lymphedema is 20% higher in those who undergo a complete axillary lymph node dissection in comparison to those who undergo a sentinel lymph node biopsy, whose risk is approximately 5.6%.[21] Patients should be alert to bring any early signs of infection in the extremity to the attention of their physician for consideration of early use of antibiotics. The American Physical Therapy Association uses the maximum limb girth difference between the affected and unaffected arm to classify lymphedema (Table 13.2).[22]

Education about exercises to help the lymph fluid drain should be a part of a survivorship visit, especially for those who have undergone lymph node dissection. If needed, counseling about weight loss can also improve symptoms in survivors who develop lymphedema. Referral to physical therapy for manual lymphatic drainage, massage, and compression bandages or sleeves can yield positive results. Compression garments should be fitted by an experienced therapist, and patients should be encouraged to wear them regularly and to replace them every 6 months to maintain proper fit. Daily intermittent compression with a pneumatic compression pump is another treatment option. Complex decongestive therapy is a multimodal regimen consisting of manual lymphatic drainage, compression bandaging, exercises to enhance lymphatic drainage, and skin care.[23] Surgical and ablative procedures such as lymphovenous anastomosis, lymph node transplantation, and liposuction have yielded mixed results and should only be pursued when other treatment options have failed.[24,25]

Cardiotoxicity

In the general population, cardiovascular disease is the number-one cause of death in women.[26] Breast cancer survivors who are obese, smokers, and/or over the age of 60 years, and those with a history of hypertension, diabetes, and hyperlipidemia, have an increased risk of developing early or delayed heart disease after treatment. Cardiac issues including left ventricular dysfunction, heart failure, valvular disease, and congestive heart disease can develop over time in these patients.[27] Antiestrogen treatment with AIs can lead to the development of hypertension, hyperlipidemia, and ischemic heart disease. Survivors with a history of hormone-positive disease need ongoing surveillance for these comorbidities.[28] Breast cancer survivors should be educated about signs of cardiotoxicity, as well as have a yearly review of systems and physical examination to assess for cardiac complications. Table 13.3 lists the potential cardiotoxic effects of cancer treatment. Women on AIs should have routine lipid assessments and intervention if needed. The Heart Failure Association Cardio-Oncology Study Group has developed some guidelines for risk assessment and ongoing surveillance. In those who received treatment with anthracyclines, measurement of left ventricular ejection fraction (LVEF) is recommended 6–12 months after completion of treatment. For those who received human epidermal growth factor receptor 2–targeted therapies, LVEF plus troponins and B-type natriuretic peptide should be measured every 6 months for up to 2 years after completion of therapy.[29] ASCO has also published guidelines for cardiovascular surveillance in cancer survivors:

- Echocardiogram should be performed between 6 and 12 months after completion of cancer-directed therapy in asymptomatic patients considered to be at increased risk of cardiac dysfunction.
- Cardiac MRI or multiple-gated acquisition may be offered for surveillance in asymptomatic individuals if an echocardiogram is not available or technically feasible (e.g., poor image quality), with preference given to cardiac MRI.
- Cardio-oncology referral for asymptomatic cardiac dysfunction during routine surveillance.

TABLE 13.2	American Physical Therapy Association Lymphedema Classification
Mild lymphedema	Maximum girth difference <3 cm
Moderate lymphedema	3–5-cm difference
Severe lymphedema	Difference >5 cm

TABLE 13.3 Potential Cardiotoxic Effects of Breast Cancer Treatment

Treatment Modality	Potential Cardiovascular Effects
Anthracyclines (doxorubicin, epirubicin): doxorubicin $\geq$250 mg/m^2 or epirubicin $\geq$600 mg/m^2	Left ventricular dysfunction, myocarditis, pericarditis, atrial fibrillation, heart failure
Alkylating agents (cyclophosphamide)	Left ventricular dysfunction, heart failure, myocarditis, pericarditis, arterial thrombosis, bradycardia, atrial fibrillation, supraventricular tachycardia
Endocrine therapy (aromatase inhibitors, tamoxifen)	Venous thrombosis, thromboembolism peripheral atherosclerosis, dysrhythmia, vascular dysfunction, pericarditis, heart failure
HER-2 directed therapies	Left ventricular dysfunction, heart failure
Radiation: high-dose radiation therapy when heart is in the field of treatment; radiotherapy $\geq$30 Gy	Coronary artery disease, cardiomyopathy, valvular disease, pericardial disease, arrhythmias

HER-2, Human epidermal growth factor receptor 2.
Mehta et al, Cardiovascular Disease and Breast Cancer: Where These Entities Intersect: A Scientific Statement From the American Heart Association, Circulation, Vol. 137, No. 8, 2018, e30–e66. https://doi.org/10.1161/CIR.0000000000000556

- No recommendations can be made regarding the frequency and duration of surveillance in patients at increased risk who are asymptomatic and have no evidence of cardiac dysfunction on their 6–12-month posttreatment echocardiogram.
- Clinicians should regularly evaluate and manage cardiovascular risk factors such as smoking, hypertension, diabetes, dyslipidemia, and obesity in patients previously treated with cardiotoxic cancer therapies. A heart-healthy lifestyle, including the role of diet and exercise, should be discussed as part of long-term follow-up care.[30]

Cognitive Impairment

Between 15% and 25% of breast cancer survivors experience cancer-related cognitive impairments after treatment. They typically describe concentration problems and difficulty remembering names and numbers, word finding, or multitasking after treatment. Deficits in verbal and visuospatial abilities, as well as executive functioning and processing speed,[31,32] are the primary cognitive domains affected. Symptoms are typically mild to moderate and are often short term, although some may experience persistent impairment.[33] It is thought that these cognitive changes are multifactorial and may be impacted by

psychological issues such as cancer-related distress, depression, anxiety, and insomnia.[34] Survivors who received higher doses of chemotherapy, are postmenopausal, and/or are over the age of 65 years seem to be particularly vulnerable. Tamoxifen use may also be a contributing factor.[35]

Changes to lifestyle behaviors can often help alleviate symptoms. Survivors should be counseled about optimizing stress management, physical activity, sleep quality, and fostering supportive social relationships.[36] For those who continue to experience significant cognitive dysfunction that negatively impacts their daily activities after 12 months of completing chemotherapy or during hormone therapy, a referral to a neuropsychologist may be warranted. Neuropsychological testing can provide an in-depth assessment of objective cognitive functioning and cognitive rehabilitation can be helpful. A recent meta-analysis[37] found that meditation/mindfulness-based stress reduction, cognitive training, cognitive rehabilitation, and exercise interventions for cognitive dysfunction showed statistical significance in improving symptoms.

NCCN survivorship guidelines[38] state that currently there is no effective brief screening tool to assess cognitive dysfunction in the clinical setting and that existing tools, such as the Mini Mental State Examination (MMSE), do not strongly correlate with patient reports of cognitive dysfunction. NCCN guidelines do provide some self-management strategies for patients, as follows:

- Teach enhanced organizational strategies and utilize memory aids such as notebooks and planners, using reminder notes, and smart phone technology.
- Encourage patients to do the most cognitively challenging tasks at the time of day when energy levels are highest.
- Provide information about relaxation and stress-management skills.
- Recommend routine physical activity.
- Recommend limiting the use of alcohol and other agents that alter cognition and sleep.
- Consider meditation, yoga, mindfulness-based stress reduction, and cognitive training, including puzzles and other brain games.
- Optimize management of depression and emotional distress, as well as sleep disturbance.
- Validate the experience of cognitive dysfunction associated with cancer diagnosis and treatment, and provide reassurance that this is usually not a progressive neurologic disorder.[38]

Distress, Depression, and Anxiety

Breast cancer patients often suffer from psychological distress, which can compromise their quality of life even after their treatment is completed. Research has shown that anxiety and depression are twice as prevalent in cancer survivors as in the general population.[39] Psychosocial distress and depression should be routinely assessed at survivorship visits. There are a number of tools that are used with cancer patients to screen for distress; Table 13.4 lists some of the tools most often used.

TABLE 13.4	Depression and Distress Screening Tools	
Screening Tool	**Description**
Personal Health Questionnaire (PHQ-9)	9-item scale composed of questions that correspond to Diagnostic and Statistical Manual of Mental Disorders (DSM-IV) diagnostic criteria for a major depressive episode
Personal Health Questionnaire (PHQ-2)	The PHQ-2 consists of the two main criteria for a major depressive episode, specifically depressed mood and anhedonia within the past 2 weeks
Hopkins Symptom Checklist (HSCL)	The 25-item version consists of a subset of items focused on individual health and functioning
National Comprehensive Cancer Network – Distress Thermometer (NCCN-DT)	The NCCN-DT consists of a single item with instructions to rate distress over the past 7 days on a scale of 0–10, with higher scores indicating higher distress
Beck Depression Inventory (BDI)	The BDI–Short Form is a widely used depression scale that consists of 13 items that measure characteristic attitudes and symptoms of depression
Brief Edinburgh Depression Scale	6-item inventory rated on a four-point Likert-type scale designed to measure depression in those in the advanced stages of cancer
Brief Symptom Inventory-18 (BSI-18)	BSI-18 is a self-report scale widely used to assess psychological symptoms in cancer survivors
Profile of Moods State–Short Form (POMS-SF)	16-item survey that assesses mood states
Psychosocial Screen for Cancer (PSSCAN)	21-item tool used to identify the psychosocial needs of patients with cancer
Hospital Anxiety and Depression Scale (HADS)	14-item questionnaire that assesses anxiety and depressive symptoms in medical settings

A 2017 study that looked at 55 cancer programs in the United States and Canada found that 84% of cancer programs used the NCCN Distress Thermometer and Symptom Checklist to screen their patients for psychosocial distress.[40] NCCN distress-management guidelines are useful in outlining recommendations for supporting patients with mild distress and providing a pathway for referral to supportive psychosocial resources. Referral to an oncology social worker, financial navigator, or psychologist or psychiatrist, preferably one who has experience working with cancer survivors, can be very beneficial for patients who are experiencing depression and anxiety. Counseling and cognitive-behavioral therapy can be beneficial for cancer survivors who are dealing with distress. Pharmacologic treatment may be indicated, but if prescribing medication, it is recommended that referral and collaboration with a prescribing mental health professional be considered.

Fatigue

Fatigue is a common complaint among cancer survivors. Wang et al. found that about one-third of cancer survivors with breast, prostate, colorectal, or lung cancer diagnoses reported moderate to severe levels of fatigue after treatment.[41] Cancer-related fatigue can be difficult to quantify and is usually multifactorial, impacted by surgery, chemotherapy, and radiation.[42] It can also be caused by chronic pain, cardiovascular or endocrine comorbidities, anemia, psychosocial distress, sleep disturbances, cognitive dysfunction, and side effects from medications.[43] When breast cancer survivors complain of fatigue post-treatment, the presence of depression and anxiety should be assessed as they are the most common psychiatric comorbidities that occur in individuals with cancer-related fatigue, even after treatment.[44]

There are a number of screening tools that can be used to assess cancer-related fatigue, including the Fatigue Symptom Inventory (FSI), the Multidimensional Fatigue Inventory (MFI), and the Multidimensional Fatigue Symptom Inventory (MFSI). The ASCO guidelines recommend that all patients be screened for fatigue as clinically indicated, and at least on a yearly basis. As part of that assessment, sleep patterns should be evaluated. Carpenter et al. found that 73% of breast cancer survivors experienced poor sleep quality and high sleep disturbance.[45] There are a number of medications that can be used to treat insomnia, but they all have potential side effects, including the risk of dependence, and ideally should only be used in the short term. Meditation, yoga, acupuncture, and cognitive-behavioral stress management can also yield positive results. Cognitive-behavioral therapy sessions with a mental health therapist have been found to be beneficial and are also now available via mobile apps. Use of psychostimulants and other wakefulness agents such as modafinil should not be used in breast cancer survivors except under special circumstances. These medications can be effectively used to manage fatigue in patients with advanced disease or those receiving active treatment. However, there is limited evidence of their effectiveness in reducing fatigue in patients after active treatment who are currently disease free.[43] The American Academy of Sleep Medicine has developed guidelines for the treatment of insomnia in adults Table 13.5).[46] Nonpharmacologic interventions to help patients sleep should be recommended, including:

TABLE 13.5 A Summary of Sleep Medication Recommendations

Medication	Sleep Latency	Quality of Sleep	Side Effects	Sleep Onset vs. Sleep Latency
Eszopiclone	14 min compared to placebo for sleep onset 28–57 min of sleep improvement	Moderate to large improvement	Dizziness, dry mouth, headache, somnolence, and unpleasant taste	Onset and latency
Ramelteon	9 min compared to placebo for sleep onset	No improvement	Headache, nausea, upper respiratory infection, and nasopharyngitis	Onset
Temazepam	37 min compared to placebo for sleep onset 99 min of sleep improvement	Small improvement	Headache, blurred vision, depression, and confusion	Onset and latency
Triazolam	8 min compared to placebo for sleep onset	Moderate improvement	Somnolence	Onset
Zaleplon	10 min compared to placebo for sleep onset	No improvement	Headache, asthenia, neurasthenia, pain, fatigue, and somnolence	Onset
Zolpidem	5–12 min compared to placebo for sleep onset 29 min of sleep improvement	Moderate improvement	Amnesia, dizziness, sedation, headache, nausea, and taste perversion (altered or unpleasant taste)	Onset and latency
Doxepin	26–32 min of sleep improvement	Small to moderate	Headache, diarrhea, somnolence	Latency
Suvorexant	10 min of sleep improvement	Not reported	Somnolence	Latency
Trazodone	10 min compared to placebo 8 min of sleep improvement	No improvement	Headache, somnolence	Onset and latency

From Sateia MJ, Buysse DJ, Krystal AD, et al. Clinical practice guideline for the pharmacologic treatment of chronic insomnia in adults: an American Academy of Sleep Medicine clinical practice guideline. *J Clin Sleep Med.* 2017;13:307-349.

- Go to bed at the same time each night and get up at the same time each morning, including on the weekends.
- Keep the bedroom quiet, dark, relaxing, and at a comfortable temperature.
- Do not use any electronic devices, such as TVs, computers, and smart phones, in the bedroom.
- Avoid large meals, caffeine, and alcohol before bedtime.
- Get some exercise during the daytime.

Nutritional counseling is recommended, as dietary modifications may help some cancer survivors with their insomnia complaints. Breast cancer survivors who improved their intake of fruits and vegetables seemed to complain of less fatigue.[47] Supplementation with omega 3 and omega 6 fatty acids can also lessen fatigue, as demonstrated in the Healthy Eating Activity and Lifestyle (HEAL) study, supporting the theory that inflammation is a driving factor in postcancer fatigue.[48] Melatonin, L-tryptophan and valerian were found to provide small improvements in sleep latency and quality. They may be beneficial for some patients with mild complaints of insomnia but are generally not recommended for treatment. Bone Health

Optimal bone health is a long-term clinical challenge for breast cancer survivors. The management of patients with hormone receptor–positive breast cancer requires the use of endocrine therapy, which is associated with an increased risk of osteoporosis and fractures. Additionally, chemotherapy-induced ovarian insufficiency in premenopausal women reduces estrogen levels, leading to osteopenia and subsequent osteoporosis. Some breast cancer survivors are at increased risk of bone loss, including those who are current smokers, those with a low body mass, those with a personal or parental history of nontraumatic fracture, and patients receiving treatment for rheumatoid arthritis.[13] Survivors should be counseled about smoking cessation, decreasing alcohol consumption, and increasing weight-bearing activity. Women should take 800–1000 IU/day vitamin D3 and calcium 1200 mg/day (made up of dietary sources and supplemental calcium). Breast cancer survivors should have their vitamin D3 levels evaluated, and if deficient (10 ng/mL or less) or insufficient (11–20 ng/mL), should have this corrected.[13] In terms of treatment, Fig. 13.1 provides an algorithm to assist in the decision of whether to use pharmacologic treatment. When patients begin treatment with an AI, their risk of fracture should be assessed. Patients with a T-score less than -2.0 or with a T-score of less than -1.5 SD with one additional risk factor or two or more risk factors should be treated with bone-directed medication as long as the patient is on antiestrogen treatment.[49]

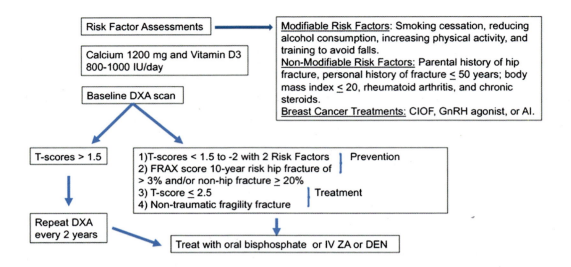

• Fig. 13.1 Algorithm for Bone Health in Women with Breast Cancer. *AI*, Aromatase inhibitor; *CIOF*, chemotherapy-induced ovarian failure; *DEN*, denosumab; *DXA*, dual-energy absorptiometry; *GnRH*, gonadotropin-releasing hormone; *IV*, intravenous; *ZA*, zoledronic acid. (From Shapiro CL. Osteoporosis: a long-term and late-effect of breast cancer treatments. Cancers. 2020; 12(11):3094. https://doi.org/10.3390/cancers12113094.)

Pain and Neuropathy

According to Forsythe et al., roughly 30% of all breast cancer survivors experience above-average pain after diagnosis and treatment.[50] Chronic pain issues in breast cancer survivors are often related to treatment. Breast surgery can damage intercostobrachial, axillary, thoracic, and cervical nerves, resulting in neuropathic pain.[51] AIs and selective estrogen receptor modulators can cause arthralgias,[52] and peripheral neuropathy is a common and distressing complication resulting from chemotherapy, specifically treatment with taxanes.[53] These symptoms may improve over time, but some patients are affected for years after treatment. Survivors who experience pain should be formally screened with visual analog pain scales and other screening tools that help to quantify their level of pain. Initially patients are often given medications such as opioids, nonsteroidal anti-inflammatories, and acetaminophen. Opioids can be used to treat acute pain for short periods of time, but for most survivors other medications and modalities should be used for long-term management. Table 13.6 provides a list of medications and supplements that may be useful in the treatment of chronic pain and neuropathy in these patients. Physical therapy and exercise programs can also offer improvement in chronic pain symptoms, specifically in survivors with AI-associated arthralgias.

Alternative and complementary therapies have a definite role in treatment. Acupuncture has been found to be useful in the treatment of neuropathy and chronic pain. Lu et al. conducted a randomized trial of breast cancer survivors with chemotherapy-induced peripheral neuropathy using acupuncture versus usual care and found a statistically and clinically significant improvement in subjective sensory symptoms, including neuropathic pain and paresthesia.[54] Hypnosis, massage therapy, myofascial release, and reflexology have also been shown to have some effectiveness in treating chronic pain in cancer survivors.[55]

TABLE 13.6 Treatment Options for Pain Management in Breast Cancer Survivors

Medications and Topical Preparations	Recommended Dosing
Gabapentin	300 mg/day to start, can titrate up to 1800 mg/day in divided doses
Venlafaxine	37.5 mg/day to start, can be increased to 75 mg/day
Amitriptyline	25 mg/day to start, can be increased to 100 mg/day
Duloxetine	30 mg/day to start, can be increased to 60 mg/day
Capsaicin topical	0.075% cream. May apply to affected areas four times a day
Arnica Montana topical	Apply up to three times daily to affected areas as needed

Infertility

Fertility preservation is an option for younger women diagnosed with breast cancer. Patient age, the condition of her eggs, and other reproductive and treatment-related factors combine to affect one's fertility after breast cancer. A consultation with a reproductive endocrinologist prior to starting treatment is recommended. Collection of eggs prior to treatment and in vitro fertilization may be an option. Other options for women after breast cancer treatment who wish to have a family include the use of donor eggs, a surrogate/gestational carrier, or adoption. The laws regarding storage of eggs and embryos, donor eggs, and surrogacy can vary depending on the state one resides in.

Sexual Health

Sexual morbidity can be defined as encompassing sexual behavior, sexual functioning, and subjective sexual satisfaction.[56] It is one of the most frequent long-term issues that a breast cancer survivor faces[57] and it should be addressed as part of their survivorship care, as changes in body image play a part in survivor distress. The Female Sexual Function Index (FSFI) is a 19 item screening tool that can be used to evaluate sexual dysfunction. Alternatively, the Female Sexual Distress Scale-Revised (FSDS-R) is a validated tool that can be used to evaluate sexually related distress.[58]

Antidepressants can negatively affect sexual desire and are commonly prescribed to women during and after cancer treatment. Selective serotonin reuptake inhibitors can cause delayed orgasm.[59] Bupropion or mirtazapine have fewer sexual side effects and may be better options for treatment of depression in these patients. Surgeries (i.e., oophorectomy) and hormonal therapy that affects estrogen can cause a decrease in libido. Vaginal dryness and vulvovaginal atrophy causing irritation can lead to painful sexual intercourse. Local estrogen creams, rings, and other preparations can be used in a subset of breast cancer survivors, although in women with hormone-positive breast cancers there is often reluctance to use these products. Vaginal moisturizers and regular use of vaginal dilators can alleviate some symptoms. The American College of Obstetricians and Gynecologists recommends that nonhormonal approaches be used as first-line choices for managing urogenital symptoms.[60] Referral to a gynecologist, or a specialist in pelvic floor rehabilitation and/or sexual health should always be a consideration. Patients may also benefit from psychologic counseling and support.

Menopausal Symptoms and Early Menopause

Most breast cancers are estrogen and/or progesterone positive,[61] so treatments to block these hormones are commonly used to prevent recurrence in many survivors. Chemotherapy can also cause early menopause for premenopausal women. Breast cancer survivors frequently complain of menopausal symptoms such as night sweats, hot flashes, vaginal symptoms, emotional lability, musculoskeletal aches and pains, and sexual issues. Although these symptoms can manifest themselves in all menopausal women, they often come on much more abruptly in patients treated for breast cancer and they can be more difficult to manage.[62] This can negatively

impact quality of life as well as patient adherence to endocrine therapy. Some symptoms, such as hot flashes, may resolve over time, but some may persist long term. Breast cancer survivors should be counseled to attempt to achieve some healthy lifestyle habits such as achieving and maintaining a healthy body mass index, limiting alcohol intake, regular exercise, and smoking cessation, which can reduce mild-to-moderate hot flashes and arthralgias.[63]

Some patients may benefit from use of the selective serotonin reuptake inhibitors and selective noradrenaline reuptake inhibitors to diminish hot flashes and emotional lability. However they can also be accompanied by sexual side effects, dry mouth, headache, nausea, and insomnia, and have potential interactions (fluoxetine and paroxetine) with tamoxifen. Venlafaxine and desvenlafaxine may be better options for breast cancer survivors. Gabapentin and clonidine have also been shown to reduce hot flashes in breast cancer patients, although they also have potential side effects and do not have an indication for relief of menopausal symptoms.[64] Integrative and psychologic modalities including paced respiration, hypnotherapy, cognitive-behavioral therapy, behavioral therapy, and mindfulness-based therapies, as well as acupuncture, have also been used with some success in these patients.[65,66]

Wellness Guidelines and Health Promotion

Discussion of diet and exercise is an important component of a survivorship visit. Obesity is known to increase the risk of developing breast cancer, and diet is a modifiable risk factor that impacts both cancer initiation and progression.[67,68] Diets that are rich in plant-based foods are associated with reduced mortality after diagnosis of breast cancer.[69] Breast cancer survivors who follow an eating pattern that is high in refined carbohydrates and sugar, as well as saturated and trans-saturated fats, and low in omega-3 fatty acids, natural antioxidants, and fiber need nutritional counseling to reduce their risk of cancer recurrence. An example of a plant-based eating pattern is the Mediterranean diet, which is high in fruit and vegetables, whole grains, nuts, legumes, fish, and monounsaturated fat (olive oil), and low in meat and saturated fats. Table 13.7 outlines basic dietary recommendations for patients.

Breast cancer survivors who choose to drink alcohol should limit consumption to less than one drink a day for women and less than two drinks a day for men. Research has shown that drinking alcoholic beverages increases the risk of cancer, specifically hormone receptor–positive breast cancer, because alcohol can increase production of estrogen in the body.[70] According to an analysis by the Collaborative Group on Hormonal Factors in Breast Cancer,[71] women who only have three alcoholic drinks per week have a 15% higher risk of breast cancer. It is estimated that a woman's risk of breast cancer goes up another 10% for each additional drink per day.[72]

In terms of physical activity, regular exercise is associated with improved survival among breast cancer survivors.[73]

TABLE 13.7 Dietary Recommendations for Breast Cancer Survivors

Healthy Eating for Breast Cancer Survivors

Maintain a healthy weight and avoid large portions of calorie-dense foods

Eat more plant foods, including vegetables, fruits, and legumes (such as beans). Aim for a minimum of 2.5 cups of fruits and vegetables every day

Make at least half of your grains whole grains, such as 100% whole-grain breads and cereals, brown rice, millet, and quinoa

Limit sugar-sweetened drinks. Choose water or unsweetened beverages instead

Drink fat-free, low-fat (1%), or plant-based milk and milk products

Choose lean proteins, such as seafood, lean meats and poultry, eggs, beans, unsalted nuts, and seeds

Cut back on sodium (salt)

Replace saturated and trans fats with "good" fats (polyunsaturated and monounsaturated fats)

Limit alcohol intake to no more than one measured drink per day and consider eliminating alcohol altogether

TABLE 13.8 Daily Activity Recommendations

Recommendations for Breast Cancer Survivors to Increase Daily Physical Activity

Take the stairs instead of the elevator

Walk or bike to your destination

Be active at lunch with your coworkers, family, or friends

Take a 20-min activity break at work to stretch or take a quick walk

Walk to visit coworkers instead of sending an email message

Wear a pedometer every day to increase your number of daily steps

Go dancing with your spouse or friends

Use a stationary bicycle or treadmill while watching TV

Survivors should aim for 30–60 minutes of moderate-to-intense physical activity on most days of the week. However, even a small increase in physical activity has benefits. Walking, swimming, bicycle riding, and participating in a sporting activity are all beneficial. Moderate-intensity activities are those that require effort equal to a brisk walk. For patients who have not been active before, they should be advised to start slowly and gradually increase the duration, frequency, and intensity over time. A cancer rehabilitation specialist can help patients design an effective and safe exercise program, and referral to these specialists should be considered. Table 13.8 outlines practical recommendations for patients who wish to increase their daily activity levels.

Survivorship Care Plans and Care Coordination

Since the Commission on Cancer began its emphasis on the need for patients to receive survivorship care plans (SCPs) and supportive services as part of patient-centered cancer care, cancer programs have worked to integrate survivorship services including the delivery of SCPs. There are a number of reasons to provide coordinated and comprehensive care to cancer survivors. The growing number of cancer survivors in the United States as well as the national healthcare provider shortages, rising costs of healthcare, and the desire to provide value-based healthcare are all changing the landscape of cancer care.[74] There is a need to design and pilot survivorship care delivery models, especially for those patients with multiple chronic conditions. Survivorship care can help to address gaps in care coordination so that care and communication can be as seamless as possible between patients, their caregivers, and their healthcare providers. There is a real need for better care coordination between oncologists and primary care practitioners. Thus it is vital that the information shared at a survivorship visit also be communicated to their primary care team. This ensures that the primary care provider knows what parts of the patient's ongoing care they will be responsible for, but also makes sure that all of their healthcare needs are addressed, above and beyond their cancer diagnosis. If a patient does not have a primary care provider, this is an excellent time to refer them to one.

The recommendation that patients completing treatment receive a SCP has been difficult for some cancer programs to implement. One of the frequent concerns reported is that there is a lack of evidence that care plans improve health outcomes and have a positive impact on care coordination. Much of the research done on SCPs has been uncontrolled and has primarily looked at feasibility and acceptability of delivering SCPs,[75] and not at outcomes that the care plans can be expected to have influence over.[76] Beyond improvement in health outcomes, if the focus is on improving issues with fragmented communication and care coordination that many cancer survivors experience, SCPs can help in improved care coordination.[77] The Patient-owned Survivorship Transition Care for Activated, Empowered survivors (POSTCARE) trial focused less on the SCP document itself and more on process, where breast cancer survivors were engaged in a one-time coaching encounter emphasizing motivational interviewing techniques as a way to better involve survivors in their own self-care. They found that when survivorship was scoped in this way, it did have a positive impact on patient outcomes, including improved self-reported health and a trend toward self-efficacy.[78] Birken and Mayer postulate that "instead of viewing SCPs as a requirement to be met, they should be viewed as an opportunity to develop systems for delivering comprehensive survivorship care, of which SCPs are just one component."[79]

Ideally, SCPs should be created from data that resides in the electronic medical record. By creating disease-specific integrated templates in the EMR, personalized treatment summaries with follow-up information and wellness recommendations can be created for patients. These documents can be housed within the EMR and should be updated as needed by the patient's multidisciplinary healthcare team. Fig. 13.2 shows the follow-up portion of a breast cancer survivorship embedded in Epic.

Models of Care

There are different models of survivorship care delivery used in community practice. Some organizations initially adopted an oncologist-led model. However, this greatly limits oncologists' capacity for seeing new and more complex patients in a rapidly evolving world of cancer treatment. Some cancer programs use nurse navigators to complete SCPs and counsel patients. There are emerging data across the country from existing survivorship programs that support the role of the nurse practitioner and/or physician's assistant as the optimal provider to carry out survivorship care. In addition to having a skill set that is particularly suited to the delivery of cancer survivorship care, advanced practice providers are able to bill for survivorship services. There are several clinical models using advanced practice providers.

An embedded model for survivorship involves a follow-up visit, ideally 3–6 months after completion of therapy, to address survivorship issues, with the oncology-based nurse practitioner or physician's assistant. This model is ideal because it increases the opportunity for the physician to focus on appropriately complex and more highly reimbursed patients. Additional follow-up visits for survivorship can continue to be embedded within the oncology follow-up schedule or can also be set as separate encounters, depending on the patient's needs (Fig. 13.3).

Another approach to survivorship care involves the use of a multidisciplinary team approach, where the patient meets with an advanced practice clinician who conducts a physical examination, reviews the treatment summary, addresses late- and long-term effects of treatment, and reviews follow-up care guidelines. Then the patient meets with other multidisciplinary specialists, such as a cancer rehabilitation specialist, dietician, sexual health specialist, and/or psychosocial counselor to address other needs and set goals. The entire multidisciplinary team emphasizes healthy living and wellness goals. This model ensures that not only are the patients' medical needs met, but also their supportive care and psychosocial needs as well. The development of other supportive care such as virtual or live support groups, educational seminars, transition workshops, and wellness-based programs (yoga, exercise, cooking classes) is also key to having a robust and comprehensive program for patients after they complete their treatment.

Some organizations have developed standalone survivorship clinics. After a patient has been disease free for 1 year, they are transitioned to the survivorship clinic, which takes over responsibility for their ongoing follow-up care. Many of these clinics are disease specific, allowing for subspecialty survivorship services. Others have launched wellness-based or primary care–led survivorship follow-up, where the primary care provider actively follows their cancer follow-up needs. There is a definite role for primary care in survivorship care, but there is a need for additional training and guidelines to fill in the gaps and to help primary care providers address the many issues that breast cancer survivors may face.

FOLLOW UP CARE

After your treatment is completed, it is very important to go to all of your scheduled follow-up appointments. During these visits, your health care provider will ask questions about any symptoms and may do physical exams and order lab tests or imaging tests as needed to look for recurrences, secondary cancers or side effects.

Follow-up Care Test	Recommendation	Provider to Contact
Medical history and physical (H&P) examination	Visit your cancer care provider every three to six months for the first three years after the first treatment, every six to 12 months for years four and five, and every year thereafter.	Dr. Haider at 262-xxx-xxxx
Post- treatment mammography	Schedule a mammogram one year after your first mammogram that led to diagnosis, but no earlier than six months after radiation therapy. Obtain a mammogram every six to 12 months thereafter based on the guidance of your physician.	Dr. Brehm at 262-xxx-xxx
Breast self-examination	Perform a breast self-examination every month. This procedure is not a substitute for a mammogram.	

• **Fig. 13.2** Snapshot of a Survivorship Care Plan in EPIC. *ERIC*, Expert recommendations for implementing change.

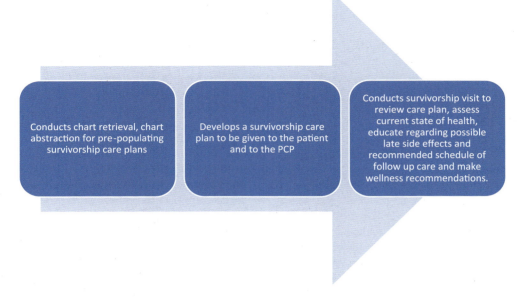

• **Fig. 13.3** Workflow of the Advanced Practice Provider in Delivering Survivorship Care. *PCP*, Primary care provider.

Barriers to Survivorship Care

There are a number of barriers that interfere with optimal survivorship care. One of the primary barriers to survivorship care is lack of survivor awareness about survivorship care and its importance. Introducing patients who are of curative intent to the concept of survivorship care early in their course of diagnosis and treatment can be helpful. At the end of their treatment, additional information and reinforcement of the importance of the visit is also beneficial. Many cancer programs offer additional programs and services to provide education and emotional support as well, which can help to keep patients engaged in the process. Survivorship programs have faltered in some cancer programs because of insufficient organizational resources, including poor integration into the electronic medical record and lack of appropriate staffing and workflow to support survivorship services.

Oncologists also need support and education, as many of them are skeptical about the need for survivorship care and feel that they already provide this care to their patients. They may be unaware that some of their patient's needs are unmet. Truant et al.[80] evaluated barriers to equity in cancer survivorship and found that, as a whole, the cancer care system prioritizes "biomedicine, evidence-based options, and care standardization," which leads to "system rigidities" that can compromise patient-centered care, especially for cancer survivors. The authors note that cancer survivorship has been "largely neglected in advocacy, clinical practice, and research."

In terms of reimbursement, there are no established billing codes specifically for survivorship care. However billable providers can bill for the total time spent examining and/or counseling survivors.

In 2017, the National Cancer Policy Forum of the National Academies of Sciences, Engineering, and Medicine held a workshop on cancer survivorship and suggested the following goals to advance cancer survivorship:
- Providing accessible, equitable, and affordable survivorship care.
- Reducing suffering and mortality for survivors while helping them return to life, work, and school.
- Testing risk-stratified care-delivery models that take into account health and social conditions in addition to cancer-specific factors.
- Improving survivorship-related education for clinicians and survivors.
- Meeting the needs of informal cancer caregivers.
- Better including diverse populations in survivorship research studies.
- Integrating psychosocial services into cancer care.
- Eliminating services where there is no benefit.
- Developing and implementing quality metrics to shape survivorship care.[81]

Program Evaluation and Metrics

The ASCO provides metrics for tracking survivorship in academic and community practice as part of its Quality Oncology Practice Initiative (QOPI) program, which measures quality cancer care and assesses adherence to recommended guidelines. Additional quality metrics may include patient-reported outcomes and feedback about their experience with survivorship care. Cost metrics are also an important component and can be assessed by determining revenue generated by survivorship visit billing and payer reimbursement. Another consideration is the assessment of downstream referrals generated from survivorship visits.

Hwang et al.[82] identified the implementation strategies that cancer programs used to achieve robust survivorship

TABLE 13.9 Expert Recommendations for Implementing Change for Cancer Survivorship Programs

Domain	ERIC Strategy[a]	Approach(es) to Consider
Survivorship care	Change record systems	Evaluate current survivorship care record system and workflow
Processes	Develop and implement tools for quality monitoring	Continuously monitor survivorship care quality (e.g., use EHRs to monitor receipt of recommended health maintenance services, psychosocial referrals, and loss to follow-up; use patient satisfaction surveys) and identify opportunities for improvement
Stakeholder involvement	Conduct local consensus discussions	Use existing stakeholder meetings as opportunities for discussion Engage patient advocates
	Use advisory boards and workgroups	Engage survivorship care staff and providers
	Identify and prepare champions	
	Identify early adopters	
Structural support	Create new clinical teams	Assess current roles and bandwidth among survivorship care providers and staff
	Revise professional roles	Ensure coverage of survivorship care roles across providers and staff, revising roles and/or hiring providers and staff as needed

[a]Moreira H, Canavarro MC. Psychosocial adjustment and marital intimacy among partners of patients with breast cancer: a comparison study with partners of healthy women. *J Psychosoc Oncol*. 2013;31(3):282-304.

EHR, Electronic health record; *ERIC*, Expert Recommendations for Implementing Change.

From Hwang S, Bozkurt B, Huson T, et al. Identifying strategies for robust survivorship program implementation: a qualitative analysis of cancer programs. *JCO Oncol Pract*. 2022;18(3):e304-e312.

programs, distinguishing them from programs that were found to be "cursory." Strategies fell into three domains: (1) establishing survivorship care processes, (2) stakeholder buy-in and engagement, and (3) organization-level support for staff hiring and role division and clarity. They found that robust survivorship programs designed "clear systems" of providing survivorship care, including the creation of survivorship-specific staff roles, developing workflows in the electronic medical record to allow for SCP autopopulation and the identification and tracking of patients who are appropriate candidates for survivorship care. Internal auditing to facilitate improvements in survivorship care over time were also found in robust survivorship programs. Table 13.9 delineates strategies used by robust cancer programs and potential approaches for programs who strive to improve programming to consider.

Stakeholder involvement was also identified as a differentiator in robust survivorship programs, with organizations making survivorship a regular part of cancer committee and tumor board meetings, but also developing survivorship-specific subcommittees that reviewed process and improvement. They found that cancer programs with robust survivorship programs generally had higher levels of stakeholder buy-in. Less robust programs often reported higher levels of internal resistance from stakeholders, such as physicians and senior leadership.

References

1. Bray F, Ferlay J, Soerjomataram I, Siegel RL, Torre LA, Jemal A. Global cancer statistics 2018: GLOBOCAN estimates of incidence and mortality worldwide for 36 cancers in 185 countries. *CA Cancer J Clin*. 2018 Nov;68(6):394–424. https://doi.org/10.3322/caac.21492.
2. American Cancer Society. Breast cancer: facts and figures 2019-2020. https://www.cancer.org/content/dam/cancer-org/research/cancer-facts-and-statistics/breast-cancer-facts-and-figures/breast-cancer-facts-and-figures-2019-2020.pdf
3. Dafni U, Tsourti Z, Alatsathianos I. Breast cancer statistics in the European Union: incidence and survival across European countries. *Breast Care (Basel)*. 2019;14(6):344–353. https://doi.org/10.1159/000503219. Epub 2019 Oct 8. PMID: 31933579; PMCID: PMC6940474.
4. American Cancer Society. Key Statistics for Breast Cancer in Men. January 2021. https://www.cancer.org/cancer/breast-cancer-in-men/about/key-statistics.html.
5. Khatcheressian JL, Hurley P, Bantug E, et al. Breast cancer follow-up and management after primary treatment: American Society of Clinical Oncology clinical practice guideline update. *Journal of Clinical Oncology*. 2013;31(7):961–965. https://doi.org/10.1200/jco.2012.45.9859.
6. Crabtree BF, Miller WL, Howard J, et al. Cancer survivorship care roles for primary care physicians. *The Annals of Family Medicine*. 2020;18(3):202–209. https://doi.org/10.1370/afm.2498.
7. Runowicz CD, Leach CR, Henry NL, et al. American Cancer Society/American Society of Clinical Oncology breast cancer

survivorship care guideline. *CA: A Cancer Journal for Clinicians.* 2015;66(1):43–73. https://doi.org/10.3322/caac.21319.

8. Ruddy K, Partridge A. Approach to the patient following treatment for breast cancer. In: Vora SR, editor.UpToDate. *Retrieved September.* 18; 20212021. https://www.uptodate.com/contents/approach-to-the-patient-following-treatment-for-breast-cancer.

9. Chikarmane SA, Cochon LR, Khorasani R, Sahu S, Giess CS. Screening mammography performance metrics of 2D digital mammography versus digital breast tomosynthesis in women with a personal history of breast cancer. *American Journal of Roentgenology.* 2021;217(3):587–594. https://doi.org/10.2214/ajr.20.23976.

10. National Comprehensive Cancer Network. (2023). Breast Cancer. v.4.2023.https://www.nccn.org/professionals/physician_gls/pdf/breast.pdf.

11. American Cancer Society. (2021, February 19). Mammograms After Breast Cancer Surgery. Cancer.Org. https://www.cancer.org/cancer/breast-cancer/screening-tests-and-early-detection/mammograms/having-a-mammogram-after-youve-had-breast-cancer-surgery.html

12. Peshkin B, Isaacs C. Genetic testing and management of individuals at risk of hereditary breast and ovarian cancer syndromes. In: Vora SR, editor.UpToDate. *Retrieved September.* 18; 20212021.. https://www.uptodate.com/contents/genetic-testing-and-management-of-individuals-at-risk-of-hereditary-breast-and-ovarian-cancer-syndromes.

13. Shapiro CL, van Poznak C, Lacchetti C, et al. Management of osteoporosis in survivors of adult cancers with nonmetastatic disease: ASCO clinical practice guideline. *Journal of Clinical Oncology.* 2019;37(31):2916–2946. https://doi.org/10.1200/jco.19.01696.

14. Li D, Weng S, Zhong C, et al. Risk of second primary cancers among long-term survivors of breast cancer. *Frontiers in Oncology.* 2020;9. https://doi.org/10.3389/fonc.2019.01426.

15. Sánchez L, Lana A, Hidalgo A, et al. Risk factors for second primary tumours in breast cancer survivors. *European Journal of Cancer Prevention.* 2008;17(5):406–413. https://doi.org/10.1097/cej.0b013e3282f75ee5.

16. Ussher JM, Perz J, Gilbert E. Changes to sexual well-being and intimacy after breast cancer. *Cancer Nursing.* 2012;35(6):456–465. https://doi.org/10.1097/NCC.0b013e3182395401.

17. Grogan S, Mechan J. Body image after mastectomy: a thematic analysis of younger women's written accounts. *Journal of Health Psychology.* 2016;22(11):1480–1490. https://doi.org/10.1177/1359105316630137.

18. Moreira H, Canavarro MC. Psychosocial adjustment and marital intimacy among partners of patients with breast cancer: a comparison study with partners of healthy women. *Journal of Psychosocial Oncology.* 2013;31(3):282–304. https://doi.org/10.1080/07347332.2013.778934.

19. Sherman KA, Przezdziecki A, Alcorso J, et al. Reducing body image–related distress in women with breast cancer using a structured online writing exercise: results from the My Changed Body randomized controlled trial. *Journal of Clinical Oncology.* 2018;36(19):1930–1940. https://doi.org/10.1200/jco.2017.76.3318.

20. Morales-Sánchez L, Luque-Ribelles V, Gil-Olarte P, Ruiz-González P, Guil R. Enhancing self-esteem and body image of breast cancer women through interventions: a systematic review. *International Journal of Environmental Research and Public Health.* 2021;18(4):1640.. https://doi.org/10.3390/ijerph18041640.

21. DiSipio T, Rye S, Newman B, Hayes S. Incidence of unilateral arm lymphoedema after breast cancer: a systematic review and meta-analysis. *The Lancet Oncology.* 2013;14(6):500–515. https://doi.org/10.1016/s1470-2045(13)70076-7.

22. American Physical Therapy Association. APTA Clinical Practice Guideline Process Manual. VA: Alexandria; 2018.

23. Tandra P, Kallam A, Krishnamurthy J. Identification and management of lymphedema in patients with breast cancer. *Journal of Oncology Practice.* 2019;15(5):255–262. https://doi.org/10.1200/jop.18.00141.

24. Patel KM, Manrique O, Sosin M, Hashmi MA, Poysophon P, Henderson R. Lymphatic mapping and lymphedema surgery in the breast cancer patient. *Gland Surg..* 2015;4(3):244–256.

25. Dayan JH, Dayan E, Smith ML. Reverse lymphatic mapping. *Plastic and Reconstructive Surgery.* 2015;135(1):277–285. https://doi.org/10.1097/prs.0000000000000822.

26. Benjamin EJ, Blaha MJ, Chiuve SE, et al. Heart disease and stroke statistics—2017 update: a report from the American Heart Association. *Circulation.* 2017;135(10). https://doi.org/10.1161/cir.0000000000000485.

27. Mehta LS, Watson KE, Barac A, et al. Cardiovascular disease and breast cancer: where these entities intersect: a scientific statement from the American Heart Association. *Circulation.* 2018;137(8). https://doi.org/10.1161/cir.0000000000000556.

28. Blaes A, Beckwith H, Florea N, et al. Vascular function in breast cancer survivors on aromatase inhibitors: a pilot study. *Breast Cancer Research and Treatment.* 2017;166(2):541–547. https://doi.org/10.1007/s10549-017-4447-6.

29. Stone JR, Kanneganti R, Abbasi M, Akhtari M. Monitoring for chemotherapy-related cardiotoxicity in the form of left ventricular systolic dysfunction: a review of current recommendations. *JCO Oncology Practice.* 2021;17(5):228–236. https://doi.org/10.1200/op.20.00924.

30. Armenian SH, Lacchetti C, Lenihan D. Prevention and monitoring of cardiac dysfunction in survivors of adult cancers: American Society of Clinical Oncology clinical practice guideline summary. *Journal of Oncology Practice.* 2017;13(4):270–275. https://doi.org/10.1200/jop.2016.018770.

31. Jim HS, Phillips KM, Chait S, et al. Meta-analysis of cognitive functioning in breast cancer survivors previously treated with standard-dose chemotherapy. *Journal of Clinical Oncology.* 2012;30(29):3578–3587. https://doi.org/10.1200/jco.2011.39.5640.

32. Hutchinson AD, Hosking JR, Kichenadasse G, Mattiske JK, Wilson C. Objective and subjective cognitive impairment following chemotherapy for cancer: a systematic review. *Cancer Treatment Reviews.* 2012;38(7):926–934. https://doi.org/10.1016/j.ctrv.2012.05.002.

33. Joly F, Lange M, dos Santos M, Vaz-Luis I, di Meglio A. Long-term fatigue and cognitive disorders in breast cancer survivors. *Cancers.* 2019;11(12):1896.. https://doi.org/10.3390/cancers11121896.

34. Hermelink K, Voigt V, Kaste J, et al. Elucidating pretreatment cognitive impairment in breast cancer patients: the impact of cancer-related post-traumatic stress. *JNCI Journal of the National Cancer Institute.* 2015;107(7):djv099.. https://doi.org/10.1093/jnci/djv099.

35. Jebahi F, Sharma S, Bloss JE, Wright HH. Effects of tamoxifen on cognition and language in women with breast cancer: a systematic search and a scoping review. *Psycho-Oncology.* 2021;30(8):1262–1277. https://doi.org/10.1002/pon.5696.

36. Henneghan A. Modifiable factors and cognitive dysfunction in breast cancer survivors: a mixed-method systematic review. *Supportive Care in Cancer.* 2015;24(1):481–497. https://doi.org/10.1007/s00520-015-2927-y.

37. Zeng Y, Dong J, Huang M, et al. Nonpharmacological interventions for cancer-related cognitive impairment in adult cancer patients: a network meta-analysis. *International Journal of Nursing Studies.* 2020;104:103514.. https://doi.org/10.1016/j.ijnurstu.2019.103514.

38. National Comprehensive Cancer Network. NCCN Clinical Practice Guidelines in Oncology (NCCN Guideline®). Survivorship. v.3.2021. https://www.nccn.org/professionals/physician_gls/pdf/survivorship.pdf.

39. Andrykowski MA, Lykins E, Floyd A. Psychological health in cancer survivors. *Seminars in Oncology Nursing.* 2008;24(3):193–201. https://doi.org/10.1016/j.soncn.2008.05.007.

40. Zebrack B, Kayser K, Bybee D, et al. A practice-based evaluation of distress screening protocol adherence and medical service utilization. *Journal of the National Comprehensive Cancer Network.* 2017;15(7):903–912. https://doi.org/10.6004/jnccn.2017.0120.

41. Wang XS, Zhao F, Fisch MJ, et al. Prevalence and characteristics of moderate to severe fatigue: a multicenter study in cancer patients and survivors. *Cancer.* 2014;120(3):425–432. https://doi.org/10.1002/cncr.28434. PMID: 24436136; PMCID: PMC3949157.

42. Gosain R, Miller K. Symptoms and symptom management in long-term cancer survivors. *Cancer J.* 2013;19:405–409.

43. Bower JE, Bak K, Berger A, American Society of Clinical Oncology Screening, assessment, and management of fatigue in adult survivors of cancer: an American Society of Clinical oncology clinical practice guideline adaptation. *Journal of clinical oncology: official journal of the American Society of Clinical Oncology.* 2014;32(17):1840–1850. https://doi.org/10.1200/JCO.2013.53.4495.

44. Berger A, Mitchell S, Jacobsen P, Pirl W. Screening, evaluation, and management of cancer-related fatigue: ready for implementation to practice? *CA: A Cancer Journal for Clinicians.* 2015;65(3):190–211.

45. Carpenter JS, Elam JL, Ridner SH, Carney PH, Cherry GJ, Cucullu HL. Sleep, fatigue, and depressive symptoms in breast cancer survivors and matched healthy women experiencing hot flashes. *Oncol Nurs Forum.* 2004;31(3):591–5598.

46. Sateia MJ, Buysse DJ, Krystal AD, et al. Clinical practice guideline for the pharmacologic treatment of chronic insomnia in adults: an American Academy of Sleep Medicine clinical practice guideline. *J Clin Sleep Med.* 2017;13:307–349.

47. Zick SM, Colacino J, Cornellier M, Khabir T, Surnow K, Djuric Z. Fatigue reduction diet in breast cancer survivors: a pilot randomized clinical trial. *Breast cancer research and treatment.* 2017;161(2):299–310. https://doi.org/10.1007/s10549-016-4070-y.

48. Alfano CM, Imayama I, Neuhouser ML, et al. Fatigue, inflammation, and ω-3 and ω-6 fatty acid intake among breast cancer survivors. *Journal of clinical oncology: official journal of the American Society of Clinical Oncology.* 2012;30(12):1280–1287. https://doi.org/10.1200/JCO.2011.36.4109.

49. Hadji P, Aapro MS, Body JJ, et al. Management of aromatase inhibitor-associated bone loss (AIBL) in postmenopausal women with hormone sensitive breast cancer: joint position statement of the IOF, CABS, ECTS, IEG, ESCEO IMS, and SIOG. *Journal of bone oncology.* 2017;7:1–12. https://doi.org/10.1016/j.jbo.2017.03.001.

50. Forsythe LP, Alfano CM, George SM, et al. Pain in long-term breast cancer survivors: the role of body mass index, physical activity, and sedentary behavior. *Breast Cancer Research and Treatment.* 2012;137(2):617–630. https://doi.org/10.1007/s10549-012-2335-7.

51. Beederman M, Bank J. Post-breast surgery pain syndrome: shifting a surgical paradigm. *Plastic and reconstructive surgery. Global open.* 2021;9(7):e3720.. https://doi.org/10.1097/GOX.0000000000003720.

52. Burstein HJ. Aromatase inhibitor-associated arthralgia syndrome. *The Breast.* 2007;16(3):223–234. https://doi.org/10.1016/j.breast.2007.01.011.

53. Mustafa Ali M, Moeller M, Rybicki L, Moore HCF. Long-term peripheral neuropathy symptoms in breast cancer survivors. *Breast Cancer Research and Treatment.* 2017;166(2):519–526. https://doi.org/10.1007/s10549-017-4437-8.

54. Lu W, Giobbie-Hurder A, Freedman RA, et al. Acupuncture for chemotherapy-induced peripheral neuropathy in breast cancer survivors: a randomized controlled pilot trial. *The oncologist.* 2020;25(4):310–318. https://doi.org/10.1634/theoncologist.2019-0489.

55. Greenlee H, DuPont-Reyes MJ, Balneaves LG, et al. Clinical practice guidelines on the evidence-based use of integrative therapies during and after breast cancer treatment. *CA: A Cancer Journal for Clinicians.* 2017;67(3):194–232. https://doi.org/10.3322/caac.21397.

56. Levin A, Carpenter K, Fowler J, Brothers B, Andersen B, Maxwell L. Sexual morbidity associated with poorer psychological adjustment among gynecological cancer survivors. *Int J Gynecol Cancer.* 2010 Apr;20(3): https://doi.org/10.1111/IGC.0b013e3181d24ce0. 2010.

57. Grover S, Hill-Kayser CE, Vachani C, Hampshire MK, DiLullo GA, Metz JM. Patient reported late effects of gynecological cancer treatment. *Gynecologic Oncology.* 2012;124(3):399–403. https://doi.org/10.1016/j.ygyno.2011.11.034.

58. Carpenter JS, Reed SD, Guthrie KA, et al. Using an FSDS-R item to screen for sexually related distress: a MsFLASH analysis. *Sexual Medicine.* 2015;3(1):7–13. https://doi.org/10.1002/sm2.53.

59. Lorenz T, Rullo J, Faubion S. Antidepressant-induced female sexual dysfunction. *Mayo Clinic Proceedings.* 2016;91(9):1280–1286. https://doi.org/10.1016/j.mayocp.2016.04.033.

60. ACOG (2016). Committee opinion: the use of vaginal estrogen in women with a history of estrogen- dependent breast cancer. Number 659 (Reaffirmed 2020). https://www.acog.org/clinical/clinical-guidance/committee-opinion/articles/2016/03/the-use-of-vaginal-estrogen-in-women-with-a-history-of-estrogen-dependent-breast-cancer

61. Anderson WF, Chatterjee N, Ershler WB, Brawley OW. Estrogen receptor breast cancer phenotypes in the Surveillance, Epidemiology, and End Results database. *Breast Cancer Res Treat.* 2002 Nov;76(1):27–36. 2002.

62. Cusack L, Brennan M, Baber R, Boyle F. Menopausal symptoms in breast cancer survivors: management update. *The British journal of general practice: the journal of the Royal College of General Practitioners.* 2013;63(606):51–52. https://doi.org/10.3399/bjgp13X660977.

63. Fisher T, Chervenak, J. Judi L. Lifestyle alterations for the amelioration of hot flashes. *Maturitas.* 2012;Volume 71(Issue 3):217–220.

64. Hickey M, Szabo RA, Hunter MS. Non-hormonal treatments for menopausal symptoms. *BMJ*. 2017:j5101.. https://doi.org/10.1136/bmj.j5101.

65. van Driel C, Stuursma A, Schroevers M, Mourits M, de Bock G. Mindfulness, cognitive behavioural and behaviour-based therapy for natural and treatment-induced menopausal symptoms: a systematic review and meta-analysis. *BJOG: An International Journal of Obstetrics & Gynaecology*. 2018;126(3):330–339. https://doi.org/10.1111/1471-0528.15153.

66. Lund KS, Siersma V, Brodersen J, Waldorff FB. Efficacy of a standardised acupuncture approach for women with bothersome menopausal symptoms: a pragmatic randomised study in primary care (the ACOM study). *BMJ Open*. 2019;9(1):e023637.. https://doi.org/10.1136/bmjopen-2018-023637.

67. Seiler A, Chen MA, Brown RL, Fagundes CP. Obesity, dietary factors, nutrition, and breast cancer risk. *Current Breast Cancer Reports*. 2018;10(1):14–27. https://doi.org/10.1007/s12609-018-0264-0.

68. Theodoratou E, Timofeeva M, Li X, Meng X, Ioannidis JP. Nature, nurture, and cancer risks: genetic and nutritional contributions to cancer. *Annual Review of Nutrition*. 2017;37(1):293–320. https://doi.org/10.1146/annurev-nutr-071715-051004.

69. Anyene IC, Ergas IJ, Kwan ML, Roh JM, Ambrosone CB, Kushi LH. Cespedes Feliciano EM Plant-based dietary patterns and breast cancer recurrence and survival in the pathways study. *Nutrients*. 2021;13(10):3374. https://doi.org/10.3390/nu13103374.

70. McDonald JA, Goyal A, Terry MB. alcohol intake and breast cancer risk: weighing the overall evidence. *Current breast cancer reports*. 2013;5(3): https://doi.org/10.1007/s12609-013-0114-z. 10.

71. Collaborative Group on Hormonal Factors in Breast Cancer Alcohol, tobacco and breast cancer – collaborative reanalysis of individual data from 53 epidemiological studies, including 58,515 women with breast cancer and 95,067 women without the disease. *British Journal of Cancer*. 2002;87(11):1234–1245. https://doi.org/10.1038/sj.bjc.6600596.

72. Key J, Hodgson S, Omar RZ, et al. Meta-analysis of studies of alcohol and breast cancer with consideration of the methodological issues. *Cancer Causes & Control*. 2006;17(6):759–770. https://doi.org/10.1007/s10552-006-0011-0.

73. Spei ME, Samoli E, Bravi F, La Vecchia C, Bamia C, Benetou V. Physical activity in breast cancer survivors: a systematic review and meta-analysis on overall and breast cancer survival. *The Breast*. 2019;44:144–152. https://doi.org/10.1016/j.breast.2019.02.001.

74. Alfano CM, Leach CR, Smith TG, et al. Equitably improving outcomes for cancer survivors and supporting caregivers: a blueprint for care delivery, research, education and policy. *CA: A Cancer Journal for Clinicians*. 2019;69:35–49.

75. Jacobsen PB, DeRosa AP, Henderson TO, et al. Systematic review of the impact of cancer survivorship care plans on health outcomes and health care delivery. *Journal of clinical oncology: official journal of the American Society of Clinical Oncology*. 2018;36(20):2088–2100. https://doi.org/10.1200/JCO.2018.77.7482.

76. Birken SA, Urquhart R, Munoz-Plaza C, et al. Survivorship care plans: are randomized controlled trials assessing outcomes that are relevant to stakeholders. *J Cancer Surviv*. 2018;12:495–508. https://doi.org/10.1007/s11764-018-0688-6.

77. Palmer SC, Stricker CT, Panzer SL, et al. Outcomes and satisfaction after delivery of a breast cancer survivorship care plan: results of a multicenter trial. *J Oncol Pract.*. 2015;11(2):e222–e229.

78. Kvale EA, Huang CS, Meneses KM, et al. Patient-centered support in the survivorship care transition: outcomes from the patient-owned survivorship care plan intervention. *Cancer*. 2016;122:3232–3242.

79. Birken SA, Mayer DK. Survivorship care planning: why is it taking so long. *Journal of the National Comprehensive Cancer Network*. 2017;15(9):1165–1169. https://doi.org/10.6004/jnccn.2017.0148.

80. Truant TL, Lambert LK, Thorne S. Barriers to equity in cancer survivorship care: perspectives of cancer survivors and system stakeholders. *Global Qualitative Nursing Research*. 2021;8 https://doi.org/10.1177/23333936211006703. 2.

81. Kline RM, Arora NK, Bradley CJ, et al. Long-term survivorship care after cancer treatment - summary of a 2017 National Cancer Policy Forum workshop. *JNCI: Journal of the National Cancer Institute*. 2018;110(12):1300–1310. https://doi.org/10.1093/jnci/djy176.

82. Hwang S, Bozkurt B, Huson T, et al. Identifying strategies for robust survivorship program implementation: a qualitative analysis of cancer programs. *JCO Oncology Practice*. 2021;18(3):e304–e312. https://doi.org/10.1200/op.21.00357. 20.

14

Breast Cancer Palliative Care

TIMOTHY GOGGINS

Breast cancer is an incredibly complex disease, and when metastatic or terminal, it becomes even more complex. The difficulties clinicians encounter with this disease go far beyond the malignancy. It includes, in many cases, particularly young women, families, including children directly affected by the disease. The course and management in these complex situations start with therapy directed at the breast cancer, although this also includes symptom management, psychosocial issues, spiritual domains, and goals of care. Many of these are addressed by the palliative care team, although this may include other ancillary personnel such as alternative medicine practitioners, dietitians, and counselors.

Palliative Chemotherapy

The goal of palliative chemotherapy is often to improve overall survival. Median overall survival is now more than 3 years among metastatic breast cancer patients, and ranges from a few months to years.[1] Palliative care is imperative in the management of metastatic breast cancer, including improved quality of life, alleviation of symptoms, and management of side effects to the treatment.[2–4]

Treatment selection is based on clinical factors, tumor biology, and goals of care, and treatment may include systemic chemotherapy, endocrine therapy, biologic therapy, and supportive care measures.[5,6] The most important predictors of treatment response are hormone receptor status and HER2/neu overexpression. Patients with genetic alterations in breast cancer susceptibility genes 1 or 2 (BRCA) are more likely to respond to poly(ADP ribose) polymerase (PARP) inhibitors.[7] Regarding chemotherapy, consistent predictors of poor response are progression with prior chemotherapy for advanced disease, relapse within 12 months of adjuvant chemotherapy, poor performance status, and multiple disease sites including visceral disease.

Pathways create a standardized approach to the care of our patients. The National Comprehensive Cancer Network provides multiple options for the treatment of patients. Unlike the NCCN, other pathway systems provide a more standardized approach and allow medicine an enormous potential to harvest retrievable data and influence the future care of patients. (Tables 14.1 to 14.5).[8–12]

Symptom Management

The most important component of palliative management is symptom management.
- Pain
  Nonpharmacologic[13]
  The idea of mind and body healing has been around for decades. How these enter symptom management varies, typically by patient.
  Rehabilitative physical modalities include ultrasound, therapeutic exercise, occupational therapy, hydrotherapy, therapy for specific disorders such as lymphedema, and heat and cold therapies.
  Psychological therapies include psychoeducation interventions, cognitive behavioral therapy, relaxation therapy, guided imagery, other types of stress management, hypnotherapy, and other forms of psychotherapy.
  Neurostimulation includes implanted neurostimulators, both transcutaneous and transcranial.
  Additional complementary therapies include acupuncture, massage, physical/movement (e.g., yoga), music therapy, art therapy, and other ideas such as mind occupational therapy (cognitive exercises such as coloring books or games such as sudoku).
  Pharmacologic
  Nonopioid
  Treatment of cancer-related pain typically incorporates a pyramid strategy. Pain control with nonopioid measures is encouraged prior to consideration of opioids.
  Nonopioid medications include acetaminophen, nonsteroidal anti-inflammatory drugs, topical agents, antidepressants, anticonvulsants, oral local anesthetics, steroids, cannabinoids, alpha-2 agonists, and ketamine.
  Interventional therapies include nerve blocks, spinal analgesics, and surgical neuroablation.
  Opioid
  Opioids remain an integral part of the management of pain in terminally ill cancer patients. The difficulties with opioids are the serious nature of the addiction

TABLE 14.1	HER2/neu-Negative Postmenopausal or Premenopausal Receiving Ovarian Ablation or Suppression
	Aromatase inhibitor + CDK4/6 inhibitor (abemaciclib, palbociclib, or ribociclib)
	Everolimus plus endocrine therapy
	Selective estrogen receptor downregulator (fulvestrant) plus a nonsteroidal aromatase inhibitor (letrozole, anastrazole)
	Fulvestrant plus CDK4/6 inhibitor (abemaciclib, palbociclib, or ribociclib)

TABLE 14.2	HER2/neu-Positive Postmenopausal or Premenopausal Receiving Ovarian Ablation or Suppression
	Aromatase inhibitor ± trastuzumab
	Aromatase inhibitor ± lapatinib
	Aromatase inhibitor ± lapatinib + trastuzumab
	Fulvestrant ± trastuzumab
	Tamoxifen ± trastuzumab

TABLE 14.3	HER2/neu-Negative Chemotherapy
	Anthracyclines (doxorubicin, liposomal doxorubicin)[a]
	Taxanes (paclitaxel)[a]
	Antimetabolites (capecitabine, gemcitabine)[a]
	Microtubule inhibitors (vinorelbine, eribulin)[a]
	Sacituzumab govitecan[a]
	Other regimens (cyclophosphamide, docetaxel, albumin-bound paclitaxel, epirubicin, ixabepilone)[a]

[a]Combinations useful in certain circumstances.

TABLE 14.4	HER2/neu-Positive Chemotherapy	
First line		Pertuzumab + trastuzumab + docetaxel
		Pertuzumab + trastuzumab + paclitaxel
Second line		Fam-trastuzumab deruxtecan-nxki
		Ado-trastuzumab emtansine (T-DM1)
Third line		Tucatinib + trastuzumab + capecitabine
		Trastuzumab + docetaxel or vinorelbine
		Trastuzumab + paclitaxel ± carboplatin
		Capecitabine + trastuzumab or lapatinib
		Trastuzumab + lapatinib (without cytotoxic therapy)
		Trastuzumab + other agents
		Neratinib + capecitabine
		Margetuximab-cmkb + chemotherapy (capecitabine, eribulin, gemcitabine, or vinorelbine)

issues surrounding these medications, and as a result, these medications are heavily regulated.

We continue to encourage the use of opioids in situations where nonopioid measures fail to gain adequate pain control.

- Nausea/vomiting

Although nausea and vomiting continue to be important to control clinically, many patients receive adequate coverage with standard premedication for their chemotherapy.

Antiemetic medications are classified based on drug type (Table 14.6).

Each class of drug type functions better depending on the nausea that is induced. Prokinetic agents are primarily used for gastric stasis and gastrointestinal dysmotility from various causes. Antihistamines are useful for vestibular and gut receptor nausea and vomiting. They are relatively contraindicated for constipation because they may further slow the bowel. Dopaminergic agents are best used for medication- and metabolic-related nausea. Serotonin 5-HTZ receptor antagonists are used for postoperative and radiation- and chemotherapy-induced nausea. Neurokinin receptor antagonists are particularly helpful for delayed chemotherapy-induced nausea and vomiting. Benzodiazepines are useful for anticipatory or anxiety-provoked nausea. Corticosteroids are useful for hepatic capsular distension, anorexia, and increased intracranial pressure. Cannabinoids help with chemotherapy-induced nausea and vomiting. Other anticholinergics are used for motion- or movement-related nausea and vomiting.

Gabapentinoids (gabapentin and pregabalin) have been used successfully for neuropathic pain. A summary of the benefits of gabapentinoids was published in 2015. It showed improvement (50% reduction in pain intensity) for gabapentin when treating postherpetic neuralgia. The number needed to treat to harm a single patient was 25.6, demonstrating a wide therapeutic index, and gabapentin has been successfully used for cancer-related pain.[14] It does appear that if pain does not respond to one gabapentinoid, it can respond to the alternative gabapentinoid.[15]

Analgesic antidepressants have also been widely studied for varied types of chronic pain.[16–19] Duloxetine is often used in conjunction with gabapentinoids and appears to be a more powerful pain medication as an alternative to opioids in cancer-related pain. It is common for duloxetine or a similar antidepressant to be used in combination with gabapentinoids for adequate cancer-related pain control.

Opioids

The use of opioid analgesics is important to sustain control of cancer-related pain. The goal of therapy is to improve quality of life while limiting opioid-related side effects. Guidelines exist to provide a rationale for

CHAPTER 14 Breast Cancer Palliative Care

TABLE 14.5 Biomarker-Associated and Molecular Testing[a]

Breast Cancer Subtype	Biomarker	Detection	US FDA-Approved Agents
Any	BRCA1 mutation BRCA2 mutation	Germline sequencing	Olaparib Talazoparib
HR-positive/Her2-negative	PIK3CA-activating mutation	PCR (blood or tissue block if blood negative), molecular panel testing	Alpelisib + fulvestrant
TNBC	PD-L1 expression (Threshold for positivity combine score of ≥10)	IHC	Pembrolizumab + chemotherapy (albumin-bound paclitaxel, paclitaxel, or gemcitabine and carboplatin)
Any	NTRK fusion	FISH, NGS, PCR (tissue block)	Larotrectinib Entrectinib
Any	MSI-H/dMMR	IHC, PCR (tissue block)	Pembrolizumab Dostarlimab-gxly
Any	TMB-H (≥10 mut/mb)	NGS	Pembrolizumab

[a]Biomarkers associated with US FDA-approved therapies.
dMMR, Deficient DNA mismatch repair; FISH, fluorescence in situ hybridization; IHC, immunohistochemistry; MSI-H, microsatellite instability-high; NGS, next-generation sequencing; NTRK, neurotrophic tyrosine receptor kinase; PCR, polymerase chain reaction; PD-L1, Programmed cell-death ligand 1; TMB-H, tumor mutational burden-high.

TABLE 14.6 Classification of Antiemetic Medications

Prokinetic agents	Metoclopramide
Antihistamines	Diphenhydramine Hydroxyzine Promethazine
Dopamine agonists	Haloperidol Chlorpromazine Prochlorperazine Olanzapine
Serotonin 5HT3 receptor antagonists	Ondansetron Granisetron
Neurokinin receptor antagonists	Aprepitant
Benzodiazepine	Diazepam Lorazepam
Corticosteroids	Dexamethasone Prednisone
Cannabinoids	Dronabinol
Other anticholinergics	Scopolamine Hydrobromide

TABLE 14.7 Different Opioids for Effective Pain Management

Opioids for moderate intensity pain	Codeine Dihydrocodeine Tramadol
Opioids for moderate-to-severe intensity pain	
Immediate release opioids as oral or injectable	Morphine Oxycodone Hydromorphone
Sustained release opioids as oral	Morphine Oxycodone Hydromorphone Tapnetadol
Transdermal formulations	Fentanyl Buprenorphine
Opioids for specialist use only	Rapid onset transmucosal fentanyl-based formulations Methadone

drug selection, route of administration, dosing, and side effect management.[20–23]

A position paper from the EFIC (European Pain Federation) Task Force illustrated opioid use for the management of pain (Table 14.7)[24]

The World Health Organization (WHO) has published a Cancer Pain Ladder, with its steps summarized here:

Step 1: When pain is mild, it may be sufficient to start with acetaminophen, a nonsteroidal anti-inflammatory drug, or an adjuvant analgesic targeting a specific type of pain (e.g., neuropathic).

Step 2: When pain persists, increases, or presents as a mild-to-moderate pain, an opioid regimen should be considered. The choice of opioid pain medications is based on the severity of pain, as illustrated earlier by the EFIC Task Force.

Step 3: When pain persists, increases, or initially presents as moderate to severe, single-entity, pure mu-agonist opioids are administered (e.g., morphine, oxycodone, oxymorphone, hydromorphone, methadone, or fentanyl). Adjuvant analgesics may be considered as well.

Step 4: For chronic and unrelieved severe pain or intolerable opioid-related side effects, consider treatment with interventional techniques.

The WHO analgesic ladder approach selects different opioids based on moderate (e.g., codeine) or severe (e.g., morphine) pain intensity.[25] Any of the single-entity, pure mu-agonist drugs can be prescribed at doses low enough to manage safely moderate pain, which eliminates the second step of the ladder.[26]

Additionally, in some circumstances, switching opioids or opioid route of administration or opioid formulation to a different opioid regimen becomes necessary. There are any of several reasons to switch regimens, including poorly controlled pain, the development of an adverse effect, change in patient condition, formulary issues, drug shortages, or patient health beliefs. It is recommended that the drugs be switched using an opioid conversion calculator.

- Fatigue

  Many cancer patients report a decline in energy levels. Although it remains important to maximize a patient's energy, there are many variables. The most important things to patients are adequate sleep, dietary intake, and exercise.

  The management of fatigue is often cause specific when conditions known to cause fatigue can be managed. Nonpharmacologic measures include cognitive behavioral therapy, exercise therapy, nutrition, sleep therapy, and other psychosocial interventions. Pharmacologic therapy can include psychostimulants (e.g., Ritalin), antidepressants (e.g., duloxetine), steroids, and hematopoietic stimulants. Erythrocyte-stimulating agents are indicated only in the palliative care setting when dealing with a malignancy.[27,28]

- Depression and anxiety

  Up to 70% of oncology patients report depression symptoms. These symptoms are complicated in the setting of psychosocial issues often related to a patient's malignancy.

Nutrition

Nutrition is an important part of the management of a terminally ill patient. The role of low muscle mass in terminally ill patients has long been correlated with worse survival.[29–31] Additionally, patients are more likely to have severe side effects from systemic treatments when associated with poor nutrition.[32]

TABLE 14.8 Various Definitions of Cachexia

Evans[33]	• Weight loss ≥5% in the past 12 months Or
	• BMI <20 kg/m² and 3–5 of the following:
	• Decreased muscle strength
	• Fatigue
	• Anorexia
	• Low muscle mass
	• Abnormal labs (elevated inflammatory parameters, anemia, hypoalbuminemia)
Fearon et al.[34]	Pre-cachexia
	• Weight loss ≤5%
	• Anorexia (reduced food intake)
	• Metabolic changes
	Cachexia
	• Weight loss >5% the past 6 months in the absence of starvation or
	• BMI <20 kg/m² and any weight loss >2% or
	• Low muscle mass and weight loss >2%Refractory cachexia
	• Variable degree of cachexia
	• Cancer disease procatabolic and not responsive to cancer treatment
	• WHO performance status 3 or 4
	• Expected survival <3 months

BMI, Body mass index; *WHO*, World Health Organization.

The definition of cachexia was determined by an international panel of experts in 2011 and varies to some extent—Table 14.8 lists its varied definitions.[33–35]

It is a multifactorial syndrome defined as an ongoing loss of skeletal muscle mass that cannot be fully reversed by conventional nutritional support and leads to progressive functional impairment. The general diagnostic criterion for cachexia includes weight loss greater than 5%, or weight loss greater than 2% in individuals already showing reduction in body mass index or skeletal muscle mass within the previous 6 months.

Cancer cachexia has been associated with worse patient outcomes. Disease-specific differences for patients with cachexia compared with those who do not have cachexia include poorer response to cancer therapy, shorter time to disease progression, and increased toxicity of treatment.[36] Additionally, cancer cachexia is associated with decreased physical function, increased assistance with activities of daily living, increased healthcare utilization, and decreased quality of life.

The role of the dietitian in terminally ill cancer patients includes educating on good nutrition, healthy eating habits, the effects of cancer and cancer treatments on nutrition, the importance of fluid intake, and the body's needs. The dietitian will work with families, patients, and the medical team to manage the cancer patient's diet during cancer therapy.

Psychosocial

Once breast cancer metastasizes, the focus on patient care begins to expand beyond the patient. Relationship dynamics change and multiple interactions change, particularly as the disease progresses. Families, including spouses (or significant others) and children, may be involved in the cancer patient's care.

The impact on children most definitely changes with the age of the child. Children go through stages of development, and their ability to understand tends to closely correlate with chronological age. Younger children prior to the age of 8 years tend to internalize and view mom as being "sick" or as having more of a temporary illness. Children up to the age of 12 years realize that death is permanent, although they can struggle with comprehending the meaning so they tend to ask more questions. It is recommended to be honest and answer questions clearly. Story books tend to be a helpful tool for children to better comprehend death and dying.[37]

Older children and young adults partly become caretakers, or play the "See Mom, I am okay" role, or completely detach from the situation. Although children are dynamic and resilient, they require attention and often counseling regarding the disease process. The death of a parent is a major, stressful event for children and their families, and in the absence of support in the early phases of grieving, children can develop some significant psychiatric disorders.[38] Palliative care referral early in the process can identify predictors of caregiver psychology and severity of grief, often directly impacting outcome.[39]

Spouses are often impacted far beyond the role of a caretaker. Much like children, the age of the caretaker tends to directly affect their response. Spouses under the age of 60 years tend to have higher rates of complicated grief.[40,41] Significant correlations have also been found between levels of complicated grief preloss and the following psychosocial factors: perceived social support; history of depression; current depression; current annual income; annual income at time of patient's diagnosis; pessimistic thinking; and the number of moderate-to-severe stressful life events. In a multivariate analysis, pessimistic thinking and severity of stressful life events remained as important factors to developing complicated grief predeath.[42] Caregiver burden and depression significantly affected levels of complicated grief.[42,43]

Communication and Counseling

The pace of communication between the physician and patient, as well as the assistance of counseling in many cases, should be an ongoing process determined by the patient's personality, coping mechanisms, and desire to know more information.[44]

Physicians, nurses, counselors, and team members often underestimate the amount of information patients want and misinterpret the type of information they wish to receive.[44] Patients often desire information that directly affects their lives (Table 14.9).

TABLE 14.9	Information Expected by Patients
	How the disease will impact their lives
	How the disease affects family members
	How their prognosis will likely affect their future plans
	Psychologic issues related to diagnosis and prognosis
	Resources to cope with daily living

Patients find it important to be responsive to their fluctuating needs for guidance and recognition, as well as being able to receive answers to their questions.[45]

Developing an interdisciplinary team approach is imperative to the patient-physician relationship and creating an environment where the patient can seek answers to their questions. Medical management as well as the assistance of counselors and social workers helps with patient understanding of their disease process.[46] Most families do not require intensive psychotherapy, but they look for answers and direction from caregivers.

In terms of psychotherapy, counseling is also important, particularly in a population of patients where depression may be higher than 50% in the malignancy population.[47] The benefits of counseling may include:[48–50]
- learning to cope with the diagnosis
- feeling less overwhelmed
- managing anxiety and depression
- coping with side effects, including pain and fatigue
- dealing with emotional issues
- managing fears and worries.

A counselor may additionally provide assistance with:
- communicating clearly with the healthcare team
- family and relationship issues
- finding resources
- making important practical decisions
- anticipating changes to treatment.

There are varying counseling types including group and individual therapy. In one study of women with metastatic breast cancer,[51] group programs had the strongest evidence for efficacy. Group interventions had the longest intervention duration and the lowest uptake and adherence; low-intensity interventions had the shortest duration and the highest uptake and adherence.

Communication is imperative in the management of any patient, particularly one receiving palliative treatment for a terminal diagnosis.

Advance Directives/Living Will/Healthcare Power of Attorney

Advance care planning is where individuals think about their values, preferences, and the type of care they are willing to receive if and when a health condition arises. In the

• BOX 14.1 Resources for Advance Care Planning

www.nia.nih.gov/health/publication/advance-care-planning

www.prepareforyourcare.org

www.americanbar.org/groups/law_aging/resources/health_care_decision_making/consumer_s_ toolkit_for_health_care_advance_planning.html

www.acpdecisions.org

www.theconversationproject.org

Compassion & Choices | End-of-Life Resources (compassionandchoices.org)

www.elderguru.com/download-the-your-life-your-choices-planning-for-future-medical-decisions-workbook

www.agingwithdignity.org

TABLE 14.10 Discussion Points for Patient Care Goals

Patient Condition	Malignancy Diagnosis
A discussion of the goals of care has been completed with (patient, family, HCPOA) regarding the prognosis:	• Function • Mobility • Nutrition • Psychological • Social
Patient-centered goals of care	• Usual oncologic care including treatments • Focus on alleviation of signs and symptoms • Live as long as possible • Spend time with family and friends • Live to a specific date (wedding, anniversary, birth of a child)
Plan for future care	• Would be okay with chemotherapy-related side effects • Would be okay with hospitalization for care • Would be okay with ICU care
The patient has a (good, fair, poor) understanding of everything discussed above	Additional items

HCPOA, Healthcare power of attorney; *ICU*, intensive care unit.

United States, many patients who are newly diagnosed with a terminal malignancy lack advance directives. The ability to identify our wants is important, and patients can also designate a healthcare agent or durable power of attorney for healthcare. They can also document their preferences in a living will.

In 1990, the Patient Self-Determination Act was federal legislation requiring healthcare providers who participate in Medicare and Medicaid programs to provide patients with information about advance directives. This required healthcare providers to document in the medical record if patients had executed an advance directive.[52,53]

There are a number of resources available for advance care planning, some of which are listed in Box 14.1.[53]

Goals of Care

Goals-of-care discussions are imperative to good patient care. They provide an "extra" layer of support to seriously ill patients and their loved ones. They help to decrease pain and depression, improve quality of life, result in fewer emergency room visits and hospitalizations, and allow more efficient coordination of care. Important aspects to be discussed in a goal of care discussion are reviewed in Table 14.10.[54] There are also several talking maps to facilitate the conversation. This includes the concept of REMAP,[55] an acronym for Reframe, Expect Emotion, Map out the future, Align with values, Plan treatments that match values.

References

1. Caswell-Jin JL, Plevritis SK, Tian L, et al. Change in survival in metastatic breast cancer with treatment advances: meta-analysis and systemic review. *JNCI Cancer Spectr*. 2018;2(4):pky062.
2. Stockler M, Wilcken NR, Ghersi D, Simes RJ. Systemic reviews of chemotherapy and endocrine therapy in metastatic breast cancer. *Cancer Treat Rev*. 2000;26(3):151–168.
3. Osoba D. Health-related quality of life as a treatment endpoint in metastatic breast cancer. *Can J Oncol*. 1995;5(Suppl 1):47.
4. Geels P, Eisenhauer E, Bezjak A, Zee B, Day A. Palliative effect of chemotherapy: objective tumor response is associated with symptom improvement in patients with metastatic breast cancer. *J Clin Oncol*. 2000;18(12):2395–2405.
5. Pagani O, Senkus E, Wood W, et al. International guidelines for management of metastatic breast cancer: can metastatic breast cancer be cured? *J Natl Cancer Inst*. 2010;102(7):456–463.
6. Beslija S, Bonneterre J, Burstein HJ, et al. Third consensus on medical treatment of metastatic breast cancer. *Ann Oncol*. 2009;20(11):1771–1785.
7. National Comprehensive Cancer Network Systemic therapy for metastatic breast cancer. *NCCN Clinical Practice Guidelines in Oncology*. 2019. Version 2. breast.pdf (nccn.org).
8. Swenerton KD, Legha SS, Smith T, et al. Prognostic factors in metastatic breast cancer treated with combination chemotherapy. *Cancer Res*. 1979;39(5):1552–1562.
9. Hortobagyi GN, Smith TL, Legha SS, et al. Multivariate analysis of prognostic factors in metastatic breast cancer. *J Clin Oncol*. 1983;1(12):776–786.
10. Yamamoto N, Watanabe T, Katsumata N, et al. Construction and validation of a practical prognostic index for patients with metastatic breast cancer. *J Clin Oncol*. 1998;16(7):2401–2408.
11. Perez JE, Machiavelli M, Leone BA, et al. Bone-only versus visceral-only metastatic pattern in breast cancer: analysis of 150 patients. A GOCS study. Grupo Oncologico CooperativeoDel Sur. *Am J Clin Oncol*. 1990;13(4):294–298.
12. Falkson G, Gelman R, Falkson CI, Glick J, Harris J. Factors predicting for response, time to treatment failure, and survival in women with metastatic breast cancer treated with DAVTH: a prospective Easterne Cooperative Oncology Groups study. *J Clin Oncol*. 1991;9(12):2153–2161.

13. Portenoy PK. Treatment of cancer pain. *Lancet.* 2011;377(9784):2236–2247.

14. Narain T, Adcock L. *Gabapentin for Adults with Neuropathic Pain: A Review of the Clinical Efficacy and Safety.* Ottawa, ON: Canadian Agency for Drugs and Technologies in Health; 2015.

15. Tanenberg RJ, Irving GA, Risser RC, et al. Duloxetine, pregabalin and duloxetine plug gabapentin for diabetic peripheral neuropathic pain management in patients with inadequate response to gabapentin: an open-label, randomized, noninferiority comparison. *Mayo Clin Proc.* 2011;86(7):615–626.

16. Verdu B, Decostered I, Buclin T, Stiefel F, Berney A. Antidepressants for the treatment of chronic pain. *Drugs.* 2008;68(18):2611–2632.

17. Collins SL, Moore RA, McQuay HJ, Wiffen P. Antidepressants and anticonvulsants for diabetic neuropathy and postherpetic neuralgia: a quantitative systematic review. *J Pain Symptom Manage.* 2000;20(6):449–458.

18. Onghena P, Van Houdenhove B. Anidepressant-induced analgesia in chronic non-malignant pain: a meta-analysis of 39 placebo controlled studies. *Pain.* 1992;49(2):205–219.

19. Saarto T, Wiffen PJ. Antidepressants for neuropathic pain. *Cochrane Database Syst Rev.* 2007(4):CD005454.

20. Cormie PJ, Nairn M, Welsh J. Control of pain in adults with cancer: summary of SIGN guidelines. *BMJ.* 2008;337:a2154.

21. Trescot AM. Review of the role of opioids in cancer pain. *J Natl Compr Canc Netw.* 2010;8(9):1087–1094.

22. Green E, Zwaal C, Beals C, et al. Cancer-related pain management: a report of evidence-based recommendations to guide practice. *Clin J Pain.* 2010;26(6):449–462.

23. Caraceni A, Hanks G, Kaasa S, et al. Use of opioid analgesics in the treatment of cancer pain: evidence based recommendations from the EAPC. *Lancet Oncol.* 2012;13(2):358–368.

24. Bennet MI, Eisenberg E, Ahmedzal SH, et al. Standards for the management of cancer-related pain across Europe-A position paper from the EFIC Task Force on Cancer Pain. *Eur J Pain.* 2019;21:660–668.

25. World Health Organization. *Cancer Pain Relieve with a Guide to Opioid Availability.* 2nd ed. Geneva, Switzerland: World Health Organization; 1996.

26. Maltoni M, Scarpi E, Modnesi C, et al. A validation study of the WHO analgesic ladder: a two-step vs three-step strategy. *Support Care Cancer.* 2005;13(11):888–894.

27. Berger AM, Mooney K, Banerjee C, et al. *NCCN Clinical Practice Guidelines in Oncology (NCCN Guidelines) Cancer-Related Fatigue.* Fort Washington, PA: National Comprehensive Cancer Network; 2017.

28. Rao AV, Cohen HJ. Fatigue in older cancer patients: etiology, assessment, and treatment. *Semin Oncol.* 2008;33(6):633–642.

29. Rier HN, Jager A, Sleijfer S, Maier AB, Levin M-D. The prevalence and prognostic value of low muscle mass in cancer patients: a review of the literature. *Oncologist.* 2016;21(11):1396–1409.

30. Rier HN, Jager A, Sleijfer S, et al. Low muscle attenuation is a prognostic factor for survival in metastatic breast cancer patients treated with first-line palliative chemotherapy. *Breast.* 2016;31:9–15.

31. Rier HN, Jager A, Sleijfer S, van Rosmalen J. Kock MCJM, Levin M-D. Changes in body composition and muscle attenuation during taxane-based chemotherapy in patients with metastatic breast cancer. *Breast Cancer Res Treat.* 2018;168(1):95–105.

32. Yip C, Dinkel C, Mahajan A, et al. Imaging body composition in cancer patients: visceral obesity, sarcopenia and sarcopenic obesity may impact on clinical outcome. *Insights Imaging.* 2015;6:489–497.

33. Evans WJ, Morley JE, Argiles J, et al. Cachexia: a new definition. *Clin Nutr.* 2008;27:793–799.

34. Fearon K, Strasser F, Anker SD, et al. Definition and classification of cancer cachexia: an international consensus. *Lancet Oncol.* 2011;12:489–495.

35. Pearson K, Strasser F, Anker SD, et al. Definition and classification of cancer cachexia: An International Consensus. *Lancet Oncol.* 2011;12(5):489–495.

36. Prado CM, Baracos VE, McCargar LH, et al. Sarcopenia as a determinant of chemotherapy toxicity and time to tumor progression in metastatic breast cancer patients receiving capecitabine treatment. *Clin Cancer Res.* 2009;15(8):2920–2926.

37. Arruda-Colli M, Weaver M, Wiener L. Communication about dying, death, and bereavement: a systemic review of children's literature. *J Palliative Med.* 2017;20(5):548–559.

38. Kirwin K, Hamrin V. Decreasing the risk of complicated bereavement and future psychiatric disorders in children. *J Child Adolesc Psychiatr Nurs.* 2005;18(2):62–78.

39. Kelly B, Edwards P, Synott R, Neil C, Baillie R, Battistutta D. Predictors of bereavement outcome for Family Carers of cancer patients. *Psychooncology.* 1999;8(3):237–249.

40. Ball J. Widows grief: the impact of age and mode of death. *OMEGA: J Death Dying.* 1977;7(4):307–333.

41. Ellifrit J. Complicated brewreavement: a national study of potential risk factors. *Am J Hosp Palliative Care.* 2003;20(2):114–120.

42. Tomarken A, Holland J, Schachter S, et al. Factors of complicated grief pre-death in caregivers of cancer patients. *Psychooncology.* 2008;17(2):105–111.

43. Beery LC, Prigerson H, Bierhals AJ, et al. Traumatic grief, depression and caregiving in elderly spouses of the terminally ill. *OMEGA.* 1997;35(3):261–279.

44. Fitch MI. How much should I say to whom? *Journal of Palliative Care.* 1994;3(10):90–100.

45. Back AL, Trinidad SB, Hopley EK, Arnold RM, Baile WF, Ewards KA. What patients value when oncologists give news of cancer recurrence: commentary on specific moments in audio-recorded conversations. *Oncologist.* 2011;16(1):342–350.

46. Karlawish JH, Quill T, Meier DE. A consensus-based approach to providing palliative care to patients who lack decision-making capacity. *Ann Intern Med.* 1999;130(10):835–840.

47. Massie MJ. Prevalence of depression in patients with cancer. *J Natl Cancer Inst Monogr.* 2004;(32):57–71. https://doi.org/10.1093/jncimonographs/lgh014.

48. National Cancer Institute. *Coping with Cancer.* National Cancer Institute; July 2014.

49. Andersen B, Farrar WB, Golden-Kreutz DM, et al. Psychological, behavioral, and immune changes after psychological intervention: a clinical trial. *J Clin Oncol.* 2004;22(17):3570–3580.

50. Granek L, Nakash O, Ben-David M, Shapira S, Ariad S. Oncologists', nurses', and social workers' strategies and barriers to identifying suicide risk in cancer patients. *Psychooncology.* 2018;27(1):148–154. https://doi.org/10.1002/pon.4481.

51. Beatty L, Kemp E, Butow P, et al. A systematic review of psychotherapeutic interventions for women with metastatic breast cancer: Context matters. *Psychooncology.* 2018;27(1):34–42. https://doi.org/10.1002/pon.4445.

52. Meisel A., Cerminara K.L. *Right to Die: The Law of End-of-Life Decision Making.* 3rd ed. Riverwoods, IL: Aspen Publishers.

53. Vig LK, Ahronheim JC, Bell C, Vitale CA Essential Practices in Hospice and Palliative Medicine. Ethical and Legal Practice. 5th ed.

54. https://www.nccn.org

55. VonGunten CF, Ferris FD, Emanuel LL. The patient-physician relationship. Ensuring competency in end-of-life care: communication and relational skills. *JAMA.* 2000;284(23):3051.

PART 5

Related Topics for Delivery of Care Today and Tomorrow

15

Genetics and Prevention

JODI LEIGH BREHM AND DEBORAH WHAM

In the United States, one in eight women (13%) will develop invasive breast cancer during her lifetime.[1] In 2021, it was estimated that 281,550 new cases of invasive breast cancer would be diagnosed in women in the United States, and 49,250 women would be diagnosed with noninvasive or in situ disease. It was expected that 43,600 women in the United States (about twice the seating capacity of the Madison Square Garden arena in New York City) would die from breast cancer in 2021.[2] While mortality from breast cancer in women under the age of 50 has remained steady since 2007, mortality from breast cancer in women over the age of 50 has continued to decrease by a rate of 1% per year between 2013 and 2018. It is felt that this reduction in breast cancer mortality is related to earlier detection due to increased screening efforts, as well as advances in therapy.[2] Given that prognosis after breast cancer is dependent on stage, early detection or, even better, prevention can make an enormous impact for an individual. This is where risk assessment and management can make a tremendous difference.

Approximately 80% of breast cancer is considered to be sporadic and occurs in women who have little to no family history of cancer. These cancers are thought to develop secondary to acquired genetic pathogenic variants that occur because of the aging process and environmental factors. The biggest risks for breast cancer across the population are age and female sex.[1] Familial breast cancer accounts for 15% to 20% of all breast cancer, and it is thought to be caused by multiple genes and environmental factors combined. Only about 5% to 10% of breast cancer is secondary to an inherited germline pathogenic variant (Fig. 15.1).[3] There are opportunities for lifestyle modification that can decrease a woman's risk of breast cancer and should be considered for even an average-risk individual. However, there is a contingent of patients who are at elevated risk for breast cancer due to personal and family history, and who would benefit from increased screening, risk-reducing medications, risk-reducing surgery, and lifestyle modifications. The goal of this chapter is to help the clinician identify and manage the patient population that is at high risk for developing breast cancer, which is defined as a lifetime risk for breast cancer greater than 20% or a 5-year risk of breast cancer greater than 1.67%.[4] The first step in identifying a patient that is at high risk for breast cancer is looking at the individual's

genetic risk factors, personal and family risk factors, and lifestyle risk factors.

Genetic Risk Factors

The National Cancer Care Network (NCCN) guidelines for genetic assessment in patients without a history of breast cancer recommends consideration for genetic counseling and possible testing for patients with a close relative, meaning a first- or second-degree relative, with one of the following: breast cancer diagnosed before the age of 45, two breast cancer primaries in a single individual, two individuals with breast cancer primaries on the same side of the family with one of those individuals being diagnosed before the age of 50, ovarian cancer, male breast cancer, pancreatic cancer, or metastatic prostate cancer. Individuals should also be considered for genetic counseling and testing if they have a personal or family history of three or more of the following cancers: breast cancer, sarcoma, adrenal corticoid carcinoma, brain tumor, leukemia, colon, endometrial, thyroid, or kidney cancer, macrocephaly, hamartomatous gastrointestinal (GI) polyps, lobular breast cancer, diffuse gastric cancer, gastrointestinal cancer, pancreatic cancer, ovarian sex cord of testicular Sertoli cell tumors, or childhood skin pigmentation. Individuals that meet the above criteria should be referred for formal genetic assessment and counseling.

Most hereditary breast cancer is caused by pathogenic variants in the BRCA1 and BRCA2 genes (BReast CAncer gene 1 and BReast CAncer gene 2). These genes are an important component in a deoxyribonucleic acid (DNA) repair pathway called homologous recombination (HR). HR is a process in which a strand of DNA is repaired using the homologous strand as a template. Loss of function of one of the copies of either of the BRCA genes leads to a defect in HR. The resulting inability of the cell to repair the DNA leaves it open to further damage, thus increasing the risk for cancer.

Over a woman's lifetime, the cumulative risk for breast cancer in a BRCA1 pathogenic variant carrier is 55% to 72%. BRCA2 pathogenic variant carriers have a lifetime risk of 45% to 69%.[5] The range in risk has not yet been fully explained. Currently, polygenic risk scores are in

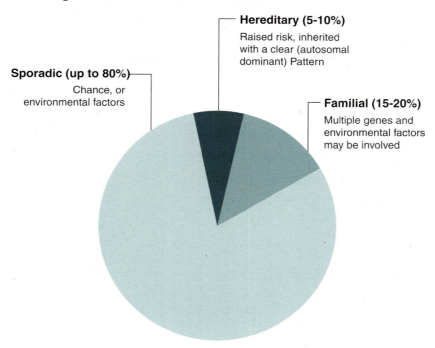

• Fig. 15.1 Categories of Breast Cancer Cases. (Source: NIH.)

development attempting to determine if otherwise benign variants in other genes modify the risk of pathogenic variants in the BRCA genes. It is likely that other nongenetic factors also influence this risk.

Women with pathogenic variants in one of the BRCA genes also have an increased risk of developing a second primary breast cancer. This risk is dependent upon the age at which the woman was when her first breast cancer was diagnosed, as well as which BRCA gene is altered. The risk for a second primary breast cancer is thought to be 21.1% within 10 years and up to 83% by age 70 in BRCA1 carriers. For BRCA2 carriers, 10.8% within 10 years and 62% by age 70.[6–9] Still, the ability to further stratify breast cancer risk by age for BRCA pathogenic variant carriers can be useful in surgical decision making. Patients can use more narrow risk assessments in determining whether they are comfortable with breast-conserving therapy versus bilateral mastectomy. Tables such as the one in Fig. 15.2[5] can be used as counseling aids in this decision-making process.

It is important to note that pathogenic variants in the BRCA genes also increase the risk for other cancers by the same HR deficiency mechanism. For women, the risk for ovarian cancer is between 39% and 44% for BRCA1 carriers and 11% to 17% for BRCA2 carriers.[5,10,11] Additionally, there are increased risks for fallopian tube cancer, primary peritoneal cancer, and pancreatic cancers. Men have an increased risk for prostate cancer.

Although the BRCA genes cause the majority of hereditary breast cancer, there are other genes in which pathogenic variants can cause varying degrees of breast cancer risk. These genes are often categorized by their lifetime risk for breast or other cancers, also known as penetrance. The genes with the highest penetrance in addition to the BRCA genes are tumor protein p53 (TP53), Cadherin 1 (CDH1), Partner and Localizer of BRCA1 (PALB2), phosphatase and tensin homolog deleted (PTEN), and serine/threonine kinase 11 (STK11). Pathogenic variants in these genes are associated with lifetime risks for breast cancer that can reach 50% or higher. The moderate penetrance genes have been more recently described, and our understanding of them is likely incomplete. Additionally, management recommendations vary for the moderate penetrance genes. For example, ataxia telangiectasia mutated (ATM), BRCA1 Associated Ring Domain 1 (BARD1), Checkpoint Kinase 2 (CHEK2), and Neurofibromatosis type 1 (NF1) all have an absolute risk for breast cancer of 15% to 40%,[12–15] and the NCCN makes recommendations for high-risk screening for breast cancer in individuals with pathogenic variants in these genes. Still, other moderate penetrance genes such as Restriction Site Associated DNA Paralog C and Paralog D (RAD51C and RAD51D) also have a lifetime risk for breast cancer in the range of 15% to 40%[16–18]; however, the NCCN recommends that screening for breast cancer be based on other factors such as family history.[19]

Genetic testing for genes related to increased risks for breast and other cancers is most commonly done via next-generation sequencing (NGS). This technology allows for the testing of multiple genes simultaneously, which renders results in a more timely manner than testing genes individually and sequentially. Still, testing multiple genes can

Years Since First Breast Cancer Diagnosis	No. of Women Contributing in Category	No. of Person-Years	No. of Events	Incidence Rate per 1000 Person-Years (95% CI)	Cumulative Risk, % (95% CI)
BRCA1					
≤5	827	2107	60	28.5 (22.1-36.7)	13 (10-16)
>5-10	618	2071	53	25.6 (19.6-33.5)	23 (20-27)
>10-15	435	1438	33	22.9 (16.3-32.3)	32 (28-36)
>15-20	236	675	17	25.2 (15.7-40.5)	40 (35-45)
>20-45	132	661	10	15.1 (8.1-28.1)	53 (44-62)
First breast cancer diagnosis at age <40 y					
≤5	370	920	31	33.7 (23.7-47.9)	15 (11-21)
>5-10	278	945	28	29.6 (20.5-42.9)	27 (21-33)
>10-15	217	739	20	27.1 (17.5-41.9)	36 (30-43)
>15-20	129	378	8	21.2 (10.6-42.3)	43 (36-50)
>20-45	70	343	6	17.5 (7.9-38.9)	60 (46-74)
First breast cancer diagnosis at age ≥40-50 y					
≤5	283	725	15	20.7 (12.5-34.3)	10 (6-16)
>5-10	225	718	19	26.5 (16.9-41.5)	21 (15-28)
>10-15	152	480	11	22.9 (12.7-41.4)	30 (23-38)
>15-20	74	222	6	27.0 (12.1-60.2)	39 (30-49)
>20-39	52	280	4	14.3 (5.4-38.1	49 (37-62)
First breast cancer diagnosis at age ≥50 y					
≤5	174	462	14	30.3 (17.9-51.2)	14 (8-22)
>5-10	115	408	6	14.7 (6.6-32.7)	20 (14-30)
>10-15	66	219	2	9.1 (2.3-36.5)	24 (16-35)
>15-20	33	75	3	40.0 (12.9-124.0)	38 (24-57)
>20-27	10	38	0	0.0	38 (24-57)
BRCA2					
≤5	565	1468	27	18.4 (12.6-26.8)	8 (6-12)
>5-10	476	1543	26	16.9 (11.5-24.8)	16 (12-21)
>10-15	285	880	11	12.5 (6.9-22.6)	21 (17-26)
>15-20	138	355	5	14.1 (5.9-33.8)	26 (20-33)
>20-43	68	290	3	10.3 (3.3-32.1)	65 (25-98)
First breast cancer diagnosis at age <40 y					
≤5	180	485	11	22.7 (12.6-41.0)	9 (5-17)
>5-10	163	542	9	16.6 (8.6-31.9)	17 (11-25)
>10-15	104	314	5	15.9 (6.6-38.2)	23 (16-32)
>15-20	58	149	4	26.9 (10.1-71.5)	31 (22-43)
>20-43	29	127	2	15.8 (3.9-63.0)	68 (29-98)
First breast cancer diagnosis at age ≥40-50 y					
≤5	206	550	7	12.7 (6.1-26.7)	6 (3-14)
>5-10	181	554	9	16.3 (8.5-31.2)	14 (8-22)
>10-15	107	322	5	15.5 (6.5-37.3)	20 (13-29)
>15-20	52	143	1	7.0 (1.0-49.6)	23 (15-35)
>20-37	29	123	1	8.1 (1.2-57.7)	28 (17-44)
First breast cancer diagnosis at age ≥50 y					
≤5	179	433	9	20.8 (10.8-40.0)	9 (5-17)
>5-10	132	447	8	17.9 (9.0-35.8)	17 (11-27)
>10-15	74	244	1	4.1 (0.6-29.1)	20 (13-30)
>15-20	28	63	0	0.0	20 (1330)
>20-30	10	40	0	0.0	20 (1330)

• **Fig. 15.2** A Reference Table Used as Counseling Aid for Surgical Decision Making.

result in complex results. Some patients may be found to have pathogenic variants in more than one gene. Patients can have variants within genes that are of unknown clinical significance. Even patients with single pathogenic variants in genes will need care beyond breast cancer risk management. It is imperative that patients understand the potential complexities of genetic testing. Because of this, the National Program of Breast Centers, the body that sets the standards and accredits breast cancer treatment centers in community care, has set a standard for genetic counseling and testing in breast cancer. Standard 2.16 says that pretest genetic counseling should be performed by a cancer genetics professional who has an educational background in genetics and cancer genetics, counseling, and hereditary cancer syndromes and can provide accurate risk assessment and empathetic genetic counseling to cancer patients and their families.[20] The National Society of Genetic Counselors has a resource to find qualified genetic counselors who can provide this evaluation both in person and virtually (https://findageneticcounselor.nsgc.org/).

Familial/Personal History/Lifestyle Risk Factors

If an individual does not meet the above criteria for genetic counseling and testing, they should then be assessed for breast cancer risk factors related to personal and family history. There are several different computer models that can be used to calculate a woman's risk of breast cancer. One of the earliest computer models to look at breast cancer risk is the modified Gail model. This model is available at the National Cancer Institute website at http://www.cancer.gov/bcrisktool/Default.aspx. The modified Gail model is based on patient age, age at menarche, age of first live birth, number of biopsies, presence of atypia (but not lobular carcinoma in-situ [LCIS]), and the number of first-degree relatives with breast cancer. The modified Gail model is only validated to use in patients age 35 or older. The NCCN Risk Reduction Panel recommends that those individuals greater than age 35 with a 1.66% or greater 5-year risk of breast cancer be considered for risk reduction strategies such as lifestyle modification and risk-reducing medication.[4] The Gail model is not without limitations. It should not be used in patients with a BRCA1, BRCA2, PTEN, or P53 mutation. It is not recommended for individuals with a strong family history of breast cancer, a history of thoracic radiation between the ages of 10 and 30, or those individuals with lobular carcinoma in situ.[4]

The Tyrer-Cuzick model is a computer-based multivariant model that considers personal history, history of atypical ductal hyperplasia (ADH), atypical lobular hyperplasia (ALH), and classical LCIS, family history of both the maternal and paternal sides and breast density. The Tyrer-Cuzick model can be found online at http://www.ems-trials.org/riskevaluator/. Individuals with a lifetime risk for breast cancer of greater than 20% based on the results of the Tyrer-Cuzick calculation can be offered increased screening with breast magnetic resonance imaging (MRI), risk-reducing medication, and recommendations regarding lifestyle modification.[4] Unlike the Gail model, the Tyrer-Cuzick risk model can be used in individuals less than 35 years of age. An analysis of the Mayo Clinic cohort demonstrated that the Gail model underestimated the risk of breast cancer in individuals with atypical hyperplasia,[21] while the Tyrer-Cuzick risk model overestimated the risk of breast cancer in individuals with a personal history of ALH/ADH.[22]

Other elements that can cause an increased breast cancer risk include being born female, increasing age, ethnicity, and race, and lifestyle factors including increased body mass index (BMI), alcohol consumption, current or prior estrogen-progesterone hormone therapy, and reproductive history.[4] The two greatest risk factors for developing breast cancer are being born female and increasing age.[1] While men can develop breast cancer, the incidence is much higher in women, and most breast cancers are diagnosed in women aged 55 and older.[3] Ethnicity and race also play a factor in breast cancer risk. Caucasian women have a slightly higher risk of breast cancer than African American women. African American women have a higher incidence of breast cancer being diagnosed before the age of 45 and are more likely to die from breast cancer at any age. Asian, Native American, and Hispanic women have a lower incidence and mortality rate from breast cancer.[1] While age, race/ethnicity, and family history are beyond the control of the individual, clinicians can educate and affect many of the breast cancer risk factors related to lifestyle.

The prevalence of obesity among adults in the United States in 2017 to 2018 was 42.4%.[23] Among women, the prevalence of obesity was 39.7% among those aged 20 to 39, 43.3% among those aged 40 to 59, and 43.3% among those aged 60 and over.[24] There is a substantial amount of evidence that overweight/obese women have a higher risk for postmenopausal breast cancer. The Nurses' Health Study suggested that women experiencing a weight gain of 25 kg or more since the age of 18 have an increased risk of breast cancer compared to those who have maintained their weight.[25] Most breast cancer diagnosed in post-menopausal individuals is hormone sensitive, specifically estrogen receptor and/or progesterone receptor sensitive. After menopause, once an individual's ovaries have stopped producing estrogen, most of the estrogen production comes from the fat tissue. Having more fat tissue increases estrogen levels and increases the risk of hormone-positive breast cancer.[23] In the same Nurses' Health Study, women who never used postmenopausal hormone replacement therapy and lost 10 kg or more after menopause and were able to keep the weight off had a significantly lower risk for breast cancer compared to those who maintain that weight.[25]

Exercise has been associated with decreased risk of breast cancer. A population, case-controlled study of 4538 patients with breast cancer and controlled patients grouped according to race demonstrated a 20% lower risk of breast cancer in both black and white women with annual lifetime activity levels greater than the median activity level when compared to inactive women.[26] The American Cancer Society recommends that adults get between 150 and 300 minutes (about 5 hours) of moderate-intensity or 75 to 150 minutes of vigorous-intensity exercise per week, with reaching 300 minutes or more of exercise per week being the ideal.[27]

There is a known correlation between alcohol intake and breast cancer risk. A population-based study of 51,847 women provided an association between alcohol consumption and an increased likelihood of developing hormone-positive breast cancer.[28] Even one drink per day can increase breast cancer risk. In an analysis of two cohort studies, there was found to be a 10% increase in risk for breast cancer for every 10 g of alcohol consumed daily.[29,30] The consensus from the NCCN risk reduction panel was to recommend less than one alcoholic beverage per day. One drink is defined as 1 oz of liquor, 6 oz of wine, or 12 oz of beer.[31]

Hormone replacement therapy can also increase an individual's risk of breast cancer. The Women's Health Initiative enrolled 161,809 women between the ages of 50 and 79 into a set of clinical trials. Two of these trials involved the use of hormone therapy in primary disease prevention. The inhibitor for risk reduction should consider cessation of the medication.

Musculoskeletal Complaints/Joint Ache

This side effect is more common with aromatase inhibitors. It is thought that patients with low vitamin D levels may have a higher incidence of joint pain/achiness when taking the aromatase inhibitors. Therefore, it is important to make sure that a patient is taking vitamin D supplementation.[45] Often these symptoms will resolve over time. However, patients can consider trying a different aromatase inhibitor to see if symptoms resolve. If symptoms do not resolve and the patient is experiencing significant difficulty, consider cessation of the medication.

Risk-Reducing Surgery

Risk-reducing mastectomy (RRM) is appropriate only for those women who are at very high risk for breast cancer. RRM is an appropriate option for individuals with pathogenic variants in high-penetrance genes, compelling family history, or prior thoracic radiation before the age of 30.[4] While RRM has been considered in the past for individuals with a personal history of LCIS, the current preferred approach is risk-reducing therapy rather than surgical intervention.[4] BRCA1/2 pathogenic variant carriers who undergo risk-reducing surgery have a substantially reduced breast cancer incidence and mortality.[52] Appropriate preoperative counseling is essential to achieve appropriate postoperative expectations. RRM candidates have the option of reconstruction, including nipple-sparing mastectomy. Prior to surgical intervention, patients should undergo clinical breast exams, mammograms, and the possible screening breast MRI. Postoperatively individuals should undergo yearly clinical breast exams. After RRM there is no recommendation for screening mammogram, ultrasound, or MRI.

Management of the High-Risk Patient

For the purposes of this chapter, the classification and subsequent management of high-risk patient is as follows:
1. Women with a history of mantle radiation between the ages of 10 and 30
2. Women with a lifetime risk of breast cancer greater than 20% based on a history of classic lobular carcinoma in situ, ADH, or ALH
3. Women with a lifetime risk greater than 20% defined by a model largely dependent on family history (i.e., Tyrer-Cuzick or Claus Model)
4. Women over the age of 35 with a 5-year breast cancer risk greater than 1.66% based on the modified Gail model
5. Women with a pedigree consistent with or having a known hereditary breast cancer syndrome

Women who underwent mantle radiation between the ages of 10 and 30 have an elevated risk for breast cancer

secondary to the radiation alone. In the Late Effects Study Group Trial, the overall risk for breast cancer for women undergoing radiation at a young age was found to be 56-fold greater than the risk for breast cancer in the general population.[53] Individuals should begin annual clinical encounters 8 years after completion of radiation. Annual screening mammograms with consideration for tomosynthesis should begin 8 years after completion of radiation therapy but not before age 30. These individuals can be recommended to begin screening breast MRI 8 years after completion of radiation therapy but not before age 25. For individuals that cannot undergo breast MRI, there is consideration for contrast-enhanced mammography or whole breast ultrasound. Patients should be counseled on lifestyle modification and risk-reducing strategies that were discussed earlier in the chapter.

Women with a personal history of classic-type lobular carcinoma in situ, ADH, or ALH should undergo a clinical breast encounter every 6 to 12 months starting at the time of diagnosis. Annual mammography with consideration for tomosynthesis should begin at the time of diagnosis of the high-risk lesion, but not before the age of 30. Patients may consider annual screening breast MRI starting at the time of diagnosis of the high-risk lesion, but not before age 25. The patient should be counseled in risk-reducing strategies such as a healthy lifestyle and risk-reducing agents.

For women with a lifetime risk of breast cancer greater than 20% based on family history models such as the Tyrer-Cuzick or Claus model, recommendations include a clinical breast exam every 6 to 12 months starting after age 21. Patients should consider annual mammograms starting 10 years prior to the age of the youngest family member with breast cancer, but not to begin before age 30. Patients may also consider an annual breast MRI, again starting 10 years younger than the age of the youngest family member as above, but not before the age of 25. Patients should be counseled regarding healthy lifestyle choices and risk-reducing medications.

Women with a calculated Gail Model 5-year risk greater than 1.66% are also recommended to consider a clinical breast exam every 6 to 12 months once they have been identified to be at increased risk. Individuals should consider annual mammography once they have been identified to be at high risk. There is not a recommendation for screening breast MRI based on Gail Model results. These individuals should also be counseled regarding healthy lifestyle and offered risk-reducing medications.

References

1. U.S Breast Cancer Statistics; 2021. Retrieved from breastcancer. org: https://www.breastcancer.org/symptoms/understand_bc/statistics
2. Cancer Facts & Figures 2021; n.d. Retrieved from Cancer.org: https://www.cancer.org/content/dam/cancer-org/research/cancer-facts-and-statistics/annual-cancer-facts-and-figures/2021/cancer-facts-and-figures-2021.pdf

3. Breast Cancer Risk Factors You Cannot Change/Genetic Risk Factors; n.d. Retrieved from cancer.org: https://www.cancer.org/cancer/breast-cancer/risk-and-prevention/breast-cancer-risk-factors-you-cannot-change.html

4. nccn.org. (n.d.). breast-risk.pdf. Retrieved from nccn.org: https://www.nccn.org/professionals/physician_gls/pdf/breast_risk.pdf

5. Kuchenbaecker KB, Hopper JL, Barnes DR, et al. Risks of breast, ovarian, and contralateral breast cancer for BRCA1 and BRCA2 mutation carriers. *JAMA*. 2017;317(23):2402–2416.

6. Graeser MK, Engel C, Rhiem K, et al. Contralateral breast cancer risk in BRCA1 and BRCA2 mutation carriers. *J Clin Oncol*. 2009;27(35):5887–5892.

7. Malone KE, Begg CB, Haile RW, et al. Population-based study of the risk of second primary contralateral breast cancer associated with carrying a mutation in BRCA1 or BRCA2. *J Clin Oncol*. 2010;28(14):2404–2410.

8. Metcalfe K, Gershman S, Lynch HT, et al. Predictors of contralateral breast cancer in BRCA1 and BRCA2 mutation carriers. *Br J Cancer*. 2011;104(9):1384–1392.

9. van den Broek AJ, Schmidt MK, van 't Veer LJ, et al. Worse breast cancer prognosis of BRCA1/BRCA2 mutation carriers: what's the evidence? A systematic review with meta-analysis. *PLoS One*. 2015;10(3):e0120189..

10. Antoniou A, Pharoah PD, Narod S, et al. Average risks of breast and ovarian cancer associated with BRCA1 or BRCA2 mutations detected in case series unselected for family history: a combined analysis of 22 studies. *Am J Hum Genet*. 2003;72(5):1117–1130.

11. Chen S, Parmigiani G. Meta-analysis of BRCA1 and BRCA2 penetrance. *J Clin Oncol*. 2007;25(11):1329–1333.

12. Marabelli M, Cheng SC, Parmigiani G. Penetrance of ATM gene mutations in breast cancer: a meta-analysis of different measures of risk. *Genet Epidemiol*. 2016;40(5):425–431.

13. Breast Cancer Association Consortium Dorling L, Carvalho S, et al. Breast cancer risk genes: association analysis in more than 113,000 women. *N Engl J Med*. 2021;384(5):428–439.

14. Cybulski C, Wokołorczyk D, Jakubowska A, et al. Risk of breast cancer in women with a CHEK2 mutation with and without a family history of breast cancer. *J Clin Oncol*. 2011;29(28):3747–3752.

15. Seminog OO, Goldacre MJ. Age-specific risk of breast cancer in women with neurofibromatosis type 1. *Br J Cancer*. 2015;112(9):1546–1548.

16. Hu C, Polley EC, Yadav S, et al. The contribution of germline predisposition gene mutations to clinical subtypes of invasive breast cancer from a clinical genetic testing cohort. *J Natl Cancer Inst*. 2020;112(12):1231–1241.

17. Couch FJ, Hart SN, Sharma P, et al. Inherited mutations in 17 breast cancer susceptibility genes among a large triple-negative breast cancer cohort unselected for family history of breast cancer. *J Clin Oncol*. 2015;33(4):304–311.

18. Li N, McInerny S, Zethoven M, et al. Combined tumor sequencing and case-control analyses of RAD51C in breast cancer. *J Natl Cancer Inst*. 2019;111(12):1332–1339.

19. National Comprehensive Cancer Network. Genetic/Familial High-Risk Assessment: Breast, Ovarian, and Pancreatic; 2021. NCCN.org, 1.2022, 1-129.

20. National Accreditation Program for Breast Centers.. *Standards Manual*. Https://Www.facs.org/Quality-Programs/Cancer-Programs/National-Accreditation-Program-for-Breast-Centers/Standards-and-Resources/: American College of Surgeons; 2018.

21. Pankratz VS, Hartmann LC, Degnim AC, et al. Assessment of the accuracy of the Gail model in women with atypical hyperplasia. *J Clin Oncol*. 2008;26:5374–5379. http://www.ncbi.nlm.nih.gov/pubmed/18854574.

22. Boughey JC, Hartmann LC, Anderson SS, et al. Evaluation of the Tyrer-Cuzick (International Breast Cancer Intervention Study) model for breast cancer risk prediction in women with atypical hyperplasia. *J Clin Oncol*. 2010;28:3591–3596. http://www.ncbi.nlm.nih.gov/pubmed/20606088.

23. Lifestyle-related Breast Cancer Risk Factors; n.d. Retrieved from cancer.org: https://www.cancer.org/cancer/breast-cancer/risk-and-prevention/lifestyle-related-breast-cancer-risk-factors.html

24. Adult Obesity Facts/Overweight and Obesity/CDC; n.d. Retrieved from cdc.gov: https://www.cdc.gov/obesity/data/adult.html

25. Eliassen AH, Colditz GA, Rosner B, et al. Adult weight change and risk of postmenopausal breast cancer. *JAMA*. 2006;296:193–201. http://www.ncbi.nlm.nih.gov/pubmed/16835425.

26. Bernstein L, Patel AV, Ursin G, et al. Lifetime recreational exercise activity and breast cancer risk among black women and white women. *J Natl Cancer Inst*. 2005;97:1671–1679. http://www.ncbi.nlm.nih.gov/pubmed/16288120.

27. American Cancer Society Guideline for Diet and Physical Activity for Cancer Prevention; n.d. Retrieved from cancer.org: https://www.cancer.org/healthy/eat-healthy-get-active/acs-guidelines-nutrition-physical-activity-cancer-prevention.html

28. Suzuki R, Ye W, Rylander-Rudqvist T, et al. Alcohol and postmenopausal breast cancer risk defined by estrogen and progesterone receptor status: a prospective cohort study. *J Natl Cancer Inst*. 2005;97:1601–1608. http://www.ncbi.nlm.nih.gov/pubmed/16264180.

29. Hamajima N, Hirose K, Tajima K, et al. Alcohol, tobacco and breast cancer—collaborative reanalysis of individual data from 53 epidemiological studies, including 58,515 women with breast cancer and 95,067 women without the disease. *Br J Cancer*. 2002;87:1234–1245. http://www.ncbi.nlm.nih.gov/pubmed/12439712.

30. Smith-Warner SA, Spiegelman D, Yaun SS, et al. Alcohol and breast cancer in women: a pooled analysis of cohort studies. *JAMA*. 1998;279:535–540. http://www.ncbi.nlm.nih.gov/pubmed/9480365.

31. NCCN Guidelines Version 1.2021 Breast Cancer Risk Reduction; March 24, 2021. Retrieved from nccn.org: https://www.nccn.org/professionals/physician_gls/pdf/breast_risk.pdf

32. Rossouw JE, Anderson GL, Prentice RL, et al. Risks and benefits of estrogen plus progestin in healthy postmenopausal women: principal results from the women's health initiative randomized controlled trial. *JAMA*. 2002;288:321–333. http://www.ncbi.nlm.nih.gov/pubmed/12117397.

33. Anderson GL, Limacher M, Assaf AR, et al. Effects of conjugated equine estrogen in postmenopausal women with hysterectomy: the Women's Health Initiative randomized controlled trial. *JAMA*. 2004;291:1701–1712. http://www.ncbi.nlm.nih.gov/pubmed/15082697.

34. Chlebowski RT, Anderson GL, Gass M, et al. Estrogen plus progestin and breast cancer incidence and mortality in postmenopausal women. *JAMA*. 2010;304:1684–1692. http://www.ncbi.nlm.nih.gov/pubmed/20959578.

35. Chlebowski RT, Kuller LH, Prentice RL, et al. Breast cancer after use of estrogen plus progestin in postmenopausal women. *N Engl J Med*. 2009;360:573–587. http://www.ncbi.nlm.nih.gov/pubmed/19196674.

36. Stefanick ML, Anderson GL, Margolis KL, et al. Effects of conjugated equine estrogens on breast cancer and mammography screening in postmenopausal women with hysterectomy. *JAMA*. 2006;295:1647–1657. http://www.ncbi.nlm.nih.gov/pubmed/16609086.

37. Rohan TE, Negassa A, Chlebowski RT, et al. Conjugated equine estrogen and risk of benign proliferative breast disease: a randomized controlled trial. *J Natl Cancer Inst*. 2008;100:563–571. http://www.ncbi.nlm.nih.gov/pubmed/18398105.

38. Colditz GA, Rosner B. Cumulative risk of breast cancer to age 70 years according to risk factor status: data from the Nurses' Health Study. *Am J Epidemiol*. 2000;152:950–964. https://www.ncbi.nlm.nih.gov/pubmed/11092437.

39. Kelsey JL, Gammon MD, John EM. Reproductive factors and breast cancer. *Epidemiol Rev*. 1993;15:36–47. https://www.ncbi.nlm.nih.gov/pubmed/8405211.

40. Rosner B, Colditz GA, Willett WC. Reproductive risk factors in a prospective study of breast cancer: the Nurses' Health Study. *Am J Epidemiol*. 1994;139:819–835. https://www.ncbi.nlm.nih.gov/pubmed/8178795.

41. Ritte R, Lukanova A, Tjonneland A, et al. Height, age at menarche and risk of hormone receptor-positive and -negative breast cancer: a cohort study. *Int J Cancer*. 2013;132:2619–2629. https://www.ncbi.nlm.nih.gov/pubmed/23090881.

42. Hsieh CC, Trichopoulos D, Katsouyanni K, et al. Age at menarche, age at menopause, height and obesity as risk factors for breast cancer: associations and interactions in an international case-control study. *Int J Cancer*. 1990;46:796–800. https://www.ncbi.nlm.nih.gov/pubmed/2228308.

43. Collaborative Group on Hormonal Factors in Breast Cancer Breast cancer and breastfeeding: collaborative reanalysis of individual data from 47 epidemiological studies in 30 countries, including 50302 women with breast cancer and 96973 women without the disease. *Lancet*. 2002;360:187–195. http://www.ncbi.nlm.nih.gov/pubmed/12133652.

44. Fisher B, Constantino JP, Wickerham DL, et al. Tamoxifen for prevention of breast cancer: report of the National Surgical Adjuvant Breast and Bowel Project P-1 Study. *J Natl Cancer Inst*. 1998;90:1371–1388.

45. American Society of Breast Surgeons; August 6, 2019. Retrieved from American Society of Breast Surgeons Official Statements. https://www.breastsurgeons.org/docs/statements/ASBrS-Resource-Guide-on-Endocrine-Therapy.pdf

46. DeCensi A, Puntoni M, Guerrieri-Gonzaga A, et al. Randomized placebo controlled trial of low-dose tamoxifen to prevent local and contralateral recurrence in breast intraepithelial neoplasia. *J Clin Oncol*. 2019 https://doi.org/10.1200/JCO.1. JC.

47. Fisher B, Constantino JP, Wickerham DL, et al. Tamoxifen for prevention of breast cancer: report of the National Surgical Adjuvant Breast and Bowel Project P-1 Study. *J Natl Cancer Inst*. 1998;90(18):1371–1388.

48. Goss P, Ingle J, Ales-Martinez J, et al. Exemestane for breast-cancer prevention in postmenopausal women. *N Engl J Med*. 2011;364:2381–2391.

49. Cuzick J, Sestak I, Forbes JF, et al. Anastrozole for prevention of breast cancer in high-risk postmenopausal women (IBIS-II): an international, double-blind, randomised placebo-controlled trial. *Lancet*. 2014;383:1041–1048. http://www.ncbi.nlm.nih.gov/pubmed/24333009.

50. Simon JA, Gaines T, LaGuardia KD. Extended-release oxybutin therapy for vasomotor symptoms in women: a randomized clinical trial. *Menopause*. 2016;23(11):1214–1221.

51. ACOG Committee Opinion No. 659 The use of vaginal estrogen in women with a history of estrogen-dependent breast cancer. *Obstet Gynecol*. 2016;127:e93–e96.

52. Li X, you R, Wang X, et al. Effectiveness of prophylactic Surgeries in BRCA 1 or BRCA 2 mutation carriers: a meta-analysis and systematic review. *Clin Cancer Res*. 2016;22(15):3971–3981.

53. Bhatia S, Yasui Y, Robison LL, et al. High risk of subsequent neoplasms continues with extended follow-up of childhood Hodgkin's disease: report from the Late Effects Study Group. *J Clin Oncol*. 2003;21:4386–4394. http://www.ncbi.nlm.nih.gov/pubmed/14645429.

16
Coping With the High Cost of Cancer

BRAD ZIMMERMAN

A breast cancer diagnosis can sometimes lead to financial hardship. The National Cancer Institute recognizes financial hardship, also known as financial distress or financial toxicity, as the negative impact of the "costs" of cancer care on the lives of cancer patients and their loved ones. There is a growing amount of research to suggest financial hardship among cancer patients is increasing in prevalence. There are many variables that contribute to financial hardship, and evidence suggests the need to recognize it during the early stages of a cancer diagnosis and to treat it much like a clinician would treat a cancer's symptoms or a treatment's side effects. This chapter will explore some of the many contributing factors to financial hardship experienced by cancer patients and various ways to reduce it.

The Significance Behind Recognizing Financial Hardship in People With Cancer

A study conducted by the National Opinion Resource Center (NORC) at the University of Chicago found that 4 in 10 people reported they fear the costs associated with a serious illness more than they fear the illness itself. Fifty-three percent of respondents said they had at least one of the following situations occur because of healthcare costs within the previous year: depleting savings (36%), credit card debt (32%), choosing between paying medical bills and affording basic necessities (30%), and an inability to add any money into savings because of healthcare costs (41%).[1] In a survey conducted by the Pink Fund, 562 female breast cancer patients responded; the results illustrated how a breast cancer diagnosis and subsequent treatment affected their personal finances, career, and well-being. In total, 46% of those surveyed reported a reduction in spending on essentials such as food, clothing, and shelter in order to pay for their out-of-pocket treatment expenses. Thirty-seven percent of those surveyed went into debt, and some reported using the majority of their assets to pay for their care (23%).[2]

As these studies identified, financial hardship for cancer patients can take many forms. Not only can it increase medical expenses and patient debt; it can also deplete savings and other assets. A cancer diagnosis can have practical implications that create financial hardship as well.

Cancer and the treatment prescribed can result in loss of economic resources and opportunities for patients and families. There are also indirect costs of cancer care including monetary losses associated with time spent receiving medical care and time lost from work or other usual activities.[3] The Pink Fund survey found that 36% of people with breast cancer reported loss of income due to loss of job or inability to perform work-related duties as a result of their treatment.[2]

Financial hardship experienced by cancer patients is a complicated matter. An initial breast cancer diagnosis can lead to a ripple effect of financial insecurities resulting from increased medical debt, a potential loss of income due to inability to work, and the possibility of losing health insurance because of the threat of the potential loss of employment. This can further lead to other troubling outcomes including housing and food insecurities, increased concerns about affording basic needs (i.e., transportation, utilities, and clothing), and a reduction in savings and other assets sometimes leading to increased debt and even bankruptcy.

The research suggests financial hardship for cancer patients can have a major impact on the quality of their lives as they receive cancer care. In a March 2019 Kaiser Family Foundation poll, more than one-fourth of US adults (26%) reported they or a household member had problems paying medical bills in the past year, and about half of this group (12%) said the bills had a major impact on their family. These same adults indicated cutting costs in other areas to pay for their medical bills, such as spending on vacations, major household purchases, and even basic household items.[4] As a result, it is very important to recognize financial hardship as a potential quality-of-life risk for cancer patients, and it should be evaluated throughout the cancer care continuum in the same way cancer treatment side effects are identified and managed.

The research also suggests that when identified early on, financial hardship can be managed or, at the very least, its negative effect on the quality of a cancer patient's life and care can be reduced. As previously noted, there are different variables that may contribute to financial hardship. Recognizing it and treating it can be a complex matter that includes a number of different intervention types. Financial hardship in cancer patients is a result of multiple layers of contributing factors. On the patient level, a cancer patient's ethnic background, socioeconomic status, and access to insurance may be factors. On the healthcare provider level, transparency of medical costs, access to charity care programs, and other financial aid for patients should be considered. On a greater societal level, public policy creation and trends in healthcare spending, particularly in cancer care, may also be contributing factors in financial hardship. In the sections that follow, we will explore some of the ways the impact of financial hardship can be reduced on each of these levels. The primary goal is to increase the quality of life of breast cancer patients as they go through the cancer care experience.

The Patient Experience

Let's Talk Health Insurance

The majority of people in the United States (91.4%) have a health insurance plan of some kind.[5] Health insurance coverage can be accessed in many ways: through an employer-sponsored plan, the federally funded marketplace, directly from private insurers, or government plans like Medicare and Medicaid. Health insurance coverage serves as the backbone of an American's experience with healthcare costs when receiving medical care. There are many elements that make up a health insurance policy that require attention and can either serve as a lifeline toward accessing life-saving breast cancer treatment or a barrier. It is extremely important for Americans using the healthcare system to understand as much about their healthcare coverage as possible, thus becoming more informed consumers of care which would lead them toward less costly outcomes.

Where Does Your Health Insurance Plan Come From?

The majority of Americans who are employed will have access to employer-sponsored health insurance plans. Employer-sponsored health plans are offered to employees and their dependents as a benefit of employment. These plans currently provide some level of health insurance coverage for approximately 160 million Americans.[6] Employers choose the plan and determine its benefit structure. Employers and employees typically share the cost of health insurance premiums.

The Affordable Care Act is a comprehensive health care reform law that was enacted in March 2010. The law's primary goal is to make affordable health insurance available to more people. The law provides consumers with subsidies that lower costs for households with incomes between 100% and 400% of the federal poverty level.[7] For Americans who do not have access to health insurance through an employer, this law has created an insurance marketplace that allows them to explore health insurance plans in their area. One can enroll in a plan during an open enrollment or special election period. Unlike commercially insured plans prior to the Affordable Care Act, insurance options available

through the marketplace do not discriminate against people who have preexisting medical conditions, including cancer.

Other government-supported plans including Medicare and Medicaid may also serve as options for Americans who meet specific qualifications. At this time, those age 65 years and older or receiving Social Security disability benefits may qualify for Medicare benefits. Medicaid is available to Americans who meet income (and sometimes asset) requirements. These income requirements may vary depending on the state in which a person resides.

There are many different types of insurance plans and different ways to enroll in one. Most importantly, it is very helpful to understand which of the options listed is the best one and to take advantage of any opportunities to secure coverage designed to reduce cancer care–related costs.

It is also necessary to understand what type of benefits are available through the health insurance plan. This is an important way to become an informed healthcare consumer. Being equipped with valuable information about available health insurance options enhances your ability to prepare for any costs stemming from the cancer care received. When understanding health insurance coverage, it is recommended to identify specific key components of a plan, including plan type, plan premium, medical deductible, maximum annual out-of-pocket costs, office visit copays, and prescription benefits. Many plans will also offer dental and vision coverage. For the purpose of this chapter, the focus is on plan benefits that will most impact coverage for breast cancer treatment-related expenses.

Plan Type

Examples of plan types as defined on healthcare.gov[8] include:

- Exclusive Provider Organization: a managed care plan where services are covered only if the patient uses doctors, specialists, or hospitals in the plan's network (except in an emergency).
- Health Maintenance Organization (HMO): a type of health insurance plan that usually limits coverage to care from doctors who work for or contract with the HMO. It generally will not cover out-of-network care except in an emergency. An HMO may require a patient to live or work in its service area to be eligible for coverage. HMOs often provide integrated care and focus on prevention and wellness.
- Point of Service (POS): a type of plan where the cost is less if the patient uses doctors, hospitals, and other healthcare providers that belong to the plan's network. POS plans require a referral from your primary care doctor in order to see a specialist.
- Preferred Provider Organization (PPO): a type of health plan where the patient pays less if they use providers in the plan's network. They can use doctors, hospitals, and providers outside of the network without a referral for an additional cost.

Plan Premiums, Deductibles, Out-of-Pocket Maximums, and Copays

A health insurance plan often includes certain components that determine the costs the insured may be responsible for throughout a year of coverage. Understanding these components will help prepare patients for potential healthcare-related costs that may be incurred as a result of a person's breast cancer care. These components are defined by healthcare.gov and are listed below:

- Insurance premium: the amount you are responsible to pay for your health insurance plan. Normally this premium is paid monthly, but some plans allow participants to pay on a quarterly or biannual schedule.
- Deductible: The amount you pay for covered health care services *before* your insurance plan starts to pay.
- Annual out-of-pocket costs: Copayments are fixed amounts paid for a covered healthcare service after the deductible is paid. Coinsurance is the percentage of costs of a covered healthcare service after the deductible is paid. The annual out-of-pocket maximum is the total (coinsurance plus copays) healthcare costs paid during the year.
- Prescription benefits: The majority of health insurance plans also come with prescription benefits. These benefits are managed by a pharmacy benefits manager, who determines the medications that are covered by the plan, as well as how much beneficiaries pay for the medication and the qualifying pharmacies where prescriptions can be filled.

It is important for cancer patients to have a good understanding of their health insurance benefits, as they will be better prepared to manage any bills that may arise due to their breast cancer care. Only considering the premium cost of an insurance policy would be detrimental to gaining the full value of an insurance plan. Over half of the respondents in one survey said they received a medical bill for a cost they thought was covered by their health insurance in the past 12 months, and a similar proportion reported receiving a medical bill saying the amount they owed was higher than expected.[1] Breast cancer treatment can be very expensive, and the care received may include a wide variety of treatments ranging from surgical procedures to chemotherapy to radiation therapy, among many other medical interventions. As a result, health insurance benefits have been proven to play an integral role in covering the costs of these treatments. It is important to understand this role along with the benefits it brings, and the potential costs stemming from any deductibles, copays, and/or coinsurance you may be responsible to pay. An understanding of health insurance coverage is one of the best ways to help reduce financial hardship in the future.

Seeking Transparency in Healthcare Costs

One way to gain a better understanding of the types of healthcare costs associated with breast cancer care is to ask questions about them. In 2009, the American Society of Clinical Oncology's (ASCO) Task Force on the Cost of Cancer Care identified patient-physician cost communication as a critical component of high-quality care. When patients were asked about their attitudes toward discussions about cost communication, 50% of patients desired these discussions but only 33% actually had them.[9] Any step a patient can take toward a better understanding of the costs associated with their healthcare is beneficial. There is also a level of consumerism associated with health care. A breast cancer patient's right to be informed of the potential side effects of treatment, along with a plan to address those side effects, is a vital part of a patient's care plan. If we begin to acknowledge that the cost of such treatment can induce side effects such as financial hardship, it should be just as important to have conversations about healthcare cost transparency. As indicated in the study mentioned earlier, it is unlikely that healthcare providers will have these kinds of conversations with patients, yet they could have a significant impact on the quality of their cancer care experience.

Look Deeper Into the Healthcare System for Financial Assistance

In most healthcare systems there are financial navigators, financial counselors, or financial advocates who are available to provide assistance to cancer patients. Some systems are more developed than others and may have a combination of these specialists. Other systems may employ just one specialist who manages all billing and insurance-related matters. In most cases, one or more of these specialists should be available to help answer questions about health insurance coverage and potential healthcare costs patients may experience when starting their cancer care journey. The same concept that applies to understanding health insurance benefits applies to understanding possible costs that stem from the gaps in coverage as they pertain to the cancer treatment plan. The more a cancer patient understands their healthcare costs, the easier it will be to explore options available to help reduce them. There are often oncology social workers, nurse navigators, or lay patient navigators and public benefits specialists who are available to help patients navigate healthcare-related expenses. Taking an active approach by inquiring about the various resources and healthcare professionals in the system who can help uncover healthcare costs and answer questions about ways to reduce these expenses will go a long way toward reducing the impact of financial hardship, especially for those at most risk to experience it.

The Role of the Healthcare Organization

Unfortunately, high healthcare costs disproportionately affect uninsured adults, Black and Hispanic adults, and those with lower incomes. Black and Hispanic adults (58% each) have reported delaying or skipping at least one type of medical care in the past year due to cost, in comparison to about half (49%) of White adults. Similarly,

63% of those with household incomes under $40,000 report delaying some sort of care due to cost, compared with 31% of those in households making $90,000 or more annually.[4] This data is quite concerning and speaks to the fact that members of minority groups are more likely to experience financial hardship in comparison to their White counterparts. This further emphasizes the systemic breakdown of how healthcare coverage and services are inequitably provided to minorities and those with lower socioeconomic status. It is imperative for healthcare organizations to recognize the large gap in their healthcare delivery services reaching minorities, the underinsured, and those with lower incomes. This argument is particularly strong when it comes to people diagnosed with cancer who frequently require multiple interventions. In the paragraphs to follow, there are some solutions to address reaching more people and helping them receive the necessary cancer treatment they need while also recognizing the financial hardship this may cause them.

It Starts With Cancer Screenings

Screening for cancer means checking for precancerous lesions or cancer in people who are experiencing no signs or symptoms. The aim is to find an abnormality at the earliest possible time in cancer development. If a cancer screening test shows a precancerous lesion is present, it can be treated or surgically removed before becoming cancer. If a test finds a cancer at an early stage of development—stage I or II—before it has spread, it is more likely that the patient can be treated successfully, resulting in cure and an increase in long-term survival. Even though the breast cancer screening rate—as defined by the percentage of women aged 50–74 years who report having had a screening mammogram in the past 2 years—for Black women is very similar to that for White women, 9% of Black women are diagnosed with breast cancer when the disease is at an advanced stage, compared with 5% of White women. The disparity in advanced stage of diagnosis is one factor contributing to the striking disparity in the breast cancer death rates for Black and White women, which are 27.3 per 100,000 and 19.6 per 100,000, respectively.[10] This is a small sample of the greater impact of healthcare disparities on minorities. However, this information also provides some direction for healthcare organizations serving the greater community to look for ways to better reach minorities and lower income families. In so doing, a number of outcomes could be achieved, including an increase in early detection of breast cancer in minorities, resulting in a decrease in death rates from cancer.

Increase Community Outreach

One way for healthcare organizations to reach more people in their communities, educating them on screening programs, and connecting them with local medical services is to incorporate a community cancer outreach program. Community outreach plays a critical role in achieving this goal by connecting with community organizations, churches and parishes, educational institutions, and other community services to gain a better understanding of the needs and interests of community members. Creating a forum within these establishments to provide education equips community members with the resources and information they need to receive necessary medical care and engagement in early detection programs. A community outreach coordinator can be that member of the oncology healthcare team who is able to develop relationships with community shareholders, aligning the needs of the people in the community with the goals and resources of the healthcare organization.

Employ a Prior Authorization Team

Healthcare organizations can also help reduce financial hardship for cancer patients by ensuring there is a preservice or prior authorization department capable of evaluating a patient's health insurance benefits, verifying coverage for prescribed medical services, and proactively recognizing potential out-of-pocket costs the patient may encounter. This department plays an integral role in ensuring cancer patients have sufficient health insurance coverage for their prescribed care. It also offers an added layer of financial protection for the healthcare organization by determining the amount of coverage available for planned treatment and securing any prior authorization approvals needed to ensure coverage is available. A preservice team can even take on added roles that can reduce the overall impact of financial hardship on both the cancer patient and healthcare organization alike. Added roles could include the ability to assess a patient's eligibility for financial assistance programs that reduce the cost of cancer care. This team can serve as the first line of defense from financial hardship. As noted earlier in this chapter, it is very important to identify any key characteristics of patients' cancer situations early on in their care. The following characteristics of a cancer patient's circumstances should trigger the need for closer examination by a member of the preservices team of a patient's potential for financial hardship:

1. Type of health insurance coverage:
   a. No health insurance or lack of coverage for prescribed treatment
   b. Limited benefits plan
   c. Medicare A and B only
   d. High deductible/high out-of-pocket maximum plan

The goal is to optimize medical insurance coverage. Understanding a patient's medical insurance coverage is a very important step toward reducing a primary cause of his/her financial distress. Medical expenses are a main driving force behind determining the potential for financial hardship that can lead to increased stress during a person's cancer treatment. A thorough evaluation of a patient's medical coverage associated with the cancer treatment plan should be completed. This evaluation incorporates the potential costs of care resulting from a patient's out-of-pocket responsibilities, which include annual deductibles, copays, and other expenses. Factoring into this evaluation are the potential costs of the treatment itself. Following this evaluation, and in the event a patient may be at greater risk for financial distress, measures should be taken to determine whether there are ways to improve the current insurance coverage or explore better alternative medical benefits.

An illustration of this process is described below:

A 72-year-old female recently diagnosed with breast cancer will soon be starting an expensive intravenous (IV) chemotherapy regimen. Upon evaluation of her medical coverage, she has been found to have only Medicare part A and B benefits. As a result of this evaluation, she is at high risk to experience significant medical expenses because these benefits include only 80% coverage for her outpatient chemotherapy treatments with no annual out-of-pocket maximum.

This patient should be evaluated to determine whether her insurance benefits can be improved. This will include assessment for additional medical coverage (i.e., Medicare supplemental policy), state benefits (i.e., secondary Medicaid insurance), or an alternative plan (i.e., Medicare Advantage plan). In this scenario, the primary goal is to increase the patient's medical coverage so to reduce the overall financial distress she may experience during her cancer care. When possible, this should be done before treatment is started.

2. Cancer diagnosis including type and stage

The impact of a cancer diagnosis, and the care plan that follows, can take many forms. It is important to take into consideration how cancer patients' lives may be impacted because of their diagnosis and future treatment course. For example, a breast cancer patient diagnosed early – stage I – may require surgical removal of the tumor and surveillance thereafter. The financial impact for this patient may look very different from a diagnosis of stage IV breast cancer that will require multiple interventions including surgery, radiation, and chemotherapy, not to mention the additional economic toll this diagnosis and subsequent treatment may bring. Proactively evaluating the potential financial impact a cancer diagnosis and treatment plan may have could ultimately lead to a reduction in the financial distress it causes the patient.

3. Treatment plan

Cancer treatment can be very expensive. Even with medical insurance coverage, high treatment costs can result from the need to pay an annual deductible, copays or out-of-pocket charges. It is important to examine breast cancer patients' treatment plans through an economic lens, as it may impact their overall financial health. There are significant differences in the cost associated with surveillance care in comparison to a surgical procedure, radiation, or oral or IV chemotherapy, particularly when considering some of the newer molecular-based therapies. Taking this a step further, it is just as important to identify patients'

direct costs, which are often dictated by the insurance plans they possess. For example, a low deductible and out-of-pocket medical policy may not significantly impact a patient's wallet if surgery, radiation, or in-office treatment is prescribed. However, this same patient may have a prescription plan that includes a high out-of-pocket responsibility. A prescription for an oral chemotherapy agent could be cost prohibitive.

4. Patient socioeconomic status

For many patients, a diagnosis of breast cancer can affect their ability to work, oftentimes causing them to decrease the hours they work or take a leave from work entirely. The added stress associated with loss of income can adversely affect the quality of their lives and their cancer care experience. In other cases, patients may be receiving a fixed income or have limited assets to afford additional medical expenses associated with their breast cancer care. Patients experiencing these circumstances should be evaluated for various financial assistance options, which can include employer-sponsored short- and long-term disability benefits, Social Security disability benefits, and other local, regional, and national financial aid resources. There may be financial assistance programs available for patients with a breast cancer diagnosis who meet certain criteria. The primary goal is to evaluate these patients and connect them to any resources for which they may qualify.

More closely examining the impact of these characteristics can reduce the impact of financial hardship by identifying risk factors early and employing resources to help those at greatest risk. A healthcare organization should employ skilled professionals who are trained in various ways to identify, assess, evaluate, and assist breast cancer patients who are at high risk for financial distress. Listed below are examples of professionals in the healthcare setting employed to support a cancer patient's financial needs.

Financial Counselors

In many healthcare organizations, financial counselors are often employed. These counselors tend to be members of the revenue cycle team and often serve as resources for cancer patients who have questions about their medical bills. They play an integral role in identifying patients who incur high medical expenses, working with them to reduce these bills or arrange payment plans.

Financial Advocates

Financial advocates often perform a similar role, providing assistance for cancer patients when billing questions arise. They also may help patients gain a better understanding of their health insurance benefits and assist patients by helping them identify alternative forms of coverage that may improve their insurance coverage (i.e., state Medicaid plans).

Financial Navigators

Financial navigators provide similar assistance to the financial counselors and advocates mentioned earlier. However, they tend to take a more holistic approach toward treating financial hardship. Financial navigators evaluate patients as a whole, recognizing that their financial hardship extends beyond cancer care and into their personal lives, including their employment background, household breadwinners, and how these factors are associated with patients' ability to manage medical debt resulting from their cancer care experiences. Navigators will work with patients to optimize insurance coverage and identify financial aid resources available to reduce the financial burden cancer care may impose.

Oncology Social Workers

Oncology social workers often play a similar role as financial navigators. Social workers also take a big-picture approach when assessing patient needs that go beyond the cancer treatment itself. Social workers can help determine whether barriers to care include indirect cancer costs like transportation needs, living expenses, and housing and food insecurities. Social workers can collaborate with patients to identify practical ways to reduce barriers for them to receive their care without creating additional financial hardship.

Public Benefits Specialists

A public benefits specialist can play an important role in supporting both the patient and the rest of the healthcare team. Public benefits specialists possess a strong knowledge of public policy and the government programs designed to provide assistance to people who meet specific requirements. These programs can include state and government-funded Medicaid benefits, food-share programs, housing assistance programs, and Social Security benefits, to name a few.

The Pharmacy Team

A pharmacist or pharmacy liaison can serve as a valuable resource for cancer patients to identify potential cost savings programs for medications which include but are not limited to medication discount programs and manufacturer co-pay cards. The pharmacy team may also be able to identify lesser costly generic alternatives for cancer patients to reduce their overall medication costs.

Financial Health Advisors

A financial health advisor is not found to be a common service provided within a healthcare organization. However, with the understanding that financial hardship extends beyond the costs of cancer care itself, a financial health advisor can be very valuable in helping cancer patients overcome some of the financial burden they face resulting from practical needs such as housing, food, and utilities, and debt incurred outside of the healthcare system (i.e., credit card debt). A good financial health advisor will more closely examine a cancer patient's overall budget as it pertains to their income, asset resources, and debts, and help them identify ways to reduce or consolidate debt to improve their budget and make it easier to manage any additional costs incurred from cancer treatment.

It truly takes a village to support cancer patients and help them reduce financial hardship. There are many healthcare professionals available that provide a unique set of skills to evaluate different aspects of a cancer patient's financial circumstances. In so doing, a broader picture is created, and through it, a more comprehensive approach toward reducing financial hardship can be implemented.

Making the Healthcare Organization's Role More Transparent

Another way healthcare organizations can reduce the financial burden experienced by many cancer patients is to be more transparent about costs of cancer care services. Cancer patients are faced with a lot of information as it pertains to the type of cancer they have, the differences in treatment options available to them, and the cancer care plan moving forward. They receive a wealth of information from their providers about their cancer: its primary location, the stage, and any other locations where it has spread; and are also given handouts and booklets detailing their cancer treatment: the mechanism of delivery (oral/IV/radiation/surgery), the length of treatment, and side effects associated with it. This is very important information for a cancer patient to understand in order to make informed decisions about the type of care they choose to receive. However, understanding a cancer patient's financial circumstances may also help determine a successful outcome for treatment, and it could be argued it is just as important for them to understand the possible costs associated with the care itself. It is not uncommon for treatment to be prescribed that the patient cannot afford. They may even skip appointments or delay treatments because of their office visit copays. A conversation about the cost of care needs to occur with cancer patients prior to their coming to a decision about their treatment. This will ensure that patients are fully informed about their treatment options and provide them with all the information necessary to make the best decision. After all, a patient's quality of life has already been impacted after receiving a breast cancer diagnosis. It is therefore imperative they receive all the information about their cancer care, which includes the potential cost burden. Without a clear understanding of this, it has the potential to negatively affect their quality of life and increase the risk of poor adherence to the treatment plan.

Charity Care

Many healthcare organizations offer charity care programs to assist cancer patients with their medical expenses. These programs take many forms. Some healthcare organizations provide a very comprehensive charity program that includes discounting the cost of medical services and even writing off medical bills for those patients who meet income/asset and other requirements. Other programs are less comprehensive and may simply provide cancer patients with the option to create a payment plan to make payments more manageable. It is important to understand the financial needs of cancer patients as a way to develop an effective charity care program. These programs sometimes serve as the one lifeline for cancer patients and their ability to access the treatment they need to survive. The healthcare organization must take a close look at the charity care available for cancer patients and how much of an impact it has on their ability to access and receive their treatment with little disruption. For example, a charity care program that only offers a payment plan for patients may not be enough for them to follow through with their treatment. If a cancer patient is unable to meet the payment arrangements set forth by the healthcare organization, the cancer patient may have no choice but to stop treatment or leave the healthcare system entirely. This would only create a greater financial burden for the patient and healthcare organization in the future in the event the patient eventually returns for care because their cancer has progressed. Charity care programs can play a very important role in ensuring that cancer patients feel comfortable adhering to their cancer treatment plan, with the understanding that they may incur costs along the way.

Understand Financial Assistance Resources

There are many national organizations, and often local ones, that offer financial assistance for breast cancer patients. These organizations receive donations from various sources including individuals, healthcare advocacy groups, and even pharmaceutical companies. Their primary goal is to support cancer patients by offering financial aid to reduce the financial burden of their cancer treatment costs. A secondary benefit of these programs is the financial aid cancer patients receive can help ensure they are able to afford the cost of their treatment, reducing financial distress and increasing the likelihood they will comply with the treatment plan. Examples of national foundations that offer financial support for breast cancer patients include CancerCare, the Patient Advocate Foundation, the Patient Access Network Foundation, and the Komen Treatment Assistance Fund. Creating a resource list that includes these foundations, and the many others available, is a first step toward connecting patients to financial assistance and lowering their financial distress.

Utilize a Software Tool to Identify Financial Assistance Funding Sources

There are some very useful software programs that healthcare organizations can utilize to more efficiently identify financial resources that are available to reduce the financial impact on breast cancer patients. Two examples, TaylorMed

and Vivor, have the ability to integrate their services with a healthcare organization's electronic medical record. The result is a proactive way to identify cancer patients who are at greater risk for financial hardship because of the coverage they possess and the treatment they will receive. The primary role of these software tools is to match cancer patients to financial assistance resources based on their health insurance benefits, cancer diagnosis, and treatment plans. Just as importantly, this matching takes place prior to a cancer patient receiving their treatment or early in their care. An illustration of the practical usefulness of these software tools is described below:

This patient was recently diagnosed with advanced breast cancer and planned therapy included an oral cyclin-dependent kinase inhibitor, palbociclib (Ibrance). An order was created by the oncologist and submitted to the prior authorization team to evaluate the patient's insurance benefits and identify the costs, if any, that they would have to acquire this medication. The patient was found to have a Medicare Advantage plan, which included Medicare prescription coverage. Following the approval of a prior authorization through their Medicare prescription plan, the prior authorization team determined the plan would cover this medication, but the first month's supply was projected to cost approximately $1200 out of pocket. Before the prior authorization team contacted the patient to provide them with this large out-of-pocket cost, the team utilized Vivor, the financial assistance software tool, to determine whether the patient might qualify for any form of financial assistance. Vivor used the medical and insurance information integrated into its platform through the healthcare organization's electronic medical record, which included the following characteristics of the patient's profile: (1) basic demographic information (address, phone number), (2) health insurance plan (i.e., commercial, government, none), (3) diagnosis (i.e., metastatic breast cancer), and (4) cancer medication list. Applying the information from this profile, Vivor was able to identify at least three different breast cancer copayment assistance funds. Unfortunately, none of the funds were open and available during the time of this investigation. With an additional click of a button, Vivor was also able to identify the manufacturer assistance program, in this case Pfizer Oncology Together, and provide the prior authorization team with all the necessary information to determine whether the patient might qualify for a free supply of their prescribed palbociclib medication.

The result: the patient was notified by the prior authorization team and informed of their high out-of-pocket cost for their palbociclib and the patient explained they would be unable to afford this cost. The conversation did not end there. The patient eventually spoke with an oncology social worker who assisted with the enrollment process to the Pfizer Oncology Together program. The patient was approved for this program and eligible to receive a free supply of palbociclib at no cost through the remaining portion of the calendar year. This situation, which could have become an extreme financial hardship for the patient, or the need for their oncologist to identify a secondary plan for treatment, was avoided with the help of Vivor. The financial assistance software tool was able to provide the healthcare team with critical information for financial support for this patient.

Utilize a Quality Metric to Identify and Evaluate Financial Assistance Need

The Commission on Cancer sets forth standards for cancer practices to ensure that they are treating cancer patients holistically. This includes Standard 5.2 Psychosocial Distress Screening, which implements a process to evaluate the psychosocial needs of a cancer patient through the use of a distress screening tool. There are a number of screening tools available, with the most common being the National Comprehensive Cancer Network (NCCN) Distress Thermometer, which provides a quick and brief opportunity to assess a cancer patient's psychosocial distress. Although this tool does recognize "finances" and "having enough food" as practical concerns, it is designed as a multifactorial screening tool. Patients who express concerns in various domains on these screening tools require additional assessment.

The development of a comprehensive financial hardship assessment, including the incorporation of a quantifiable financial distress screening metric, is beneficial not only as a means to identify those cancer patients with greatest financial distress, but to also provide targeted financial assistance support at the earliest possible point during their cancer care. The benefits of implementing a comprehensive approach to financial distress screening, including the use of a financial distress measurement tool, was highlighted by Khera, Holland, and Griffin.[11] They suggest that examining financial toxicity as an independent patient-reported outcome for all patients with cancer at multiple points during their treatment is highly advisable. In so doing, the cancer treatment team is better equipped to manage the "other" side effect of cancer care—financial hardship—by employing members of the financial assistance team to support those patients who appear to be at greatest risk for financial stress.

There are metrics available to support this process. The Comprehensive Score for Financial Toxicity, or COST tool is a validated 11-item questionnaire that was designed to provide a more thorough evaluation of the individual's financial needs and potential stressors.[12] Another financial hardship assessment tool is the Breast Cancer Finances Survey Inventory, a 42-item questionnaire assessing cancer-related economic burden including potential work-related changes, causes for financial hardship and out-of-pocket expenses.[13] These are two example metrics that can help provide a clearer financial wellness picture of cancer patients in a healthcare setting.

As identified throughout this chapter, the need to develop strategies to reduce financial hardship for cancer patients can play an integral role in the effectiveness and success of their treatment. Utilizing a financial hardship screening process and combining it with a metric that can identify the greatest areas of financial stress will provide the healthcare organization with the information and resources to best serve those patients with the greatest needs.

The Impact of Financial Hardship on the Country

Cancer and the treatments prescribed can result in the loss of economic resources and opportunities for patients, families, employers, and society as a whole. These losses include financial loss, morbidity, reduced quality of life, and premature death.[3] Excess financial burden for patients with cancer continues to grow as the costs of cancer care has increased dramatically in the past decades, with many new cancer drugs priced at $100,000 or higher annually. Emerging use of targeted therapies and their dramatic rise in cost over the past decade highlights the issue of increased out-of-pocket costs and financial burden for cancer patients. Compounding this problem, health insurance companies are increasingly shifting costs of care to patients through higher deductibles, copayments, and coinsurance.[9] Because most health insurance plans require some form of cost sharing for drug therapy, patients and their families with health insurance may face a significant increase in medical bills.[3] The overall economic impact of healthcare costs in this country is significant. During a 10-year period between 1999 and 2009, for example, US healthcare spending nearly doubled, climbing from $1.3 trillion to $2.5 trillion. In 2009, while the rest of the US economy plunged into a recession, healthcare costs, including cancer care expenses, grew by 4%.[14] Sadly, on average, the United States spends about twice as much per person on healthcare compared to other industrialized countries, yet three-quarters of people surveyed by the National Opinion Resource Center do not think Americans get good value for their healthcare dollar. This is especially true among those who say they have experienced financial hardships due to healthcare costs.[1] This is a very complex problem and needs to be examined on a societal level. Since most health insurance in the United States is employment-based in the working-age population, its relationship with the economic burden of cancer survivorship is complex. A cancer diagnosis can limit employment opportunities, which in turn may lead to a loss of health insurance. One must also take into consideration family obligations, and responsibilities for the patient may limit a caregiver's ability to hold a full-time position in order to maintain health insurance through their employer.[3] Conversely, working-age cancer patients who are unable to maintain employment, and their caregivers alike, create a decline in economic resources for employers and the country as a whole. For example, more than 90% of employed breast cancer survivors who had health insurance through their job stated they were working to maintain their health insurance coverage, which highlights the critical role employers play in the lives of cancer survivors.[9]

Cancer Policy Advocacy

Many studies have exposed the impact of high cancer costs on cancer patients and healthcare systems alike. As identified throughout this chapter, patient financial hardship has taken many forms including loss of income, loss of health insurance, increased medical expenses, and increased debt. The financial hardship cancer care can cause for patients spills over to the healthcare organization, with increased costs for revenue cycle and sustained debt due to unpaid or delayed bill payments. More recently, there have been conversations throughout the country looking at ways to create cancer care reform that improves the quality of care provided and reduces resources utilized and costs incurred.

In 2019, a study entitled "*The impact of provider payment reforms and associated care delivery models on cost and quality in cancer care*" and published in the Public Library of Science conducted a thorough review of literature published in PubMed, Embase, and Cochrane library between 2007 and 2019. The primary goal of this study was to identify the impact of cancer care reform on resource use, cost, and quality of care, including clinical outcomes. Reports on some of the research follows:

Three reviewed studies reported the impact of provider payment reform implemented as part of the Medicare Modernization Act and determined it was effective in switching treatment patterns and chemotherapy use.

Eleven studies reported data on care delivery reforms, including adoption of clinical pathways and participation in patient-centered medical homes, accountable care organizations, or oncology care model programs. The adoption of clinical pathways was consistently associated with reductions in resource use and costs for a variety of cancer types. The impact of the Community Oncology Medical Home program on cancer care spending was compared with Fee for Service Medicare beneficiaries diagnosed with various cancer types. Implementing a patient-centered medical home was found to be associated with significantly reduced emergency department visits resulting in a cost savings per patient. The evaluations of accountable care organizations in cancer care found mixed results, with Medicare Pioneer accountable care organizations demonstrating some reduction in utilization of certain low-value services in the first year of implementation.

Findings from this thorough study of payment reform and care delivery research suggest promising improvements in resource utilization and cost control after the transition to prospective payment models. However further research is needed to apply more robust measures of performance and quality to ensure that providers are delivering high-value care to their patients while reducing costs.[15]

Conclusion

The diagnosis of breast cancer can bring with it serious financial ramifications. Financial hardship, also known as financial toxicity or financial distress, is a real side effect of cancer care. Because financial hardship is a potential outcome, it should be evaluated and addressed, optimally during the earliest stages of a cancer patient's care. Research demonstrates the great impact financial hardship has on the overall quality and effectiveness of care cancer patients receive. Financial hardship can be very complicated and multifaceted, and is best approached by a multidisciplinary team. This chapter provided a wide range of causes of financial hardship but also explores different techniques to manage it, including enlisting different members of the cancer care and financial assistance teams.

Implementing a multidisciplinary approach will allow for a more thorough investigation of the causes of financial hardship for cancer patients. After identifying these causes, this chapter has also provided programs and resources that can be utilized to reduce financial hardship or at least make it more manageable for the cancer patient. By doing this, the goals are to improve the cancer care experience, increase adherence to cancer care treatment, and, most importantly, reduce the distress patients may experience from costs associated with their cancer care journeys. A collaborative effort employed to reduce financial hardship will help breast cancer patients receive the most appropriate treatment and improve their quality outcomes.

References

1. Americans' Views of Healthcare Costs, Coverage and Policy. https://www.norc.org/PDFs/WHI%20Healthcare%20Costs%20Coverage%20and%20Policy/WHI%20Healthcare%20Costs%20Coverage%20and%20Policy%20Issue%20Brief.pdf March 2018.
2. pinkfund.org. https://pinkfund.org/wp-content/uploads/2018/09/TPF_Survey20172018.pdf.
3. Yabroff KR, Lund J, Kepka D, Mariotto A. Economic burden of cancer in the United States: estimates, projections, and future research. *Cancer Epidemiol Biomarkers Prev.* 2011 Oct;20(10):2006–2014. https://doi.org/10.1158/1055-9965.EPI-11-0650. PMID: 21980008; PMCID: PMC3191884.
4. Montero A, Kearney A, Hamel L, Brodie M. Americans' Challenges with Health Care Costs. https://www.kff.org/health-costs/issue-brief/americans-challenges-with-health-care-costs/ July 14, 2022.
5. Census.gov. https://www.census.gov/library/publications/2021/demo/p60-274.html
6. Kaiser Family Foundation. https://www.kff.org/other/state-indicator/total-population/?dataView=1&currentTimeframe=0&selectedDistributions=employer&sortModel=%7B%22colId%22:%22Location%22,%22sort%22:%22asc%22%7D
7. Healthcare.gov Subsidy Requirements. https://www.healthcare.gov/glossary/subsidized-coverage/
8. Healthcare.gov Plan Types. https://www.healthcare.gov/choose-a-plan/plan-types/
9. Yabroff KR, Bradley C, Shih YT. Understanding financial hardship among cancer survivors in the United States: strategies for prevention and mitigation. *J Clin Oncol.* 2020 Feb 1;38(4):292–301. https://doi.org/10.1200/JCO.19.01564. Epub 2019 Dec 5. PMID: 31804869; PMCID: PMC6994250.
10. American Association for Cancer Research. https://cancerprogressreport.aacr.org/disparities/

11. Khera N, Holland JC, Griffin JM. Setting the stage for universal financial distress screening in routine cancer care. *Cancer*. 2017 Nov 1;123(21):4092–4096. https://doi.org/10.1002/cncr.30940. Epub 2017 Aug 17. PMID: 28817185.

12. de Souza JA, Yap BJ, Hlubocky FJ, et al. The development of a financial toxicity patient-reported outcome in cancer: the COST measure. *Cancer*. 2014;120(20):3245–3253. https://doi.org/10.1002/cncr.28814

13. Given BA, Given CW, Stommel M. Family and out of pocket costs for women with breast cancer. *Cancer Practice*. 1994;2(3):187–193.

14. Auerbach David I, Arthur L Kellermann. *How Does Growth in Health Care Costs Affect the American Family?* Santa Monica, CA: RAND Corporation, RB-9605, 2011. As of July 21, 2022. https://www.rand.org/pubs/research_briefs/RB9605.html

15. Nejati M, Razavi M, Harirchi I, Zendehdel K, Nejati P. The impact of provider payment reforms and associated care delivery models on cost and quality in cancer care: a systematic literature review. *PLoS ONE*. 2019;14(4):e0214382. https://doi.org/10.1371/journal.pone.021438

17

Expectations for the Future

AMY BOCK AND JAMES L. WEESE

There will be continual evolution of the management of breast cancer. All fields of medicine that touch patients who have or will develop breast cancer have changed and will continue to do so, currently on a much more frequent basis than we have ever seen in the past. Changes have occurred and will continue in all disciplines with increasing knowledge in prevention, genetics, diagnosis, treatment, and survivorship.

According to the National Institutes of Health Cancer Trends progress report published in April 2022, in the United States the total cost of treating female breast cancer in 2015 was $26.8 billion and in 2022 it was $29.8 billion, an increase of over 11%. From the perspective of the individual patient, in their initial year after diagnosis the cost was $34,979.50; for continuing care, the annual cost was $3,539.60; in their last year of life, it was $76,101.20.[1–3] As providers who care for these patients, we must continue to ask if we are providing patients with the best quality and value that they deserve for these expenditures. Moving forward, the value of the programs we provide to patients will be an increasingly critical concern—are we providing the highest-quality, evidence-based, innovative, and cost-effective care for the patients under our guidance?

In the preceding chapters of this book, the history and current state of breast cancer management have been well reviewed. There has been extensive progress from historical unimodality treatment, with evolution toward evidence-based and integrated multidisciplinary care. The importance of clinical trials and the value of standardization of management based on evidence-based pathways cannot be overstressed.[4–13] Cancer treatment is outrageously expensive, and the costs will continue to increase, but from the perspective of the patient and their loved ones, it is money well spent. From the perspective of society, we must continually make progress in preventing cancer, diagnosing it earlier when the chance for cure is greatest and the treatment should be the least expensive, refining therapy to provide the best care for the correct patient in whom it will have the greatest chance for success, creating supportive care to allow patients to successfully navigate the trials of therapy, encouraging the use of the best clinical trials to move the field forward, developing plans for life after cancer to encourage patients to return to a vibrant and successful lifestyle, and, finally, identifying those patients in whom further aggressive therapy is futile, and support and prepare them appropriately.

Surgery for breast cancer will continue to evolve into the future. Because of the rapid changes in the approach to breast cancer, there will need to be improved methods to keep surgeons and the entire multidisciplinary team alerted to these changes. This should reinforce the use of clinical pathways and multidisciplinary conferences and clinics. Although most breast cancer surgery is done by general surgeons, these patients will likely migrate to surgeons who evaluate and treat a larger volume of breast cancer patients. Certainly, the trends from radical procedures to much more conservative surgery have progressed slowly; however the transition to nipple-sparing mastectomies, conservative lumpectomies, sentinel node biopsies, oncoplastic techniques, and new biopsy and reconstructive techniques have occurred in a much shorter timeframe. These changes best occur with frequent multidisciplinary discussions, well-designed clinical trials, and thorough evaluation of the data. Although often presented at national meetings, it will become increasingly important for these multidisciplinary discussions to occur at the local and regional levels. Many improvements have come about by surgeon participation in clinical trials and a focus on local organizational excellence, such as National Cancer Institute-supported clinical trial groups and National Accreditation Program for Breast Centers participation.

Although we believe there will continue to be a reduction in the number of mastectomies performed, there will be increased involvement by plastic surgeons. Many breast surgeons are trained in oncoplastic techniques, but others will continue to collaborate with their plastic surgery colleagues to improve the appearance of a patient's breast after cancer surgery. Advances in plastic surgery have resulted in improved postoperative appearance after reconstructive surgery. Improvement in implants as well as tissue transfer techniques have led to better, more natural-appearing post-treatment cosmesis. Techniques such as lymph node transfer and lymphatic channel reanastomosis have become more commonplace in the treatment and prevention of lymphedema, and we believe these will have an expanded role in the future. Similarly, it will be increasingly important for the plastic surgeon to become an integral part of the multidisciplinary breast cancer team whose services should be offered to patients undergoing major procedures for breast cancer.

Although we see movement toward universal screening and prevention, there will always be patients who procrastinate and present with later-stage disease. We hope and expect that this will become a smaller group in the future, but the field must still be prepared to deal with these patients appropriately. As we have seen, although surgery will most likely become less relevant in those patients who present with metastatic disease, it will still have an impact on those presenting with locally advanced disease. The patient who presents with extensive, even ulcerated, and necrotic cancers on the chest wall will continue to be a therapeutic challenge. Newer molecular therapies and enhanced use of hormonal manipulation have continued to give this group of patients extended survival when compared to the past; however society will need to find better ways to encourage patients to seek help earlier in the course of their disease. Innovative multidisciplinary care has come a long way, but patients will always need to be willing participants in their care to maximize their chance for cure and longevity.

Radiation therapy will continue to have a role in the treatment of breast cancer. As technology has advanced and creative treatment routines have become more commonplace, the historical nightmare of severe burns and long-term toxicity of treatments have been greatly reduced. For breast cancer, prone treatments to reduce cardiotoxicity, breath holding, and electrons to treat more superficial lesions have all been used to generate maximal treatment effect with limited toxicity. Creative planning will continue to evolve. There has already been a marked reduction in the length of treatment courses to deliver comparable radiation doses without a reduction in the chance for control of the disease on the chest wall and for cure. Routine whole-breast radiation can currently be safely administered in half the time that was required as recently as 5 years ago. Techniques such as interstitial radiation and intraoperative radiation therapy have evolved and have been shown to have appropriate value in highly selected patients.

Game-changing technologies will continue to be discovered. Although proton therapy allows very precise planning for treatment, its limitations of great cost and limited sites have not made it a consideration for breast cancer, and whether it will have a role in the future of breast cancer treatment remains to be seen. Treatment planning based on magnetic resonance imaging is in further evolution but has not been shown to have a major role in limiting breast cancer at this time. There is evolving technology based on positron emission tomography activity, which could provide benefit for appropriate patients in the future.

In addition, local therapy approaches, particularly for smaller lesions, such as microwave, radiofrequency ablation, and cryoablation, continue to be explored.[14–19] Studies have suggested an immunomodulatory effect of ablative

procedures in breast cancer.[20,21] Whether they will play a major role in the future has yet to be determined.

The field of medical oncology will continue to evolve significantly. Although the use of chemotherapy has improved the cure rate of many patients with breast cancer, it has also created significant morbidity or even mortality. Better understanding of complications of therapy such as cardiotoxicity from anthracyclines, Herceptin, and other cancer treatment drugs is needed. Focus on a genetic predisposition to develop toxicity will improve prevention of side effects.[22] Combinations of cytotoxic drugs will continue to evolve to create maximal cancer cell destruction with protection of normal cells. Precision medicine, the development of drugs directed toward specific genetic mutations within tumor cells, will continue to expand and become more refined. Although the cost of these new, often oral agents can be prohibitive, appropriate selection of patients who have the highest likelihood of a prolonged positive response can be quite dramatic. Similarly, harnessing real-world data to identify those mutations that should offer a response to a drug but do not must also be determined. Avoiding costly medications that will not be effective is an equally important part of the equation.

The National Comprehensive Cancer Network (NCCN) has provided a valuable reference source to select therapy for patients with a given stage of disease and tumor characteristics.[4] Unfortunately, the selection of possible drug regimens is so vast that it can be counterproductive to appropriate drug selection. This is particularly true when trying to develop treatment for a large group of patients within a healthcare system—treating a significant number of patients according to evidence-based guidelines yields much more valuable information regarding the response to therapy. Large numbers of patients treated the same way is often the best method to truly assess the effectiveness of a given treatment. There are distinct advantages to well-designed, evidence-based pathways. Our personal bias is to select pathways determined by groups of both academic and community-based oncologists, which can be selected to prioritize clinical trials and then ordered based on efficacy, toxicity, and cost. We are quite wary of pathways determined by insurance providers, whose selection criteria are often prioritized by cost. Although appropriate consideration of cost is very important, we believe it should not be the driving force in determination of therapy unless it provides patients with the best chance for cure.

The importance of clinical trials cannot be overlooked. Well-controlled clinical trials have been largely responsible for the tremendous improvement in the management of breast and other cancers, and encouraging more patients to participate, particularly minority and underserved patients, should be a goal of all oncologists. The special characteristics of this group of patients needs to be a focus of clinical trials moving forward.

Immunotherapy, described by Ehrlich in the late 1800s as the magic bullet, has moved into a new place in cancer therapy.[23] Combined with chemotherapy, or even as a standalone therapy often based on genetic testing, immunotherapy has been shown to significantly prolong survival even in patients with widely metastatic disease. As further refinement is accomplished, we anticipate greater use of this modality in the treatment of breast and other cancers.

Until cancer is ultimately eradicated, clinical trials need to be a mainstay of therapy. Unfortunately, less than 1 in every 20 cancer patients finds an appropriate clinical trial in which to participate, and all practitioners must work to improve that ratio.[24] Some organizations believe that trials can only be performed at a centralized home site. Although this might be true for experimental phase I trials, most trials can be appropriately offered in the community—close to where patients live and where most patients prefer to be treated. Unfortunately, performing clinical trials carries an extra cost and burden of additional personnel to be successful, but this is a cost that many feel is worth adding to make progress in the field. Investment in clinical trials research is a critical need to move all cancer treatment forward. Much work needs to be done to make the necessary improvements to increase access and improve diversity and inclusion in clinical trials by government, pharmaceutical companies, insurance companies, and individual institutions in this quest for investment. Although the cost to develop new drugs can be quite high, the ultimate goal needs to be the eradication of cancer, and its continual impact on the individuals affected, and on society in general, must always be considered. All of us will be much better served by the elimination of this deadly disease.

As we look at the practice of oncology, we must be prepared for transitions in the workforce. Oncologists as a group are aging, and the current supply of younger oncologists is not keeping up with demand. In addition, as the complexity of the field continues to evolve, it is increasingly hard for anyone to keep up with the expanding knowledge base of new treatments that grow exponentially. We will need to see a greater reliance on advanced practice clinicians, nurse practitioners, and physician assistants as the number of patients continues to rise.[25] When advanced practice clinicians are effectively incorporated into the multidisciplinary care model, they can increase patient satisfaction, accessibility, and productivity. In addition, the use of telemedicine with remote monitoring and facilities to work with home care teams staffed by Oncology Certified Nurse will be required to expand the reach to care for cancer patients.

Despite multiple successes and refinements in the past, what can be expected for the future? There will continue to be changes in all aspects of care for patients who have developed or are at increased risk of developing breast cancer. Diagnostic techniques will need to improve along with prevention studies. We will need to identify those patients who are developing or likely to develop the earliest breast cancers and be able to intervene in their course even before the cancers are clinically apparent. This will require increasing the depth of investigation into cancer genetics and carcinogenesis. Certainly, those patients at genetic risk to develop breast cancer should have availability of improved

and increased screening to identify the presence of cancer as early as possible. Progress in cancer genetics will also help identify family members of cancer patients who may be at greatest risk for developing the disease. This will need to be done in the least invasive and readily available manner to make such screening available and cost effective. Trials looking for shed cancer cells in the blood are currently underway and could provide the potential to enhance early diagnosis. These should be followed closely.

The cost of cancer care has continued to rise to an unacceptable share of our gross national product. In addition to this toll nationally, the financial hardships caused to patients and their families leave tragic stories of financial ruin.[26] As the human genome has been unraveled, there are increasing data suggesting that new genetic aberrations increase the risk to develop breast cancer. Currently patients with known genetic markers such as *BRCA1* and *BRCA2* may be offered the option of surgery (bilateral mastectomy) to reduce their risk of developing breast cancer. They may be offered oophorectomy to reduce their risk of developing ovarian cancer as well, but unfortunately these operations are not an absolute guarantee of a cure and take a significant emotional toll. Mastectomies do not remove all microscopic breast tissue, and although this procedure can markedly reduce the risk of developing breast cancer, it is not a 100% guarantee. In addition, patients with these genetic aberrations are at increased risk of developing cancer at other sites, in both females and males, some of which cannot be prevented with an operation alone. We expect advances in genetics and the cancer genome to be our best hope for cancer prevention in the future. As understanding of the genome increases and the increased use of viral vectoring or CRISPR technology can focus on individual genes or base pair anomalies, we will enter a more exciting era of cancer prevention long before tumor cells manifest themselves.[27,28] Unfortunately, we are in the very preliminary stages of this technology, but we believe it will have a much greater role in the future. In the field of cancer, we can all be assured that change will be the only constant.

References

1. National Cancer Institute. https://progressreport.cancer.gov/after/economic_burden.
2. Yabroff KR, Mariotto A, Tangka F, et al. Annual Report to the Nation on the Status of Cancer, Part 2: Patient Economic Burden Associated With Cancer Care. JNCI: Journal of the National Cancer Institute. 2021;113(12):1670–1682. https://doi.org/10.1093/jnci/djab192.
3. Mariotto Angela B, Enewold Lindsey, Zhao Jingxuan, Zeruto Christopher A, Robin Yabroff K. Medical care costs associated with cancer survivorship in the United States. *Cancer Epidemiol Biomarkers Prev*. 2020 Jul;29(7):1304–1312. https://doi.org/10.1158/1055-9965.EPI-19-1534.
4. NCCN Guidelines. https://www.nccn.org/guidelines/nccn-guidelines.
5. Markham MJ, Wachter K, Agarwal N, et al. Clinical cancer advances 2020: annual report on progress against cancer from the American Society of Clinical Oncology [published

correction appears in J Clin Oncol. 2020 Sep 10;38(26):3076]. *J Clin Oncol*. 2020;38(10):1081. https://doi.org/10.1200/JCO.19.03141.

6. Weber JS, Levit LA, Adamson PC, et al. American Society of Clinical Oncology policy statement update: the critical role of phase I trials in cancer research and treatment. [published correction appears in J Clin Oncol. 2019 Feb 1;37(4):353]. *J Clin Oncol*. 2015;33(3):278–284. https://doi.org/10.1200/JCO.2014.58.2635.

7. Hirsch BR, Califf RM, Cheng SK, et al. Characteristics of oncology clinical trials: insights from a systematic analysis of ClinicalTrials.gov. *JAMA internal Medicine*. 2013;173(11):972–979.

8. Somkin CP, Ackerson L, Husson G, et al. Effect of medical oncologists' attitudes on accrual to clinical trials in a community setting. Journal of Oncology Practice. 2013;9(6):e275–e283. https://doi.org/10.1200/JOP.2013.001120.

9. Zon Robin T, Stephen B Edge, Page Ray D, et al. American Society of Clinical Oncology criteria for high-quality clinical pathways in oncology. *Journal of Oncology Practice*. 2017;13(no. 3): 207–210.

10. Daly Bobby, Zon Robin T, Page Ray D, et al. Oncology clinical pathways: charting the landscape of pathway providers. *Journal of Oncology Practice*. 2018;14(3):e194–e200. https://doi.org/10.1200/JOP.17.00033.

11. Weese JL, Citrin L, Shamah CJ, Bjegovich-Weidman M. Implementation of treatment pathways in a large integrated health care system. *Journal of Clinical Oncology*. 2016;34(15):6613–6613. https://doi.org/10.1200/JCO.2016.34.15_suppl.6613.

12. Weese JL, Shamah CJ, Sanchez FA, et al. Use of treatment pathways reduce cost and decrease ED utilization and unplanned hospital admissions in patients (pts) with stage II breast cancer. *Journal of Clinical Oncology*. 2019;37(15_suppl): e12012-e12012.

13. Jackman DM, Zhang Y, Dalby C, et al. Cost and survival analysis before and after implementation of Dana-Farber clinical pathways for patients with stage iv non-small-cell lung cancer. *J Oncol Pract*. 2017 Apr;13(4):e346–e352. https://doi.org/10.1200/JOP.2017.021741.

14. Fleming Margaret M, Holbrook Anna I, Newell Mary S. Update on image-guided percutaneous ablation of breast cancer. *Am JRoentgenol*. 2017;208(2):267–274. https://doi.org/10.2214/AJR.16.17129.

15. Pan H, Qian M, Chen H, et al. Precision breast-conserving surgery with microwave ablation guidance: a pilot single-center, prospective cohort study. Front. Oncol., 26 May 2021 Sec. Breast Cancer. https://doi.org/10.3389/fonc.2021.680091.

16. Xia L, Hu Q, Xu W. Efficacy and safety of radiofrequency ablation for breast cancer smaller than 2 cm: a systematic review and meta-analysis. Front. Oncol., 03 May 2021 Sec. Radiation Oncology. https://doi.org/10.3389/fonc.2021.651646.

17. Kinoshita T, Yamamoto N, Fujisawa T, et al. Radiofrequency ablation for early-stage breast cancer: results from 5 years of follow-up in a prospective multicenter study. *Journal of Clinical Oncology*. 2017;35(15_suppl):e12098-e12098.

18. Ward RC, Lourenco AP, Mainiero MB. Ultrasound-guided breast cancer cryoablation. *American Journal of Roentgenology*. 2019;213:716–722. https://doi.org/10.2214/AJR.19.21329.

19. Yu J, Han ZY, Li T, et al. Microwave ablation versus nipple sparing mastectomy for breast cancer ≤5 cm: a pilot cohort study. *Front Oncol*. 2020 Oct 7;10:546883. https://doi.org/10.3389/fonc.2020.546883.

20. Yu M, Pan H, Che N, et al. Microwave ablation of primary breast cancer inhibits metastatic progression in model mice via activation of natural killer cells. *Cell Mol Immunol*. 2021;18:2153–2164. https://doi.org/10.1038/s41423-020-0449-0.

21. Zhou W, Yu M, Pan H, et al. Microwave ablation induces Th1-type immune response with activation of ICOS pathway in early-stage breast cancer. *Journal for Immunotherapy of Cancer*. 2021;9:e002343. https://doi.org/10.1136/jitc-2021-002343.

22. Schneider BP, Shen F, Gardner L, R, et al. Genome-wide association study for anthracycline-induced congestive heart failure. *Clin Cancer Res*. 2017 Jan 1;23(1):43–51. https://doi.org/10.1158/1078-0432.CCR-16-0908.

23. Piro A, Tagarelli A, Tagarelli G, Lagonia P, Quattrone A. Paul Ehrlich: the Nobel Prize in physiology or medicine 1908. *Int Rev Immunol*. 2008;27(1-2):1–17. https://doi.org/10.1080/08830180701848995.

24. Unger Joseph M, Cook Elise, Tai Eric, Bleyer Archie. The role of clinical trial participation in cancer research: barriers, evidence, and strategies. *Am Soc Clin Oncol Educ Book*. 2016;35:185–198. https://doi.org/10.14694/EDBK_156686.

25. Bruinooge Suanna S, Pickard Todd A, Vogel Wendy, et al. Understanding the role of advanced practice providers in oncology in the United States. *Journal of Oncology Practice*. 2018;14(9):e518–e532.

26. Banegas MP, Guy GP Jr, deMoor JS, et al. For working-age cancer survivors medical debt and bankruptcy create financial hardships. *Health Affairs*. 2016;35(1):54–61. https://doi.org/10.1377/hlthaff.2015.8030.

27. Sabit H, Abdel-Ghany S, Tombuloglu H, et al. New insights on CRISPR/Cas9-based therapy for breast Cancer. *Genes and Environ*. 2021;43:15–28. https://doi.org/10.1186/s41021-021-00188-0.

28. Karn V, Sandhya S, Hsu W, et al. CRISPR/Cas9 system in breast cancer therapy: advancement, limitations and future scope. *Cancer Cell Int*. 2022;22:234. https://doi.org/10.1186/s12935-022-02654-3.

Index

Note: Page numbers followed by *f* indicate figures, *t* indicate tables, and *b* indicate boxes.

A

Abemaciclib, 120
ABUS. *See* Automated breast ultrasound
ACS. *See* American Cancer Society
Acute curative radiation, cancer rehabilitation after, 141*t*–142*t*
ADI. *See* Area Deprivation Index
Adjuvant bisphosphonate therapy, 118
Adjuvant chemotherapy, 115
Adjuvant therapy, for breast cancer, 110–119
  adjuvant bisphosphonate therapy, 118
  adjuvant chemotherapy, 115
  adjuvant endocrine therapy, 111–112
  after neoadjuvant treatment, 109–110
  aromatase inhibitors, 112–113
  duration of endocrine therapy, 113
  HER2-positive subtypes, 115–116
  hormone receptor and HER2-negative subtype, 117–118, 117*f*
  hormone receptor-positive and HER2-negative subtype, 110
  multigene assays, 110–111
  role of cyclin-dependent kinase 4 and 6 inhibitors, 113–115, 114*f*
  role of ovarian suppression in premenopausal women, 112
  role of PARP inhibitors in patients with BRCA mutation, 118
  special considerations, 118–119
  tamoxifen, 113
  treatment of smaller HER2-positive tumors, 116
Advance directives, for breast cancer, 183–184, 184*b*, 184*t*
Advanced practice clinicians (APC), 4
ALA. *See* Alpha-linoleic acid
Alcohol intake, breast cancer and, 191
ALND. *See* Axillary lymph node dissection
Alpha-linoleic acid (ALA), in flaxseed, 161
American Cancer Society (ACS), 11
American Society of Breast Surgeons (ASBrS), 46
American Society of Clinical Oncology (ASCO), 151
Amitriptyline, 170*t*
Analgesic antidepressants, for nausea and vomiting, 180
Anastrozole aromatase inhibitors, 193
Anthracyclines, sequential use of, 115
Anticholinergics, for nausea and vomiting, 180
Antiemetic medications, 181*t*
Anti-HER2 therapy, for breast cancer, 137
Antihistamines, for nausea and vomiting, 180
Anti-inflammatory diet, 161–163, 162*f*
Anxiety
  breast cancer and, 167–168, 168*t*
  management of, 182

APC. *See* Advanced practice clinicians
Area Deprivation Index (ADI), COVID-19 and, 42
Arm lymphedema
  nonsurgical management of, 61
  surgical management of, 61, 62*f*
Arnica Montana topical, 170*t*
Aromatase inhibitors, 112–113
ASCO. *See* American Society of Clinical Oncology
Atypical hyperplasia, 63
Authorization team, in healthcare organization, 200
Automated breast ultrasound (ABUS), 30
Average-risk women, breast cancer screening guidelines for, 22–25, 24*f*, 24*t*
Axilla, management of, 54–61, 109
  after neoadjuvant chemotherapy, 57–58
  axillary reverse mapping in, 58, 58*f*
  lymphatic microsurgical preventive healing approach in, 58–59, 59*f*
Axillary dissection, 53
Axillary lymph node dissection (ALND), 57
  cancer rehabilitation after, 141*t*–142*t*
Axillary reverse mapping (ARM), 58, 58*f*

B

Background parenchymal enhancement (BPE), 28, 29*f*
Basal-like subtype, of breast cancer, 133–134, 136*f*
Batwing mastopexy, 67, 69*f*
Beck Depression Inventory (BDI), 168*t*
Benzodiazepines, for nausea and vomiting, 180
Biennial screening, for breast cancer, 23, 24*t*
Biomarker testing, for precision oncology, 135–138
Biopsy techniques, for breast cancer, 46–49
  considerations in, 47
  fine needle aspiration *versus* core needle biopsy, 46
  historical context of, 46
  indications of, 46
  magnetic resonance biopsy in, 48, 48*f*
  palpable lesions *versus* nonpalpable lesions in, 46–47
  postbiopsy considerations and concordance in, 48
  stereotactic biopsy in, 47, 47*f*
  types of needles and devices in, 46
  ultrasound biopsy in, 47–48, 48*f*
BI-RADS. *See* Breast Imaging-Reporting and Data System
Body image, breast cancer and, 166
Bone density testing, 165
Bone marrow support drugs, cancer rehabilitation after, 141*t*–142*t*

Bone-modifying agents, 124
BPE. *See* Background parenchymal enhancement
BPNC. *See* Breast Patient Navigator Certification
BRCA mutations, 26
  role of PARP inhibitors in, 118
BRCAPRO model, 27
Breast cancer
  adjuvant treatment of, 110–119
    adjuvant bisphosphonate therapy, 118
    adjuvant chemotherapy, 115
    adjuvant endocrine therapy, 111–112
    aromatase inhibitors, 112–113
    duration of endocrine therapy, 113
    HER2-positive subtypes, 115–116
    hormone receptor and HER2-negative subtype, 117–118, 117*f*
    hormone receptor-positive and HER2-negative subtype, 110
    multigene assays, 110–111
    role of cyclin-dependent kinase 4 and 6 inhibitors, 113–115, 114*f*
    role of ovarian suppression in premenopausal women, 112
    role of PARP inhibitors in patients with BRCA mutation, 118
    special considerations, 118–119
    tamoxifen, 113
    treatment of smaller HER2-positive tumors, 116
  biopsy techniques for, 46–49
    considerations in, 47
    fine needle aspiration *versus* core needle biopsy, 46
    historical context of, 46
    indications of, 46
    magnetic resonance biopsy in, 48, 48*f*
    palpable lesions *versus* nonpalpable lesions in, 46–47
    postbiopsy considerations and concordance in, 48
    stereotactic biopsy in, 47, 47*f*
    types of needles and devices in, 46
    ultrasound biopsy in, 47–48, 48*f*
  clinical trials for, 3–4
  in community, 1–5
  contemporary surgical approaches to, 54–61
    breast reconstruction in, 64, 72–78
    ductal carcinoma in situ, lobular carcinoma in situ, other high-risk lesions in, 62–64
    oncoplastic breast reconstruction in, 64
  coping with the high cost of, 197–206
    cancer policy advocacy, 205
    health insurance plan in, 205
    healthcare system for financial assistance, 199
    impact of financial hardships on the country, 204–205

211

Index

Breast cancer (*Continued*)
  recognizing financial hardships in, 197–198
  role of healthcare organization in, 199–204
  seeking transparency in, 199
 evaluation and treatment of, in underserved community, 40–44
  from theory to practice, 42–43, 43f
 expectations for the future, 207–210
 genetics and prevention of, 187–196, 189f
  familial/personal history/lifestyle risk factors in, 191–192
  genetic risk factors in, 188–191, 190f
  management of high-risk patient in, 194
  risk-reducing interventions in, 192–193
  risk-reducing surgery in, 194
 guidelines on, 2
 HER2-positive, 121–122, 122f
 in males, 118–119
 metastatic, 119–124
  biology of metastatic disease, 119
  chemotherapy, 123–124, 124f
  HER2-positive breast cancer, 121–122, 122f
  hormonal therapy, 119–120, 121f
  triple-negative breast cancer, 122–123
 molecular classification of, 132–134
  basal-like subtype, 133–134, 136f
  HER2-positive/HER2-enriched subtype, 133
  luminal subtypes, 133, 134f–135f
 multidisciplinary team approach for, 6–10, 7f
  ancillary services in, 9
  components of, 6
  decisions on testing prior to, 8
  high-risk patient evaluation and management in, 8–9
  implementation of, 6
  patients in, 8
  shared decision making in, 9
  value of, 6–8
 neoadjuvant therapy for, 101–110
  adjuvant therapy after neoadjuvant treatment, 109–110
  current goals of, 101–102
  historical perspective, 101
  management of residual disease after, 116–117
  neoadjuvant systemic therapy, 103–109
  patient selection for, 102–103
  post-treatment assessment and management, 109
  preoperative evaluation, 103
 nutrition for, 158
  medical nutrition therapy, 158–161
  oncology dietitians in, role of, 158, 159f
 oncology nurse navigation in, 11–16
  accreditation of, 11–12
  addressing barriers to care, 14
  history of, 11
  knowledge and skills requirements for, 13, 13t
  literature review of, 12–13
  in multidisciplinary team, 14, 15f
  psychosocial screening and support in, 14
  role development in, 13
  specialty certification in, 13–14
  in survivorship and end of life, 14–15
 outcomes and quality indicators, 33–39, 36t–37t
  for breast cancer treatment, 38–39
  framework for, 33, 34t

Breast cancer (*Continued*)
  management team, implementation of, 38
  measures, examples, 38
  system initiatives and management of quality, 33–36, 35f
 palliative care for, 179–185
  advance directives/living will/healthcare power of attorney in, 183–184, 184b, 184t
  communication and counseling in, 183, 183t
  goals of, 184, 184t
  palliative chemotherapy, 179–183, 180t, 181t
  psychosocial, 183
 pathology of, for precision oncology, 131–138
  biomarker testing for, 135–138
  hormone receptors, 131–132, 132f, 133f
  human epidermal receptor-2 in, 131–132, 133f
  molecular prognostic tests for, 134–135
 physical therapy for, 139–155
  during chemotherapy, efficacy of, 147–149, 148f
  efficacy of, 143
  goals of, 144
  impairments and dysfunctions of, 143b
  implications for, 143–147
  interventions for, 145
  introduction to, 139–140
  late and end-stage metastatic, 151
  late effects of, 152–153
  long-term side effects of, 152
  metastatic, implications for, 150–151
  objective examination of, 144–145
  overview of, 140, 141t–142t
  plan of care, 145
  during radiation therapy, overview of, 149
  referral to, 143–144
  referring to, 140–143
  rehabilitation assessment of, 145
  resolving, 145
  subjective history of, 144
  survivorship, implications for, 151–153
  treatment of, 145, 146f
 during pregnancy, 119
 radiation therapy, 87–100
  assessing patients appropriate for, 90
  background, 87–88, 88f
  biology, 90–91
  definitions of, 88–89, 89f
  ductal carcinoma in situ, 92–93
  general clinical, 91–92
  intraoperative, 94–99
  invasive, 93
  other indications, 94
  post mastectomy, 93–94, 94f
  side effects following treatment of breast cancer, 91
  technical definitions, 91–92, 92f
 screening, 17–32
  after recent vaccination, 26t, 28
  for average-risk women, 22–25, 24f, 24t
  for higher-than-average risk populations, 24f, 24t, 25–27, 26t
  for LGBTQ, 26t, 28
  magnetic resonance imaging for, 28–29, 29f
  for male, 26t, 27–28
  mammography for, 18
  during pregnancy/lactation, 26t, 28
  ultrasound for, 29–30
 surgical options for, 49–54

Breast cancer (*Continued*)
  after neoadjuvant chemotherapy, 54
  axillary dissection in, 53
  breast conservation in, 50–51, 51f
  complications in, 53
  future directions of, 54
  historical context of, 49
  localization of biopsied lesion in, 49–50, 50f
  margins following breast-conserving surgery in, 51
  mastectomy in, 51–52
  sentinel node biopsy in, 52–53, 53f
 surgical techniques for, 3
 systemic therapy for, 101–130
 treatment for, 2
 triple-negative, 122–123
 tumor marker testing, 165
Breast cancer survivorship, in community oncology practice, 164–178
 assessment and management of physical and psychosocial long-term and late effects of, 166–171
  body image, 166
  cardiotoxicity, 166–167, 167t
  cognitive impairment, 167
  distress, depression, and anxiety, 167–168, 168t
  fatigue, 168–170, 169t, 170f
  infertility, 170–171
  lymphedema, 166, 166t
  menopausal symptoms and early menopause, 171
  pain and neuropathy, 170, 170t
  sexual health, 171
 imaging for, 164–165
  breast cancer tumor marker testing, 165
  genetics, 165
  mammography, 164–165
 screening for secondary cancers in, 165–166
 surveillance for, 164, 165t
 wellness guidelines and health promotion for, 171–175, 172t
  barriers to survivorship care, 174
  models of care, 173–174, 174f
  program evaluation and metrics, 174–175, 175t
  survivorship care plans and care coordination, 172–173, 173f
Breast cancer–related lymphedema (BCRL), 54
Breast conservation, 50–51, 51f
 margins following, 51
Breast Imaging-Reporting and Data System (BI-RADS), 19, 46
Breast irradiation, partial, 60, 60f
Breast Patient Navigator Certification (BPNC), 13
Breast reconstruction, 64, 72–78
 cancer rehabilitation after, 141t–142t
 complications of, 74–75, 77f, 77t
 implant-based reconstruction, technical aspects of, 74, 77f, 77t
 oncoplastic, 64
  basic oncoplastic approach of, 65–66
  level 2 and extreme oncoplastic procedure in, 71
  level 1 oncoplastic procedure in, 66–67
  in lower pole, 67–68, 70f, 71f
  preoperative considerations of, 64–65, 65f, 66f, 67f
  in upper pole, 67–72, 68f
 patient selection for, 74, 77t
 tissue-based reconstruction, 75–78

Index

Breast-conserving adjuvant radiation treatment, 93
Breast-conserving therapy (BCT), 94
Brief Edinburgh Depression Scale, 168t
Brief Symptom Inventory-18 (BSI-18), 168t

C

Cachexia, definition of, 182, 182t
Calculation models, 8
Cancer Pain Ladder, 181–182
Cancer policy advocacy, 205
Cancer Registrars, 38
Cancer rehabilitation, 139, 141t–142t, 142f
Cancer risk assessment, 135–138
Cancer survivorship
    anti-inflammatory diet for, 162
    issues of, cancer rehabilitation for, 141t–142t
    lifestyle intervention for, 159f
    physical therapy for, 151–153
Cannabinoids, for nausea and vomiting, 180
Capsaicin, topical, 170t
Cardiac events, risk-reducing medications and, 193
Cardiotoxicity, breast cancer and, 166–167, 167t
CBCN. See Certified Breast Care Nurse
Cellulitis, breast cancer–related lymphedema and, 56
Centers for Medicare and Medicaid Services (CMS), quality measures by, 38
Certified Breast Care Nurse (CBCN), 13–14
Charity care, 202–203
CHEK2 mutations, 27
Chemotherapy, for breast cancer, 3, 38
    metastatic, 123–124, 124f
    palliative, 179–183, 180t, 181t
        nutrition in, 182, 182t
        symptom management of, 179–182
    physical therapy during, efficacy of, 147–149, 148f
Chemotherapy-induced peripheral neuropathy (CIPN), physical therapy for, 152
CIPN. See Chemotherapy-induced peripheral neuropathy
Circumareolar (donut) mastopexy, 67, 70f
CISNET models, for breast cancer, 23
Claus model, 27
Clinical trials, for breast cancer, 3–4, 208
CMS. See Centers for Medicare and Medicaid Services
Cognitive impairment, breast cancer and, 167
Communication, for breast cancer, 183, 183t
Community outreach
    health equity and, 42
    increase, in healthcare organization, 200
Community passion, connecting to, 40
Complementary and integrative medicine therapies, 9
Comprehensive Cancer Network, 111
Contemporary surgical approaches, to breast cancer, 54–61
    biopsy techniques in, 46–49
    breast reconstruction in, 64, 72–78
    ductal carcinoma in situ, lobular carcinoma in situ, other high-risk lesions in, 62–64
    oncoplastic breast reconstruction in, 64
    surgical options in, 49–54
Coping, with high cost of cancer, 197–206
    cancer policy advocacy, 205
    health insurance plan in, 205
    healthcare system for financial assistance, 199
    impact of financial hardships on the country, 204–205

Coping, with high cost of cancer (Continued)
    recognizing financial hardships in, 197–198
    role of healthcare organization in, 199–204
    seeking transparency in, 199
Corticosteroids, for nausea and vomiting, 180
Counseling, for breast cancer, 183, 183t
COVID-19
    vaccination for, in community, 42, 43f
Cranio-caudal (CC) view, in screening mammogram, 19, 20f, 21f
Crescent mastopexy, 67, 69f
Cyclin-dependent kinase 4 and 6 inhibitors, role of, 113–115, 114f
Cytotoxic chemotherapy
    cancer rehabilitation after, 141t–142t
    physical therapy during, 147

D

DBT. See Digital breast tomosynthesis
Deductibles, in health insurance plan, 199
De-escalating axillary surgery, 57
Depression
    breast cancer and, 167–168, 168t
    management of, 182
Diet, anti-inflammatory, 161–163, 162f
Dietitians, oncology, role of, 158, 159f
Digital breast tomosynthesis (DBT), 18–19, 21–22
Distant relapse-free survival (DRFS), 111
Distress, breast cancer and, 167–168, 168t
Dopaminergic agents, for nausea and vomiting, 180
Dose-dense data, choice of, 115
Doxepin, 169t
Ductal carcinoma in situ (DCIS), 62–64, 92–93
    diagnosis of, 62
    epidemiology of, 62
    future perspectives of, 63
    natural history of, 62
    pathology of, 62
    prognostic scores of, 63
    recurrence of, 63
    treatment for, 62–63
Duloxetine, 170t
    for nausea and vomiting, 180
Dyspareunia, risk-reducing medications and, 193

E

Early Breast Cancer Trialists' Collaborative Group (EBCTCG), 93
EBCTCG. See Early Breast Cancer Trialists' Collaborative Group
Elderly, omit radiation in, 60–61
Electron radiotherapy, intraoperative, intraoperative radiation therapy versus, 97t
Empathy, in community, 41
Endocrine therapy
    adjuvant, 111–112
    for breast cancer, 135–136
    duration of, 113
    neoadjuvant systemic therapy, 108
End-stage disease, cancer rehabilitation for, 141t–142t
Ensuring Quality Cancer Care, 33
Estrogen receptor (ER), in breast cancer, 131, 132f
Eszopiclone, 169t
Evidence-based pathways, 2
Exaggerated cranio-caudal (XCCL) view, in screening mammogram, 19, 21f
Exemestane, 193
Exercise, for breast cancer, 144, 147, 148f
External beam radiation therapy (EBRT), 60

F

Family cancer genetics program, 8
Fatigue, cancer-related, 168–170, 169t, 170f
    exercise for, 147
    management of, 182
Fatty acids, omega-3
    in flaxseed, 161
Financial advocates, 201
Financial assistance
    healthcare system for, 199
    resources, 203
    software tool for, 203–204
Financial counselors, 201
Financial hardships
    impact of, 204–205
    significance behind recognizing, 197–198
Financial health advisors, 202
Financial navigators, 12t, 202
Fine needle aspiration, core needle biopsy versus, 46
Flaxseed, 161
Freeman, Dr. Harold, 11

G

Gabapentin, 170t
    for nausea and vomiting, 180
Gabapentinoids, for nausea and vomiting, 180
Gail model, modified, 191
70-gene assay (MammaPrint), 111
Genetics and prevention, 187–196, 189f
    in breast cancer survivorship, 165
    familial/personal history/lifestyle risk factors in, 191–192
    genetic risk factors in, 188–191, 190f
    management of high-risk patient in, 194
    risk-reducing interventions in, 192–193
        exemestane/anastrozole aromatase inhibitors, 193
        raloxifene, 192–193
        side effect management for, 193–194
        tamoxifen, 192
    risk-reducing surgery in, 194
Genistein, in soy, 160–161

H

Halsted, William, 2–3
Health insurance plan, 198
    copays, 199
    deductibles, 199
    out-of-pocket maximums, 199
    plan premiums, 199
    source of, 198
    types of, 198–199
Healthcare accreditation, 11–12
Healthcare organization, role of, 199–204
    authorization team in, 200
    cancer screenings in, 200
    charity care in, 202–203
    as financial advocates, 201
    as financial counselors, 201
    as financial health advisors, 202
    as financial navigators, 202
    increase community outreach in, 200
    as oncology social workers, 202
    optimize patient's insurance coverage in, 200–201
    as public benefits specialists, 202
    quality metric for, 204
    software tool for, 203–204
    transparency of, 202
    understand financial assistance resources in, 203

Index

Hemi-batwing mastopexy, 67, 69f
HER2-negative breast cancer, 110
HER2/neu-positive disease, 102–103
HER2/neu-targeted therapy, 104–107, 105f–107f, 107f
HER2-positive breast cancer, 121–122, 122f, 133
Higher-than-average risk populations, breast screening for, 24f, 24t, 25–27
  calculated individual risk in, 27
  family history/genetic risk factors in, 25–27
  personal history in, 25, 26t
  race in, 27
  radiation history in, 27
Homologous recombination (HR), 188
Homologous recombination deficiency (HRD), 137
Hopkins Symptom Checklist (HSCL), 168t
Hormonal therapy
  cancer rehabilitation after, 141t–142t
  of metastatic breast cancer, 119–120, 121f
Hormone receptor-positive breast cancer, 110
Hormone receptors
  in breast cancer, 131–132, 132f, 133f
  HER2-negative subtype and, 117–118, 117f
Hormone replacement therapy, breast cancer and, 191–192
Hospital Anxiety and Depression Scale (HADS), 168t
Hot flashes or vasomotor symptoms, side effect management for, 193–194
  cardiac events, 193
  musculoskeletal complaints/joint ache, 194
  osteopenia/osteoporosis, 193–194
  uterine cancer, 193
  vaginal atrophy/dyspareunia, 193
HPV. *See* Human papilloma virus
HRD. *See* Homologous recombination deficiency
Human epidermal receptor-2 (HER2), in breast cancer, 131–132
  immunohistochemistry for, 132, 133f
Human papilloma virus (HPV), vaccination rates of, 41, 41t

I

IBIS. *See* International Breast Cancer Intervention Study
Immunotherapy, 208–209
IMRT. *See* Intensity-modulated radiation therapy
In situ breast cancer, 9
In situ hybridization (ISH), analysis of, 132
Infertility, breast cancer and, 170–171
Insurance premium, 199
Intensity-modulated radiation therapy (IMRT), 88
International Breast Cancer Intervention Study (IBIS) tool, 27
Intraoperative electron radiotherapy, intraoperative radiation therapy *versus*, 97t
Intraoperative radiation therapy (IORT), 94–99
  APBI clinical results: orthovoltage (50-kV X-rays) prospective randomized results, 98–99
  as boost, 95
  clinical results
    for IOERT as a boost, 95–96, 96t
    for IORT as a boost, 96, 97t
    for IORT/IOERT APBI, 98
    versus intraoperative electron radiotherapy, 97t
  as the sole radiation treatment (IORT APBI), 96–98
Invasive breast cancer, 93

IORT. *See* Intraoperative radiation therapy
ISH. *See* In situ hybridization
Isoflavones, in soy, 160–161

J

Joint ache, risk-reducing medications and, 194

K

Ki-67, 132

L

Lactation, breast cancer screening during, 26t
Lapatinib, adjuvant, role of, 116
Lay navigator, 12t
LGBTQ, breast cancer screening for, 26t, 28
Lifestyle intervention, for cancer survivor, 159f
Li-Fraumeni syndrome, 26
LINACs. *See* Linear accelerators
Linear accelerators (LINACs), 87, 88f
Living will, 183–184, 184b, 184t
Lobular carcinoma in situ (LCIS), 63
Lobular neoplasia, 25
Luminal subtypes, of breast cancer, 133, 134f–135f
Lymph node-positive disease, 102
Lymph nodes, assessment of, 103
Lymphatic microsurgical preventive healing approach (LyMPHA), 58–59, 59f
Lymphedema, 161
  arm
    nonsurgical management of, 61
    surgical management of, 61, 62f
  breast cancer and, 166, 166t
  less radiation to prevent, 60
  management of, 54–61
  omit radiation in elderly and neoadjuvant responders with, 60–61
  post treatment for, 61
  preoperative assessment and surveillance of, 55–56, 56f
  reduction of risk of, 56–57
  risk reduction and risk reduction education for, 145–147
  stages of, 54–57, 55f

M

Magnetic resonance biopsy, 48, 48f
Magnetic resonance imaging (MRI)
  for breast cancer screening, 28–29, 29f
Male breast cancer, 94, 118–119
  screening for, 26t, 27–28
MammaPrint, for breast cancer, 134–135
Mammography, 164–165
  early use of, for cancer detection, 18
Mammoplasty
  split wise pattern reduction, 72, 75f, 76f
  wise pattern reduction, 72, 73f, 74f
Management team, outcomes and quality, implementation of, 38
Manual therapy, for breast cancer, 145
Mastectomy
  cancer rehabilitation after, 141t–142t
  radical, 2–3
MBC. *See* Metastatic breast cancer
MDCC. *See* Multidisciplinary care centers
Medical nutrition therapy (MNT), 158–161
  flaxseed, 161
  soy, 160–161
Medio-lateral oblique (MLO) view, in screening mammogram, 19, 20f, 21f
Metastatic breast cancer (MBC), 119–124

Metastatic breast cancer (MBC) (*Continued*)
  biology of metastatic disease, 119
  chemotherapy, 123–124, 124f
  HER2-positive breast cancer, 121–122, 122f
  hormonal therapy, 119–120, 121f
  physical therapy for, implications for, 150–151
  triple-negative breast cancer, 122–123
Metastatic disease, biology of, 119
Microsatellite instability (MSI), testing, for breast cancer, 137
Mindful eating, 161–162
MNT. *See* Medical nutrition therapy
Modified Gail model, 27, 191
MonarchE, 113–114
MRI. *See* Magnetic resonance imaging
MSI. *See* Microsatellite instability
Multidisciplinary care centers (MDCC), 6
Multidisciplinary care program, 6–10, 7f
  ancillary services in, 9
  components of, 6
  decisions on testing prior to, 8
  high-risk patient evaluation and management in, 8–9
  implementation of, 6
  patients in, 8
  shared decision making in, 9
  value of, 6–8
Multidisciplinary clinic conferences, 6
Multidisciplinary tumor boards, 6
Multigene assays, 110–111
Musculoskeletal complaints, risk-reducing medications and, 194

N

NAPBC. *See* National Accreditation Program for Breast Centers
National Accreditation Program for Breast Centers (NAPBC), 11–12, 140
National Comprehensive Cancer Network (NCCN), 2, 179, 208
  cancer rehabilitation and, 140, 147
  Distress Thermometer, 168t
  Risk Reduction Panel, 191
National Institutes of Health Cancer Trends, 207
Nausea, management of, 180
NCCN. *See* National Comprehensive Cancer Network
Neoadjuvant chemotherapy, cancer rehabilitation after, 141t–142t
Neoadjuvant responders, omit radiation in, 60–61
Neoadjuvant systemic therapy, 103–109
  chemotherapy, 103–104
  endocrine therapy, 108
  HER2/neu-targeted therapy, 104–107, 105f–107f, 107f
  immunotherapy, 108
  principles of radiation in, 109
  principles of surgery in, 109
Neoadjuvant therapy
  for breast cancer, 101–110
    adjuvant therapy after neoadjuvant treatment, 109–110
    current goals of, 101–102
    management of residual disease after, 116–117
    neoadjuvant systemic therapy, 103–109
    patient selection for, 102–103
    post-treatment assessment and management, 109
    preoperative evaluation, 103
    patient selection for, 102–103

Neoadjuvant therapy (*Continued*)
  HER2/Neu-positive disease, 102–103
  lymph node-positive disease, 102
  primary tumor, 102
  timing of surgery, 103
Neratinib, 122
  adjuvant, role of, 116
Neurokinin receptor antagonists, for nausea and vomiting, 180
Neuropathy, breast cancer and, 170, 170*t*
Next generation sequencing (NGS), 189–190
Non-anthracycline regimens, 115
Nonopioid, management of, 179–180
Nulliparity, breast cancer and, 192
Nurse navigator, in breast cancer, 8
Nutrition, 158
  medical nutrition therapy, 158–161
    flaxseed, 161
    soy, 160–161
  oncology dietitians in, role of, 158, 159*f*

O

Objective data, in community, 41
Omega-3 fatty acids, in flaxseed, 161
OMH. *See* Oncology Medical Home
Oncology dietitians, role of, 158, 159*f*
Oncology Medical Home (OMH) standards, 12
Oncology nurse navigation, 11–16
  accreditation of, 11–12
  addressing barriers to care, 14
  history of, 11
  knowledge and skills requirements for, 13, 13*t*
  literature review of, 12–13
  in multidisciplinary team, 14, 15*f*
  psychosocial screening and support in, 14
  role development in, 13
  specialty certification in, 13–14
  in survivorship and end of life, 14–15
Oncology nurse navigator (ONN), 11
  knowledge and skills requirements for, 13, 13*t*
  role of, 12, 12*t*
Oncology Nursing Society (ONS), 11
Oncology practitioners, referring to breast cancer physical therapy, 140
Oncology, precision, 131–138
  biomarker testing for, 135–138
  hormone receptors, 131–132, 132*f*, 133*f*
  molecular prognostic tests for, 134–135
Oncology social workers, 202
Oncoplastic breast reconstruction, 64
  basic oncoplastic approach of, 65–66
  level 2 and extreme oncoplastic procedure in, 71
  level 1 oncoplastic procedure in, 66–67
  in lower pole, 67–68, 70*f*, 71*f*
  preoperative considerations of, 64–65, 65*f*, 66*f*, 67*f*
  in upper pole, 67–72, 68*f*
OncotypeDx assay, 111, 134–135
ONN. *See* Oncology nurse navigator
ONS. *See* Oncology Nursing Society
Opioid, management of, 179–182, 181*t*
Osteopenia, risk-reducing medications and, 193–194
Osteoporosis, risk-reducing medications and, 193–194
Outcome indicators, 33–39
  for breast cancer treatment, 38–39
  framework for, 33, 34*t*
  management team, implementation of, 38
Out-of-pocket maximums, 199

P

Pain
  breast cancer and, 170, 170*t*
  management of, 179
Palbociclib, 113, 120
Palliative care, for breast cancer, 179–185
  advance directives/living will/healthcare power of attorney in, 183–184, 184*b*, 184*t*
  communication and counseling in, 183, 183*t*
  goals of, 184, 184*t*
  palliative chemotherapy, 179–183, 180*t*, 181*t*
    nutrition in, 182, 182*t*
    symptom management of, 179–182
  psychosocial, 183
Palliative chemotherapy, for breast cancer, 179–183, 180*t*, 181*t*
  nutrition in, 182, 182*t*
  symptom management of, 179–182
Palpable lesions, nonpalpable lesions *versus*, 46–47
Partial breast irradiation, 60, 60*f*
Partial mastectomy, cancer rehabilitation after, 141*t*–142*t*
Patient Navigator and Chronic Disease Prevention Act, 11
Patient prioritization, for vaccination, 42
Patient Self-Determination Act, 184
PD-L1 testing, for breast cancer, 137
Pegfilgrastim, cancer rehabilitation after, 141*t*–142*t*
Pembrolizumab, 123
PENELOPE-B, 113
Personal Health Questionnaire (PHQ-2), 168*t*
Personal Health Questionnaire (PHQ-9), 168*t*
Pertuzumab, adjuvant, role of, 116
Photons, 91
PHSA. *See* Public Health Service Act
Physical therapy, for breast cancer, 139–155
  during chemotherapy, efficacy of, 147–149, 148*f*
  efficacy of, 143
  goals of, 144
  impairments and dysfunctions of, 143*b*
  implications for, 143–147
  interventions for, 145
  introduction to, 139–140
  late and end-stage metastatic, 151
  late effects of, 152–153
  long-term side effects of, 152
  metastatic, implications for, 150–151
  objective examination of, 144–145
  overview of, 140, 141*t*–142*t*
  plan of care, 145
  during radiation therapy, overview of, 149
  referral to, 143–144
  referring to, 140–143
  rehabilitation assessment of, 145
  resolving, 145
  subjective history of, 144
  survivorship, implications for, 151–153
  treatment of, 145, 146*f*
Phytonutrients, 160
PIK3CA gene, in breast cancer, 136–137
Plastic surgery, for breast cancer, 207–208
Post curative radiation, cancer rehabilitation after, 141*t*–142*t*
Post mastectomy radiation therapy, 93–94, 94*f*
Power of attorney, 183–184, 184*b*, 184*t*
Precision Medicine program, 4
Precision oncology, 131–138
  biomarker testing for, 135–138
  hormone receptors, 131–132, 132*f*, 133*f*
  molecular prognostic tests for, 134–135

Pregabalin, for nausea and vomiting, 180
Pregnancy, breast cancer during, 119
  screening for, 26*t*, 28
Premenopausal women, role of ovarian suppression in, 112
Prescription benefits, 199
Primary tumor, management of, 109
Profile of Moods State–Short Form (POMS-SF), 168*t*
Progesterone receptor (PR), in breast cancer, 131
Prognostic biomarker studies, for breast cancer, 8
Prokinetic agents, for nausea and vomiting, 180
Psycho social distress, 14
Psychosocial Screen for Cancer (PSSCAN), 168*t*
PTEN mutation, 26–27
Public benefits specialists, 202
Public Health Service Act (PHSA), 11

Q

Quality indicators, 36–38, 36*t*–37*t*
  for breast cancer treatment, 38–39
  framework for, 33, 34*t*
  management team, implementation of, 38
  measures, examples, 38
  system initiatives and management of quality, 33–36, 35*f*
Quality measure dashboard, 35, 35*f*

R

Radiation therapy, 87–100, 208
  assessing patients appropriate for, 90
  background, 87–88, 88*f*
  biology, 90–91
  definitions of, 88–89, 89*f*
  ductal carcinoma in situ, 92–93
  general clinical, 91–92
  intraoperative, 94–99
    APBI clinical results: orthovoltage (50-kV X-rays) prospective randomized results, 98–99
    as boost, 95
    versus intraoperative electron radiotherapy, 97*t*
    as the sole radiation treatment (IORT APBI), 96–98
  other indications, 94
  physical therapy during, overview of, 149
  post mastectomy, 93–94, 94*f*
  side effects following treatment of breast cancer, 91
  technical definitions, 91–92, 92*f*
Radiation-induced sarcomas, 91
Radical mastectomy, 2–3
Radiologic studies, for breast cancer, 8
Raloxifene, 192–193
Ramelteon, 169*t*
Rehabilitation, for breast cancer, 9, 139
  comprehensive, 142*f*
  indications for, 141*t*–142*t*
  during radiation therapy, 149
Report to the Nation on Cancer in the Poor, 11
Ribociclib, 120
Risk-reducing mastectomy (RRM), 194

S

Sacituzumab govitecan, 123
Sarcomas, radiation-induced, 91
Screening, breast cancer, 17–32
  after recent vaccination, 26*t*, 28
  for average-risk women, 22–25, 24*f*, 24*t*
  cost of, 200

Screening, breast cancer (*Continued*)
  for higher-than-average risk populations, 24*f*, 24*t*, 25–27, 26*t*
  for LGBTQ, 26*t*, 28
  magnetic resonance imaging for, 28–29, 29*f*
  for male, 26*t*, 27–28
  mammography for, 18
  during pregnancy/lactation, 26*t*, 28
  ultrasound for, 29–30
Screening mammography
  for average-risk women, 22–25, 24*f*, 24*t*
  benefits of, 18
  characterizing breast tissue density in, 19–21, 22*f*
  limitations/incorporation of tomosynthesis in, 21–22, 23*t*
  patient positioning in, 19, 20*f*, 21*f*
  risks of, 18–19
  standardization of, 19
SDG. *See* Secoisolariciresinol diglucoside
Secoisolariciresinol diglucoside (SDG), in flaxseed, 161
Seed localization, 49–50, 50*f*
Selective estrogen receptor modulator (SERM), 111
Sentinel lymph node biopsy (SLNB), 52–53, 53*f*
  cancer rehabilitation after, 141*t*–142*t*
Sentinel Node Biopsy Following Neoadjuvant Chemotherapy (SN FNAC), 57
Serotonin 5-HTZ receptor antagonist, for nausea and vomiting, 180
Sexual health, breast cancer and, 171
Shared decision making, in breast cancer management, 9
SLNB. *See* Sentinel lymph node biopsy
Smaller HER2-positive tumors, treatment of, 116
Social vulnerability index (SVI), COVID-19 and, 43
Social work navigator, 12*t*
Social workers, 9
Soy, 160–161
Split wise pattern reduction mammoplasty, 72, 75*f*, 76*f*
Stage IV disease, cancer rehabilitation for, 141*t*–142*t*

Staging studies, for breast cancer, 8
Stereotactic biopsy, 47, 47*f*
Subclinical edema, breast cancer–related lymphedema and, 56
Subjective feedback, in community, 41
Supplement pills, 160
Support groups, 9
Surgical options, for breast cancer, 49–54
  after neoadjuvant chemotherapy, 54
  axillary dissection in, 53
  breast conservation in, 50–51, 51*f*
  complications in, 53
  future directions of, 54
  historical context of, 49
  localization of biopsied lesion in, 49–50, 50*f*
  margins following breast-conserving surgery in, 51
  mastectomy in, 51–52
  sentinel node biopsy in, 52–53, 53*f*
Suvorexant, 169*t*
SVI. *See* Social vulnerability index

T
Tamoxifen, 192
  adjuvant endocrine therapy, 111
  aromatase inhibitors and, 113
  flaxseed and, 161
Targeted intraoperative radiation (TARGIT-IORT), 60
Taxanes, choice of, 115
Team Phoenix, 153
Temazepam, 169*t*
Therapeutic exercise, for breast cancer, 145
Tissue density, 19–21, 22*f*
Tissue-based reconstruction, 75–78
  complications of, 78
  patient selection for, 75–77, 77*t*, 78*f*
  technique for, 77–78, 78*f*
TMB. *See* Tumor mutational burden
Total breast mastectomy, 93
TP53 mutation, 26
Trastuzumab, 116
Trastuzumab emtansine (TDM1), 104
Trazodone, 169*t*
Treatment-related nausea and vomiting, 9

Triangle mastopexy, 70*f*
Triazolam, 169*t*
Triple-negative breast cancer, 122–123
Tumor mutational burden (TMB), testing, for breast cancer, 137
Tyrer-Cuzick model, 191
Tyrosine kinase inhibitors (TKIs), 122

U
Ultrasound biopsy, 47–48, 48*f*
Ultrasound, for breast cancer screening, 29–30
Underserved community, evaluation and treatment in, 40–44
  from theory to practice, 42–43, 43*f*
Upper pole, oncoplastic breast reconstruction of, 67–72, 68*f*
Uterine cancer, risk-reducing medications and, 193

V
Vaccination
  breast cancer screening after, 26*t*, 28
  for COVID-19
  in community, 42
  rates, of human papilloma virus, 41, 41*t*
Vaginal atrophy, risk-reducing medications and, 193
Venlafaxine, 170*t*
Vertical cancer quality program structure, 34, 35*f*
Vertical mastopexy, 71, 71*f*, 72*f*
Virtual telemedicine, 3
Vivor, 203
Vomiting, management of, 180

W
Warren, Stafford, 18
Weight, loss of, in survivorship nutrition, 163
Weighted tool, for quality measures, 36, 36*t*–37*t*
Wire localization, 49, 50*f*
Wise pattern reduction mammoplasty, 72, 73*f*, 74*f*

Z
Zaleplon, 169*t*
Zolpidem, 169*t*